Vaccine Adjuvants

METHODS IN MOLECULAR MEDICINE™

John M. Walker, SERIES EDITOR

46. **Angiogenesis:** ***Reviews and Protocols,*** **edited by** *J. Clifford Murray*, 2000
45. **Hepatocellular Carcinoma Methods and Protocols, edited by** *Nagy A. Habib*, 2000
44. **Asthma:** ***Mechanisms and Protocols,*** **edited by** *K. Fan Chung and Ian Adcock*, 2000
43. **Muscular Dystrophy:** ***Methods and Protocols,*** **edited by** *Katherine B. Bushby and Louise Anderson*, 2000
42. **Vaccine Adjuvants:** ***Preparation Methods and Research Protocols***, edited by *Derek T. O'Hagan*, 2000
41. **Celiac Disease:** ***Methods and Protocols***, edited by *Michael N. Marsh,* 2000
40. **Diagnostic and Therapeutic Antibodies,** edited by *Andrew J. T. George and Catherine E. Urch*, 2000
39. **Ovarian Cancer:** ***Methods and Protocols***, edited by *John M. S. Bartlett*, 2000
38. **Aging Methods and Protocols,** edited by *Yvonne A. Barnett and Christopher P. Barnett*, 2000
37. **Electrically Mediated Delivery of Molecules to Cells**, edited by *Mark J. Jaroszeski, Richard Heller, and Richard Gilbert,* 2000
36. **Septic Shock Methods and Protocols**, edited by *Thomas J. Evans*, 2000
35. **Gene Therapy of Cancer:** ***Methods and Protocols***, edited by *Wolfgang Walther and Ulrike Stein*, 2000
34. **Rotavirus Methods and Protocols**, edited by *James Gray and Ulrich Desselberger*, 2000
33. **Cytomegalovirus Protocols,** edited by *John Sinclair*, 2000
32. **Alzheimer's Disease:** ***Methods and Protocols,*** edited by *Nigel M. Hooper*, 1999
31. **Hemostasis and Thrombosis Protocols:** ***Methods in Molecular Medicine,*** edited by *David J. Perry and K. John Pasi*, 1999
30. **Vascular Disease:** ***Molecular Biology and Gene Therapy Protocols,*** edited by *Andrew H. Baker,* 1999
29. **DNA Vaccines:** ***Methods and Protocols,*** edited by *Douglas B. Lowrie and Robert Whalen,* 1999
28. **Cytotoxic Drug Resistance Mechanisms,** edited by *Robert Brown and Uta Böger-Brown,* 1999
27. **Clinical Applications of Capillary Electrophoresis,** edited by *Stephen M. Palfrey,* 1999
26. **Quantitative PCR Protocols,** edited by *Bernd Kochanowski and Udo Reischl,* 1999
25. **Drug Targeting,** edited by *G. E. Francis and Cristina Delgado,* 1999
24. **Antiviral Methods and Protocols,** edited by *Derek Kinchington and Raymond F. Schinazi,* 2000
23. **Peptidomimetics Protocols,** edited by *Wieslaw M. Kazmierski,* 1999
22. **Neurodegeneration Methods and Protocols,** edited by *Jean Harry and Hugh A. Tilson,* 1999

METHODS IN MOLECULAR MEDICINE™

Vaccine Adjuvants

Preparation Methods and Research Protocols

Edited by

Derek T. O'Hagan

Chiron Corporation
Emeryville, CA

Humana Press Totowa, New Jersey

999 Riverview Drive, Suite 208
Totowa, New Jersey 07512

This publication is printed on acid-free paper. ∞
ANSI Z39.48-1984 (American Standards Institute) Permanence of Paper for Printed Library Materials.

Cover art: Poly(lactide co-glycolide) microparticles. The PLG microparticles were prepared by Manmohan Singh. Photo courtesy of Derek O'Hagan.

Cover design by Patricia F. Cleary.

For additional copies, pricing for bulk purchases, and/or information about other Humana titles, contact Humana at the above address or at any of the following numbers: Tel: 973-256-1699; Fax: 973-256-8341; E-mail: humana@humanapr.com, or visit our Website at www.humanapress.com

Printed in the United States of America. 10 9 8 7 6 5 4 3 2 1
Library of Congress Cataloging-in-Publication Data

Vaccine adjuvants: preparation methods and research protocols / edited by
Derek T. O'Hagan.
p. ; cm. -- (Methods in molecular medicine ; 42)
Includses bibliographical references and index.
ISBN 0-89603-735-5 (alk. paper)
1. Immunological adjuvants. 2. Vaccines. I. O'Hagan, Derek T. II.
Series.
[DNLM: Vaccines--immunology. 2. Adjuvants, Immunologic. QW
805 V1154 2000]
QR187.3. .V33 2000
615′.372--dc21

99-088373

Preface

Vaccine Adjuvants: Preparation Methods and Research Protocols was developed to promote the optimal use of immunological adjuvants in preclinical studies. The book's primary focus is on the use of adjuvants in vaccination studies in order to induce potent immune responses against either antigens derived from infectious organisms or cancer-associated antigens. In general, our work should be of interest and significant value to researchers who need to induce potent immune responses against their respective antigens, including those involved in the development of vaccines for infectious diseases, cancers, fertility regulation, and autoimmune disorders. In addition, the book should also be valuable for those involved in the selective manipulation of the immune response, including virologists, bacteriologists, parasitologists, and immunologists. Each chapter describes a single approach, but includes suggestions as to why the specific adjuvant might be preferred for a given antigen, depending on which type of immune response is desired. Alternative adjuvant approaches are presented in detail in such a manner as to permit researchers to choose those most efficacious for their specific indications.

The main focus of *Vaccine Adjuvants: Preparation Methods and Research Protocols* is on the use of adjuvants in vaccines, since it is already clear that the new generation of vaccines—based on recombinant proteins, synthetic peptides, or DNA— will require adjuvants for optimal efficacy. Each chapter describes in detail the preparation and characterization of an adjuvant or an adjuvant formulation, including recommended protocols for its in vivo evaluation in preclinical studies. Whenever possible, detailed adjuvant preparation and characterization methods are presented in each chapter by the individuals who originally invented or developed the approaches, including specific examples for guidance. The preparation methods described range from simple mixing of an antigen with a preformed adjuvant, to a complex formulation process requiring the antigen to be physically associated within, or entrapped within, an adjuvant formulation. In all chapters, practical advice and guidance is provided to allow optimal adjuvant preparation. Each chapter also includes detailed notes, which highlight important practical points, and warns against potential pitfalls and problems. Following adjuvant preparation, steps are often necessary to characterize the vaccine/adjuvant formulation, to ensure that the preparation was successful, and to allow quantitative estimation of important parameters, including antigen incorporation or association, and antigen integrity. Whenever necessary, these steps are described in detail, with full practical guidance and examples of the expected results. In addition, an overview chapter describing the evaluation of novel adjuvants in clinical studies is included. Also included is a chapter describing recommended guidelines to evaluate the safety of novel adjuvants and adjuvant formulations.

Derek T. O'Hagan

Contents

Contributors

ROBERT EDELMAN • *Center for Vaccine Developmzent, Department of Medicine (Geographic Medicine), University of Maryland School of Medicine, Baltimore, MD*
JIA-HWA FANG • *Chiron Corporation, Emeryville, CA*
MARTIN A. GIEDLIN • *Chiron Corporation, Emeryville, CA*
SARAH C. GILBERT • *The Wellcome Trust Centre for Human Genetics, University of Oxford, Oxford, UK*
GREGORY M. GLENN • *Department of Membrane Biochemistry, Walter Reed Army Institute of Research, Washington, DC*
SUSAN GOULD-FOGERITE • *Department of Laboratory Medicine and Pathology, University of Medicine and Dentistry–New Jersey Medical School, Newark, NJ; BioDelivery Sciences, Inc.*
REINHARD GLÜCK • *Head, Virology, Swiss Serum and Vaccine Institute Berne, Berne Switzerland*
GREGORY GREGORIADIS • *Center for Drug Delivery Research, The School of Pharmacy, University of London, London, UK*
RAJESH K. GUPTA • *Wyeth Lederle Laboratories, Vaccines, Pearl River, NY*
MANINDER HORA • *Chiron Corporation, Emeryville, CA*
CHARLOTTE READ KENSIL • *Adjuvant and Drug Delivery Research, Aquila Biopharmaceuticals, Inc., Framingham, MA*
JÖRG KREUTER • *Institut für Pharmazeutische Technologie, Johann Wolfgang Goethe-Universität, Biozentrum, Frankfurt am Main, Germany*
DEBORAH M. LIDGATE • *Roche, Palo Alto, CA*
ERIK B. LINDBLAD • *Superfos Biosector, Production, Frederikasund, Denmark*
KARIN LÖVGREN-BENGTSSON • *Section of Virology, Department of Veterinary Microbiology, Swedish University of Agricultural Sciences, Uppsala, Sweden*
RAPHAEL J. MANNINO • *University of Medicine and Dentistry—New Jersey Medical School, Newark, NJ; and BioDelivery Sciences, Inc.*
BRENDA MCCORMACK • *Center for Drug Delivery Research, The School of Pharmacy, University of London, London, United Kingdom*

Bror Morein • *Section of Virology, Department of Veterinary Microbiology, Swedish University of Agricultural Sciences, Uppsala, Sweden*
Jason A. Neidleman • *Chiron Corporation, Emeryville, CA*
Mark J. Newman • *Epimmune, San Diego, CA*
David C. Neujahr • *Division of Rheumatology, Allergy and Clinical Immunology, Duke University Medical Center, Durham, NC*
Mia Obrenovic • *Center for Drug Delivery Research, The School of Pharmacy, University of London, London, UK*
Derek T. O'Hagan • *Chiron Corporation, Emeryville, CA*
Gary Ott • *Chiron Corporation, Emeryville, CA*
Yvonne Perrie • *Center for Drug Delivery Research, The School of Pharmacy, University of London, London, UK*
David S. Pisetsky • *Division of Rheumatology, Allergy and Clinical Immunology, Duke University Medical Center, Durham, NC*
Ramachandran Radhakrishnan • *Chiron Corporation, Emeryville, CA*
Bradford E. Rost • *Massachusetts Biological Laboratories, University of Massachusetts Medical Center, Boston, MA*
Roghieh Saffie • *Center for Drug Delivery Research, The School of Pharmacy, University of London, London, UK*
Tanya Scharton-Kersten • *Department of Membrane Biochemistry, Walter Reed Army Institute of Research, Washington, DC*
Manmohan Singh • *Chiron Corp., Emeryville, CA*
Charles W. Todd • *Vaxcel, Inc., Norcross, GA*
Duncan E. S. Stewart-Tull • *Division of Infection and Immunity, Institute for Biomedical and Life Sciences, University of Glasgow, UK*
J. Terry Ulrich • *Adjuvant Evaluation, Corixa Corporation, Hamilton, MT*
Russell Vassell • *Department of Membrane Biochemistry, Walter Reed Army Institute of Research, Washington, DC*

1

An Overview of Adjuvant Use

Robert Edelman

1. Introduction

Adjuvants have been used to augment the immune response to antigens for more than 70 years. Ramon first demonstrated that it was possible to increase levels of diphtheria or tetanus antitoxin by the addition of bread crumbs, agar, tapioca, starch oil, lecithin, or saponin to the vaccines *(1)*. In this chapter, an overview is provided of modern vaccine adjuvants as background for more detailed discussions of promising adjuvants in chapters to follow. After a more general discussion of adjuvants including their definition, mechanisms of action, safety, ideal characteristics, impediments to development, and preclinical and clinical regulatory issues, examples will be provided of experimental vaccine adjuvants that have entered clinical trial to enhance a variety of licensed and experimental vaccines in humans. For additional expositions on this complex subject and for a historical perspective, the reader is referred to recent textbooks on vaccine adjuvants *(2–4)* and a selection of useful review articles published over the past 18 years *(5–10)*.

Interest in vaccine adjuvants is growing rapidly for several reasons. First, dozens of new vaccine candidates have emerged over the past decade for prevention or treatment of infectious diseases, cancer, fertility, and allergic and autoimmune diseases. Many of these candidates require adjuvants. Second, vaccines have become commercially more profitable in the past few years. Third, the Children's Vaccine Initiative (CVI) initiated in 1990 has helped to energize political and public health interest in vaccine adjuvants by establishing ambitious goals for enhancing present vaccines and for developing new ones *(11)*. Fourth, refinements in the fields of analytical biochemistry, macromolecular purification, recombinant technology, and improved understanding

From: *Methods in Molecular Medicine, Vol. 42: Vaccine Adjuvants: Preparation Methods and Research Protocols*
Edited by: D. T. O'Hagan © Humana Press, Inc., Totowa, NJ

of immunological mechanisms and disease pathogenesis have helped to improve the technical basis for adjuvant development and application. Finally, the development of experimental adjuvants has been driven by the failure of aluminum compounds (1) to enhance many vaccines in man, (2) to enhance many subunit vaccine antigens in animals, and (3) to stimulate cytotoxic T-cell responses.

2. Definitions

The discussion of vaccine adjuvants will be facilitated by a definition of terms. The term "adjuvant" (from the latin, adjuvare = help) was first coined by Ramon in 1926 for a substance used in combination with a specific antigen that produces more immunity than the antigen used alone *(12)*. The enormous diversity of compounds that increase specific immune responses to an antigen and thus function as vaccine adjuvants makes any classification system somewhat arbitrary. Adjuvants in **Table 1** are grouped according to origin rather than according to mechanism of action, because the mechanism for most adjuvants are incompletely understood. Cox and Coulter *(10)* have recently classified adjuvants into two broad groups, particulate or nonparticulate. Within each group, an adjuvant may act in one or more of five ways, based on current knowledge; namely, immunomodulation, presentation, induction of CD8+ cytotoxic T-lymphocyte (CTL) responses, targeting, and depot generation. These five basic mechanisms will change or increase as our immunological knowledge expands.

2.1. Examples of Modern Vaccine Adjuvants Used in Animals and Man

Agents listed in **Table 1** are examples of the many varieties of immunopotentiators used during the past 30 years. The majority of adjuvants are being developed and tested by industry. The list of adjuvants is incomplete, because I have not conducted an exhaustive literature search, because the results have appeared in abstracts in nonindexed publications, and because many studies are proprietary.

The adjuvants marked by an asterisk in **Table 1** have completed trial in man, or they are now undergoing clinical trial. Promising adjuvants not yet tested in humans are also listed. In some instances, adjuvants have been combined in an adjuvant formulation hoping to gain a synergistic or additive effect.

2.1.1. Vaccine Adjuvants vs Nonspecific Enhancers of Immunity

Agents listed in **Table 1** enhance specific antigens and are administered concurrently with the antigen. Adjuvants not administered in a single dose, at or near the time of antigen injection, and into the same injection site as the antigen, are not listed. Thus, adjuvants administered repeatedly as nonspecific enhancers of immune response are largely excluded. Immunopotentiating agents administered to humans separately in time or location from the vaccine may be impractical for vaccinating large numbers of persons, and potentially unsafe because of their physiological effects on the entire body. They may have a role, however, in immunizing a small number of high-risk, immunoincompetent individuals, such as renal dialysis patients at risk for hepatitis B or the very elderly at risk of influenza. Examples of such "whole body" adjuvants used in humans to augment vaccines include Na diethyldithiocarbamate ***(13)***, thymosin alpha one ***(14)***, loxoribine ***(15)***, granulocyte-macrophage stimulating factor ***(16,17)***, cimetidine ***(18)***, and dehydroepiandrosterone sulfate ***(19)***. The results of such trials to date have been disappointing.

2.1.2. Carriers, Vehicles, and Adjuvant Formulations

Several terms used in **Table 1** need to be defined. A "carrier" has several meanings: it is an immunogenic protein bound to a hapten or a weakly immunogenic antigen ***(20)***. Carriers increase the immune response by providing T-cell help to the hapten or antigen. A carrier may also be a living organism (or vector) bearing genes for expression of the foreign hapten or antigen ***(21,22)***. A DNA vaccine is a carrier in the sense that, like some living vectors, it carries a plasmid-based DNA vector encoding the production of the protein antigen upon inoculation into the host ***(23)***.

A "vehicle" provides a substrate for the adjuvant, the antigen, or the antigen-carrier complex. Vehicles are not immunogenic (unlike carriers), but most vehicles can enhance antigens. Their immunostimulatory effects are often augmented by the addition of conventional adjuvants to constitute "adjuvant formulations."

Examples of adjuvant formulations tested in humans with a variety of antigens include monophosphoryl lipid A and cell wall skeleton of *Mycobacterium phlei* adjuvants in a squalane-in-water emulsion vehicle ***(24)***, monophosphoryl lipid A adjuvant in a liposome vehicle ***(25)***, threonyl-muramyl dipeptide adjuvant and Pluronic L-121 block polymer adjuvant in a vehicle emulsion of squalane and Tween-80 ***(26)***, muramyl tripeptide-dipalmitoyl phosphatidylethanolamine adjuvant in a squalene-in-water emulsion vehicle ***(27)***, and monophosphoryl lipid A and QS-21 adjuvants in a proprietary oil-in-water emulsion ***(28)***.

2.1.3. Adjuvants for Mucosal Vaccines

Recent advances in vaccinology have created an array of vaccines that can be delivered to mucosal surfaces of the respiratory, gastrointestinal, and genitourinary tracts using intranasal, oral, and vaginal routes ***(29)***. Well-tolerated

Classes of Modern Vaccine Adjuvants

1. *Mineral Salts*
   - Aluminum ("Alum")
     - Aluminum hydroxide*
     - Aluminum phosphate*
   - Calcium phosphate*
2. *Surface-Active Agents and Microparticles*
   - Nonionic block polymer surfactants*
   - Virosomes*
   - Saponin (QS-21)*
   - Meningococcal outer membrane proteins (Proteosomes)*
   - Immune stimulating complexes (ISCOMs)*
   - Cochleates
   - Dimethyl dioctadecyl ammonium bromide (DDA)
   - Avridine (CP20,961)
   - Vitamin A
   - Vitamin E
3. *Bacterial Products*
   - Cell wall skeleton of *Mycobacterium phlei* (Detox®)*
   - Muramyl dipeptides and tripeptides
     - Threonyl MDP (SAF-1)*
     - Butyl-ester MDP (Murabutide®)*
     - Dipalmitoyl phosphatidylethanolamine MTP*
   - Monophosphoryl lipid A*
   - *Klebsiella pneumonia* glycoprotein*
   - *Bordetella pertussis**
   - Bacillus Calmette-Guérin*
   - *V. cholerae* and *E. coli* heat labile enterotoxin*
   - Trehalose dimycolate
   - CpG oligodeoxynucleotides
4. *Cytokines and Hormones*
   - Interleukin-2*
   - Interferon-α*
   - Interferon-γ*
   - Granulocyte-macrophage colony stimulating factor*
   - Dehydroepiandrosterone*
   - Flt3 ligand*
   - 1,25-dihydroxy vitamin D_3
   - Interleukin-1
   - Interleukin-6
   - Interleukin-12
   - Human growth hormone
   - β2-microglobulin
   - Lymphotactin
5. *Unique Antigen Constructs*
   - Multiple peptide antigens attached to lysine core (MAP)*
   - CTL epitope linked to universal helper T-cell epitope and palmitoylated at the N terminus (Theradigm-HBV)*
6. *Polyanions*
   - Dextran
   - Double-stranded polynucleotides

Table 1 *(continued)*

7. *Polyacrylics*
   - Polymethylmethacrylate
   - Acrylic acid crosslinked with allyl sucrose (Carbopol 934P)
8. *Miscellaneous*
   - N-acetyl-glucosamine-3yl-acetyl-L-alanyl-D-isoglutamine (CGP-11637)*
   - Gamma insulin + aluminum hydroxide (Algammulin)*
   - Transgenic plants*
   - Human dendritic cells*
   - Lysophosphatidyl glycerol
   - Stearyl tyrosine
   - Tripalmitoyl pentapeptide
9. *Carriers*
   - Tetanus toxoid*
   - Diphtheria toxoid*
   - Meningococcal B outer membrane protein (proteosomes)*
   - Pseudomonas exotoxin A*
   - Cholera toxin B subunit*
   - Mutant heat labile enterotoxin of enterotoxigenic *E. coli**
   - Hepatitis B virus core*
   - Cholera toxin A fusion proteins
   - CpG dinucleotides
   - Heat-shock proteins
   - Fatty acids
10. *Living Vectors*
    - Vaccinia virus*
    - Canarypox virus*
    - Adenovirus*
    - Attenuated *Salmonella typhi**
    - Bacillus Calmette-Guérin*
    - *Steptococcus gordonni**
    - Herpes simplex virus
    - Polio vaccine virus
    - Rhinovirus
    - Venezuelan equine encephalitis virus
    - *Yersinia enterocolitica*
    - *Listeria monocytogenes*
    - *Shigella*
    - *Bordetella pertussis*
    - *Saccharomyces cerevisiae*
11. *Vehicles*
    - Water-in-oil emulsions
      - Mineral oil (Freund's incomplete)*
      - Vegetable oil (peanut oil)*
      - Squalene and squalane*
    - Oil-in-water emulsions
      - Squalene + Tween-80 + Span 85 (MF59)*
    - Liposomes*
    - Biodegradable polymer microspheres
      - Lactide and glycolide*
      - Polyphosphazenes*
      - Beta-glucan
      - Proteinoids

*Identifies adjuvants administered to humans.

adjuvants that enhance such vaccines will play a important role in mucosal immunization. Some of the more promising adjuvants completed, in or near clinical trial include microspheres *(30)*; proteosomes *(31)*, liposomes *(32)*, CpG DNA *(33)*, cochleates *(34)*, and virus-like particles *(35)*. Cholera toxin and the closely related heat-labile enterotoxin (LT) of enterotoxigenic *Escherichia coli* are powerful adjuvants that augment the local and systemic serum antibody response to coadministered antigens *(36)*. Mutant toxin molecules have been engineered that show greatly reduced toxicity but sufficient retained adjuvanticity to enhance local IgA, systemic IgG, and cellular immune responses to coadministered vaccine antigens. Clinical trials using mutant LT toxins as adjuvants of nonliving vaccine antigens are in progress *(29)*. Surprisingly, cholera toxin applied to the skin of volunteers allowed transdermal immunization with tetanus toxoid *(37)*. Attenuated recombinant bacteria *(38,39)* and viruses *(40)*, administered orally as live vectors of cloned genes encoding protective antigens of other pathogens, have undergone phase I trials to stimulate immune effector responses. Most of these early attempts to stimulate mucosal immune responses in volunteers using mucosal adjuvants have been only marginally successful. The first attempt to immunize volunteers against LT encoded in a transgenic plant and administered as an edible vaccine was more successful *(41)*. It remains to be seen if other protein antigens (e.g., HBsAg) when given via transgenic plants will be immunogenic or will instead induce tolerance to the antigen.

3. Mechanisms of Adjuvant Action

To date, most subunit vaccines are poor antigens, whether or not they are natural products, recombinant products, or synthetic peptides. Subunit antigens fail for a variety of reasons, such as incorrect processing by the immune system, rapid clearance, stimulation of inappropriate immune response, and lack of critical B-cell or T-cell epitopes. Potentially, some of these failures can be overcome by administering subunit antigens with adjuvants. It should be remembered, however, that the best adjuvant will never correct the choice of the wrong (nonprotective) epitope.

Traditional live vaccines or whole-cell inactivated microbial vaccines are generally better immunogens than subunit vaccines. Live and inactivated whole organisms are structurally more complex than subunit vaccines, and so contain many redundant epitopes that offer more opportunity to bypass genetic restriction of the vaccinee. Such vaccines also provide a larger antigen mass than subunit vaccines, particularly if they replicate in vivo. Their antigens are larger molecules, portions of which may serve as carrier proteins and thus function as intrinsic adjuvants to enhance immunogenicity by providing T-cell help. Finally, bacterial DNA may directly stimulate the host's immune system

Table 2
Some Mechanisms of Adjuvant Action

- Stabilizes epitope conformation.
- Generates a depot at the site of inoculation with slow release of antigen.
- Targets the antigen to antigen-presenting cells by formation of multimolecular aggregates, or by binding antigen to a cell-surface receptor on APCs.
- Directs antigen presentation by MHC class I or MHC class II pathways, by means of fusion or disruption of cell membranes, or by direct peptide exchange on surface MHC molecules.
- Preferentially stimulates Th1 or Th2 $CD4^+$ T-helper cells or $CD8^+$ cytotoxic T lymphocytes, by modulation of the cytokine network in the local microenvironment.

because of its large content of unmethylated CpG dinucleotides *(42)*, and whole bacterial vaccines may contain CpG DNA.

3.1. Specific Immune Mechanisms

Some mechanisms of adjuvant action are discussed below, and which are summarized in **Table 2**. Vaccine adjuvants can (1) increase the potency of small, antigenically weak synthetic or recombinant peptides. (2) They can enhance the speed, vigor, and persistence of the immune response to stronger antigens. For example, aluminum adjuvants used with licensed pediatric vaccines (e.g., DTP) elicit early and higher antibody response after primary immunization than do unadjuvanted preparations. (3) Adjuvants can increase the immune response to vaccines in immunologically immature, immunosuppressed, or senescent individuals. (4) Adjuvants can select for, or modulate humeral or cell-mediated immunity, and they can do this in several ways. First, antigen processing can be modulated, leading to vaccines that can elicit both helper T cells and cytotoxic lymphocytes (CTL) (reviewed in *[7,43]*). Second, depending upon the adjuvant, the immune response can be modulated in favor of MHC class I or MHC class II response *(7,43)*. For example, the QS-21 adjuvant can elicit MHC class I CTL responses when mixed with protein antigens, peptides, or inactivated viruses *(44,45)*. Many other adjuvants elicit principally MHC class II antibody responses when combined with protein antigens or inactivated organisms *(7,43)*. Third, adjuvants can modulate the immune response by preferentially stimulating T-helper type 1 (Th1) or Th2 CD4(+) T-helper cells (reviewed in *[7,43]*). The Th1 response is accompanied by secretion of interleukin-2 (IL-2), interferon-gamma (IFN-γ), and TNF-beta leading to a CMI response, including activation of macrophages and CTL and high levels of IgG2a antibodies in mice. The Th2 response is modulated by secretion of IL-4, IL-5, IL-6, and IL-10 which provide better help for B-cell

Table 3
Beneficial Effects of Vaccine Adjuvants

- Increase the potency of antigenically weak peptides.
- Enhance the speed, vigor, and persistence of the immune response to stronger antigens.
- Modulate antibody avidity, specificity, quantity, isotype, and subclass.
- Select for or enhance the cytotoxic T-cell response.
- Increase the immune response to vaccines in immunologically immature, suppressed, or senescent individuals.
- Decrease the amount of antigen required, thus reducing the cost and the likelihood of antigen competition in combination vaccines.

responses, including those of IgG1, IgE, and IgA isotypes in mice. Aluminum salts principally stimulate the Th2 response ***(46)***, while the Th1 response is stimulated by many adjuvants, such as muramyl dipeptide, monophosphoryl lipid A, and QS-21 ***(7,47)***. (5) Vaccine adjuvants can modulate antibody avidity, specificity, quantity, isotype, and subclass against epitopes on complex immunogens ***(8,48,49)***. For example, only certain adjuvants, vehicles and adjuvant formulations can induce the development of the protective IgG2a antibody isotype against *Plasmodium yoelii* ***(8)***. (6) Vaccine adjuvants can decrease the amount of antigens in combination vaccines, thus reducing the liklihood of antigen competition and carrier-specific epitope suppression. In addition, by reducing the quantity of antigen needed to protect, adjuvants can decrease the cost and increase the availability of vaccines. On the other hand, the high cost of some modern adjuvants may offset the savings realized by the reduced antigen requirement, thereby paradoxically driving up vaccine cost overall.

One must remember that in vivo, most adjuvants have complex and multifactorial immunological mechanisms, often poorly understood. The immunological mechanisms utilized by many adjuvants are under investigation. The discussion of the promising adjuvants in this book will include what is known about their immunological mechanisms. Such information will include answers to some of the following questions. Does the adjuvant induce humoral or cell mediated immunity? Which IG isotypes dominate? Which cytokines are induced? Are CD4(+) T-helper cells or CD8(+) cytotoxic T-lymphocytes induced? The list of such questions is extensive, and grows in proportion to our understanding of immunological mechanisms.

4. Advantages of Adjuvants

Vaccine adjuvants influence the immune response to our benefit in one or more ways (*see* **Table 3**). The ability of adjuvants to influence so many parameters of the immune response greatly complicates the process of finding an

Table 4
Modulators of Vaccine Adjuvant Effects

- Route
- Timing
- Dose
- Adjuvant Formulation
- Antigen Construct
- Host Species
- Intraspecies Genetic Variation
- Immune Status of the Host

effective adjuvant. This is because our knowledge of how any one adjuvant operates on a cellular level is insufficient to support a completely rational approach for matching the vaccine antigen with the proper adjuvant. Consequently, many investigators advocate an empirical approach for antigen selection based on the balance between toxicity, adjuvanticity in animals, and whether one wishes to stimulate a cellular (Th1) response, a humeral (Th2) response, or a balance of the two responses.

5. Modulation of Adjuvant Activity

The effect of adjuvants are modulated strongly by the immunization schedule, the substances administered, and by the host (*see* **Table 4**). The modulation of adjuvanticity by such variables will be discussed in chapters devoted to individual adjuvants.

6. Safety

The most important attribute of any adjuvanted vaccine is that it is more efficacious than the aqueous vaccine, and that this benefit outweighs its risk. During the past 70 years many adjuvants have been developed, but they were never accepted for routine vaccination because of their immediate toxicity and fear of delayed side effects. The current attitude regarding risk-benefits of vaccination in our Western society favors safety over efficacy when a vaccine is given to a healthy population of children and adults. In high-risk groups, including patients with cancer and AIDS, and for therapeutic vaccines, an additional level of toxicity may be acceptable if the benefit of the vaccine was substantial.

Unfortunately, the absolute safety of adjuvanted vaccines, or any vaccine, cannot be guaranteed, so we must minimize the risks. The concern about adjuvant safety has encouraged continued use of aluminum adjuvants because of their long record of relative safety in children. Safety concerns have helped justify the development of unique synthetic antigen constructs and DNA vac-

Table 5
Real and Theoretical Risks of Vaccine Adjuvants

1. Local acute or chronic inflammation with formation of painful abscess, persistent nodules, ulcers, or draining lymphadenopathy.
2. Influenza-like illness with fever.
3. IgE-type immediate hypersensitivity to vaccine antigen, including anaphylaxis.
4. Chemical toxicity to tissues or organs.
5. Induction of hypersensitivity to host tissue, producing autoimmune arthritis, amyloidosis, anterior uveitis.
6. Cross-reactions with human tissue antigens, causing glomerulonephritis or meningoencephalitis.
7. Immune suppression or oral tolerance.
8. Carcinogenesis.
9. Teratogenesis or abortogenesis.
10. Spread of a live vectored vaccine to the environment.

cines not dependent on adjuvants. For example, large polymerized monomers of haptens and peptides have been linked together in a multimeric form designed to increase intrinsic adjuvanticity (multiple antigen peptide systems [MAPs]) *(50,51)*. The first phase 1 trial of a DNA-based vaccine showed it to be safe *(23)*. It remains to be seen if MAPs, DNA vaccines, and other unique antigen constructs will retain enough inherent adjuvanticity to avoid the small risk of administering them with extraneous chemical or biological adjuvants to humans.

The real or theoretical risks of administering vaccine adjuvants have been discussed in detail *(5,6,52,53)* and are summarized in **Table 5**. Undesirable reactions can be grouped as either local or systemic.

6.1. Local Reactions

The most frequent adverse side effect associated with adjuvanted vaccines is the formation of local inflammation with signs of swelling and erythema, and symptoms of tenderness to touch and pain on movement. Such reactions occur more frequently in preimmune individuals, or after repeated immunization *(24)*. The inflammation is thought to be the result of formation of inflammatory immune complexes at the inoculation site by combination of the vaccine antigen with preexisting antibodies and complement, resulting in an arthus-type reaction. Such reactions tend to occur more frequently after adjuvanted vaccines than after aqueous vaccines because of the high antibody titers induced by adjuvants.

Painful abscesses and nodules at the inoculum site are less frequently seen [reviewed in *(5)*]. Possible mechanisms for such local reactions include (1) contamination of the vaccine at the time of formulation with reactogenic chemicals and microbial products, (2) instability of the vaccine on storage with breakdown into reactogenic side products, and (3) poor biodegradability of the adjuvanted vaccine resulting in prolonged persistence in the tissues and reactive granuloma formation. Such local reactions are of special concern for depot-type adjuvants, such as aluminum salts, oil emulsions, liposomes, and biodegradable polymer microspheres. Severe local reactions in humans have followed injections of FIA (Freund's Incomplete Adjuvant) [reviewed in ***(5)***], DETOX™ (monophosphoryl lipid A + cell wall skeleton of *Mycobacterium phlei* + squalane oil vehicle + Tween-20 emulsifier) ***(24,54)***, and muramyl tripeptide covalently linked to dipalmitoyl phosphatidylethanolamine [(MTP)-PE] in a squalene-in-water emulsion ***(55)***.

We have noted development of local ulceration for as long as 70 d after intradermal inoculation of volunteers with a recombinant BCG-OspA Lyme disease vaccine; the open sores drained viable rBCG-OspA before they spontaneously healed ***(39)***. Development of similar draining sores occur commonly in adults after intradermal inoculation with standard BCG vaccine ***(56,57)***. We and others have observed immediate swelling, hives, and intense pruritis in volunteers associated with inoculation of different malaria synthetic peptide vaccines adsorbed to alum (Edelman et al., unpublished data), ***(58,59)***. The reactions occur in the inoculated arm or in the previously inoculated contralateral arm within 20 min after the third injection. The reactions resemble an unusual variant of an immediate-type hypersensitivity response, and seem to be associated with high-titered IgE serum antibody (Edelman et al., unpublished data).

6.2. Systemic Reactions

Anterior chamber uveitis has been reported with MDP and several MDP analogues in rabbits ***(60)*** and monkeys ***(61)***. Anterior uveitis has been systematically sought in at least one adjuvant vaccine study involving 110 volunteers, but it was not found ***(62)***. A slit lamp examination of volunteers to detect subclinical uveitis is not commonly performed. Adjuvant-associated arthritis ***(63–65)*** has not been reported in humans, even after long-term follow-up ***(66–69)***. More theoretical risks include the induction of autoimmunity or cancer. Fortunately, in 10- and 18-yr follow-up studies, the incidence of cancer, autoimmune and collagen disorders in 18,000 persons who received oil-emulsion influenza vaccine in the early 1950s was not different from that in persons given aqueous vaccines ***(11,68,70)***. A 35-yr follow-up of these vaccinees again failed to demonstrate higher mortality associated with a variety of chronic diseases ***(69)***. It requires decades of expensive and time-consuming follow-up to identify low-incidence reactions, and at present a mechanism for the systematic, active follow-up of vaccinees given experimental adjuvants is not available.

To date, the largest and most systematic published investigation of the safety of vaccine adjuvants in humans involves HIV-negative, healthy volunteers followed on average for 2.4 yr as part of the NIAID-sponsored AIDS Vaccine Evaluation Group trials *(71)*. This informative report includes safety data from 1398 volunteers immunized with seven recombinant, two synthetic peptide and two live poxvirus-vectored HIV-1 vaccines in 25 randomized, double-blind studies conducted between 1988 and 1997 *(71)*. The adjuvants tested alone or in combination included several aluminum preparations, deoxycholate, MF-59, QS-21, monophosphoryl lipid A, liposomes, muramyl tripeptide-PE, muramyl dipeptide, SAF/2, and recombinant vaccinia and canarypox. Safety data was compiled for 1711 person-years of follow-up among vaccine recipients, and 308 person-years among placebo recipients. The mean duration of protocols was 1.5 yr, and the mean number of immunizations was 3.5 yr. The candidate vaccines without adjuvant were generally well tolerated. The only adverse effects clearly related to vaccination were associated with moderate to severe local pain or inflammation, self-limited in nature, that were associated with the adjuvants, particularly alum plus deoxycholate, (MTP)-PE, and QS-21. (MTP)-PE was also associated with severe, self-limited febrile reactions similar to that reported for (MTP)-PE and influenza virus vaccine *(55)*. No serious adverse laboratory toxicities and no evidence of significant immunosuppressive events occurred after immunization. A few volunteers experienced rash, hemolytic anemia, or arthralgia that might relate to an underlying immunopathologic mechanism, but such reactions were mild and quite infrequent. Eleven volunteers were diagnosed with malignancies, which was within the 95% confidence interval of the number of cases predicted by the National Cancer Institute for the general population *(71)*.

7. Characteristics of an Ideal Adjuvant

It is likely that the "ideal" adjuvant does not and will not exist, because each adjuvant and its targeted antigen will have their unique requirements. Nevertheless, the generic characteristics summarized in **Table 6** would be desirable. To date, no adjuvant meets all of these goals.

8. Impediments to Rational Adjuvant Development

As already discussed, safety of new adjuvants is a major concern, particularly of those rare reactions that occur once in several thousand doses and that may not be detected until late in the development program. But other impediments exist that retard orderly development of adjuvants; those impediments proposed by Gupta and Siber are discussed below *(9)*.

Table 6
Characteristics of the Ideal Adjuvant

1. It must be safe, including freedom from immediate and long-term side effects.
2. It should be biodegradable or easily removed from the body after its adjuvant effect is exhausted to decrease the risk of late adverse effects.
3. It should elicit a more robust protective or therapeutic immune response combined with the antigen than when the antigen is administered alone.
4. It must be defined chemically and biologically, so that there is no lot-to-lot variation in the manufactured product, thereby assuring consistent responses in vaccinees between studies and over time.
5. Efficacy should be achieved using fewer doses and/or lower concentrations of the antigen.
6. It should be stable on the shelf to be commercially and clinically useful.
7. The adjuvant should be affordable.

8.1. Limited Adjuvanticity

Most adjuvants are effective with some antigens, but not others. For example, aluminum compounds failed to augment vaccines against whooping cough *(72)*, typhoid fever *(73)*, trachoma *(74)*, adenovirus hexon antigens *(75)*, influenza hemagglutinin *(76)*, and *Haemophilis influenzae* type b capsular polysaccharide conjugated to tetanus toxoid *(77)*. It is not always possible to predict compatible and incompatible adjuvant-vaccine combinations early in development, before the late stages of preclinical or early clinical development. This situation is especially common when there are no reliable animal models. Although ovalbumin is often used as a "model antigen" for preliminary screening, doses used are often too high to discriminate between small differences among adjuvant formulations *(78)*, and no functional antibody assays are available for this nonpathogenic antigen. If possible, initial preclinical studies should be done with the antigen destined for clinical studies at minimal threshold concentrations for preliminary evaluation of adjuvants *(9,52)*.

8.2. Suboptimal Use of Aluminum Adjuvants

Aluminum salts have become the reference preparations for evaluation of new adjuvants for human vaccines. Therefore, it is important that aluminum adjuvants be used optimally to allow correct evaluation of the experimental adjuvant *(5,9,79)*. Aluminum adjuvants are difficult to manufacture in a physicochemically reproducible way, and this failure affects immunogenicity. Thus, during the adsorption of antigens on aluminum adjuvants, attention must be paid to the chemical and physical characteristics of the antigen, type of aluminum adjuvant, conditions of adsorption, and concentration of adjuvant

(9,79–82). Although these adjuvants are commonly called "alum" in the literature, referring to all aluminum adjuvants as "alum" is misleading. Alum is $Al(SO_4)_2.12H_2O$, and not all aluminum salts labeled "alum" are equally effective. For instance, aluminum hydroxide is more potent than aluminum phosphate *(79)*. To minimize the variations and to avoid nonreproducible results owing to use of different preparations of aluminum compounds, it has been recommended that a specific preparation of aluminum hydroxide such as Alhydrogel from a single manufacturer be chosen as a scientific standard for evaluation of new adjuvant formulations *(3)*.

8.3. Animal Models

Different animal species, and different strains within a species, may behave differently to the same adjuvant. Intraspecies variation in immune response to adjuvants and vaccines is particularly true among mouse strains *(9,83)*. For this reason, preclinical studies in one strain of a single animal species should be interpreted with caution. Again and again, we have discovered that biological differences between animal models and humans have led to the failure of formulations in clinical trials after showing great promise in preclinical studies.

Guinea pigs have been used widely for vaccine quality control, and guinea pigs may be the animal of choice for evaluating adjuvant formulations *(3)*, although the absence of reagents to analyze guinea pig cytokines and IgG subclasses may impede full utilization. Recently, a useful rabbit model has been described by FDA and NIH investigators to evaluate the toxicity and adjuvanticity of adjuvant formulations *(52)*. The rabbit model provides a new and much needed standard protocol linking preclinical assessment of adjuvant formulations with phase I trials. The wide availability of murine cytokine and Ig subclass reagents, low husbandry costs, and ease of handling will still insure the continued use of mice despite their inconsistent responses to adjuvants. It is recommended that at least two strains of mice with different haplotypes be utilized, in addition to rabbits or guinea pigs. Vaccine alone, adjuvant alone, and vaccine-adjuvant combinations should be studied for toxicity and immunogenicity, and their concentrations should mimic and exceed human doses *(9,52)*.

8.4. Immunoassays

In addition to measuring antibodies by ELISA or other antigen-antibody binding assays, one should measure antibody function by neutralization, opsonophagocytic, or bacteriocidal assays, if available. However, the most decisive test is protection against experimental challenge. For example, many adjuvant formulations induced high-titer antibody against malarial *(8)* and SIV antigens *(84)*, but antibody titers were not sufficient to predict protection even when the antigen contained protective epitopes and protection was mediated by antibody. The induction of protective immunity depended upon the quality rather the quantity of antibody, that is, induction of antibody of the appropriate isotype and fine-epitope specificity. This induction was dependent upon unique, poorly understood interactions between the adjuvant, the antigen, and the host. The conclusions from such experience suggests that the search for an effective vaccine must involve both antigens and adjuvants from the start of preclinical development, and that no adjuvant can be considered a gold standard *(8)*.

9. Selection of Vaccine/Adjuvant Candidates for Clinical Trial

The decision to begin human trials of vaccines and adjuvanted vaccines is complex and depends on a number of criteria *(85)*.

1. The vaccine/adjuvant candidate must address a public health need, and it must be a logical means to prevent or treat the disease of interest.
2. The vaccine/adjuvant must have been designed with a sound scientific rationale.
3. There must be an expectation of safety, as discussed in the section above on safety.
4. There must be animal studies demonstrating the immunogenicity of the product when given in the appropriate dose and route. If an appropriate animal model exists, it should be used to demonstrate protective or therapeutic efficacy against challenge with the virulent organism.
5. The vaccine/adjuvant should be prepared in a practical formulation for phase 1 studies, if possible. Response to a pilot vaccine adjuvant formulation can change after manufacturing scale up or after a more practical formulation is introduced.
6. Unless subsidized by the government, clinical development of a new vaccine/ adjuvant formulation must attract industrial funding. A company is unlikely to enter into expensive commercial development unless the vaccine/adjuvant formulation is protected by worldwide patent or commercial license.

10. Preclinical and Phase I Clinical Trial Design Issues

10.1. U.S. Food and Drug Administration Regulations

No detailed or specific guidelines exist in the United States for assessing the safety of adjuvant preparations for use in humans. Only two guidelines refer to adjuvants. The first guideline formally issued by the FDA, which includes adjuvanted vaccines *(86)*, refer to tests of the final container lot of all biological products. These FDA standards are paraphrased in **Table 7** for ease of understanding. It is unclear if adjuvants, such as QS-21, which are added to the vaccine immediately before inoculation, are subject to the final container assay.

The second FDA regulation simply states that, "An adjuvant shall not be introduced into a product unless there is satisfactory evidence that it does not

Table 7
Standards Used to Test Clinical Lots of Biological Products. 21 CFR 610.11

1.	Safety:	Contains no extraneous toxic contaminants causing unexpected, unacceptable biological activity. (No weight loss over 7 d in two mice and two guinea pigs.)
2.	Sterility:	Contains no contaminating bacteria or yeast. (Sterile aerobic and anaerobic cultures.)
3.	Purity:	Contains no extraneous matter, such as pyrogens or chemicals. (Negative pyrogenicity assay in eight rabbits.)
4.	Potency:	The biological can do what is claimed for it. (Measure by laboratory or clinical tests.)
5.	Identity:	The biological is what you say it is. (Characterize by physical or chemical tests, microscopy, culture, or by immune assay.)

affect adversely the safety or potency of the product." (Code of Federal Regulations, 21 CFR, Part 610.15). Because the definition of "satisfactory evidence" is rather vague, investigators should interact with the professional staff of the Center for Biologics Evaluation and Research, FDA, in order to reach a consensus definition. Incidentally, aluminum compounds alone are not licensed. Aluminum compounds are not considered to be "investigational adjuvants" because they are components in already licensed vaccines. Thus, antigen-adjuvant formulations are licensed for clinical use, but adjuvants alone are not *(52)*.

10.2. Center for Biologics Evaluation and Research (CBER), FDA

The CBER, FDA, Rockville, MD is responsible for regulating vaccines and other biologics in the United States. In addition to meeting the general standards before public release (**Table 7**), each vaccine and adjuvant are tested for safety on a case by case basis, preferably with the help and guidance of the CBER as noted before. Such guidance, informal in nature but quite helpful, was published in 1993 in response to the needs of HIV-1 vaccine development *(52)*. The principles laid down by that publication can be adapted to the needs of other vaccines. It is recommended that as a general principle, all novel (nonaluminum) vaccine/adjuvant formulations be discussed earlier rather than later in preclinical development with the staff of the CBER. The principles are summarized in the next few paragraphs. These and other preclinical and clinical trial study design issues have been discussed in some detail *(52,53)*.

1. Extensive experience with aluminum compounds have shown them to be safe. Therefore, for vaccines with aluminum adjuvants, postinjection observation of the animal and injection site is generally adequate for preclinical safety without

the need for formal toxicology study of the combined product, unless there is some special concern about the antigen.

2. For other adjuvants, additional tests are necessary. These include reactogenicity and toxicology tests of the adjuvant alone and the antigen-adjuvant combination in a manner that is relevant to the intended clinical use, including route of administration, injection volume, and clinical formulation. A standard safety assessment protocol in rabbits should be utilized, but only if the rabbit is thought to be sensitive to the biological effects of the vaccine. This standard safety assessment protocol provides a bridging study that links preclinical and clinical development.
3. Early in clinical development, the FDA recommends inclusion of a control group of volunteers given antigen alone and/or antigen adsorbed to aluminum as comparison groups. Results of the immunological assessments obtained from such early phase 1 studies should be combined with the safety profile to help define the risk/benefit of proceeding to further clinical studies.

10.3. Clinical Framework Required for Trials of Vaccines and Vaccine/Adjuvant Formulations

The successful clinical development of a vaccine depends upon an number of clinical components or principles *(85,87)*. Most of these principles are shared by vaccine-adjuvant formulations. They include

1. Phase 1, 2, 3, and 4 studies,
2. Inpatient and outpatient facilities for testing vaccines in volunteers,
3. Good Clinical Practice (GCP, the name given by pharmaceutical companies to the set of federal regulations and guidelines for conducting clinical trials designed to support an application for licensure of a biological or drug),
4. Investigational new drug application (IND),
5. Institutional review board (IRB),
6. Product License Application (PLA) and Establishment License Application (ELA). Laboratory-based investigators concerned with preclinical development should be familiar with these components of clinical development.

The steps along the clinical development route leading to the use of a licensed vaccine by the public has been nicely summarized by Davenport *(87)*.

11. Comparative Vaccine Adjuvant Trials

11.1. Animal Studies

Modern studies have compared up to 24 investigational adjuvants individually mixed with one antigen in a single protocol [reviewed by Edelman *(88)*]. The single protocol controls for confounding test variables, such as antigen, dose, schedule, animal species, and immunological assays. These variables make comparisons between two or more separately conducted studies difficult, if not impossible. When adjuvants provide equally good immunogenicity in such comparison trials, adjuvant choice may depend upon other factors. These include cost, commercial availability, reactogenicity, mode of action, and induction of the desired arm of the immune response. Nevertheless, results of comparative trials may fail to identify the best adjuvant or adjuvants. For example, two comparative trials of simian immunodeficiency virus (SIV) vaccines combined with different adjuvants were conducted in macaques ***(84,89)***. The results were disappointing in that the mechanism of immunity could not be clearly delineated, and the large number of primates (80 and 98 animals) was still insufficient to allow meaningful statistical comparison of protection between all adjuvant groups.

11.2. Studies in Humans

Two large clinical trials have compared adjuvanted HIV vaccines ***(62,71)*** and adjuvanted malaria vaccines ***(28)*** in healthy young adult volunteers. These trials illustrate results that can be obtained from comparative adjuvanted vaccine trials in volunteers using similar clinical protocols. In a phase 1, double-blind, randomized, placebo-controled trial in healthy adults, 50 µg of HIV gp120 was combined with one of seven adjuvants ***(62)***. The summary of side effects caused by these vaccines and additional HIV vaccine using similar protocols ***(71)*** was discussed in **Subheading 6.2.** Each adjuvanted vaccine was injected into 15 persons at 0, 2, 6, and 18 mo. The adjuvants included: aluminum hydroxide, MPL®, liposome- encapsulated MPL® with aluminum, MF59, MF59/MTP-PE, SAF, and SAF/threonyl-MDP. The group that received SAF/threonyl-MDP was significantly more likely to experience moderate or severe local and systemic reactions compared to all other groups combined, but this group and the SAF/threonyl-MDP group developed the highest geometric mean HIV-1 neutralizing antibody titers. All adjuvant groups except MPL® induced neutralizing antibody in 80% or more of volunteers after the third dose. The aluminum group had the lowest geometric mean antibody titers. CD8(+) CTL responses were not measured. The results illustrate the common association of high reactogenicity and high adjuvanticity observed in many adjuvant trials.

Numerous attempts have been made to adjuvant the circumsporozoite and blood-stage proteins of *P. falciparum* and to use the adjuvanted proteins as vaccines to protect the majority of vaccinees against experimental or natural malaria challenge. Adjuvants used included aluminum ***(90–93)***, aluminum plus *Pseudomonas aeruginosa* detoxified toxin A carrier ***(94,95)***, aluminum plus fusion protein of HBsAg and MPL ***(28,96)***, fusion protein of HBsAg in a proprietary oil-in-water emulsion ***(28)***, aluminum plus liposomes and MPL ***(97)***, Detox™ (MPL, cell wall skeleton of mycobacteria, and squalane) ***(24)***, recombinant vaccinia virus ***(21)***, and recombinant *Salmonella typhi* ***(38)***. All attempts were unsuccessful until Stout et al. *(28)*, using three adjuvant formulations developed over a decade of trial and error, protected six of seven volunteers with one of them. The successful formulation was composed of CSP protein fused to a HBsAg peptide and adjuvanted with an oil-in-water proprietary emulsion (SmithKline Beecham Biologicals) plus monophosphoryl lipid A (MPLA) and QS-21. The vaccine formulation was administered repeatedly at 0, 4, and 24–28 wk. The two less-protective formulations were composed of CSP-HBsAg in the oil-in-water emulsion, and CSP-HBsAg in a formulation containing alum and MPLA. The results demonstrate that strong, complex adjuvant formulations were required, that a protective adjuvant formulation cannot be deduced from animal studies, that the more robust adjuvants produced more severe local and systemic reactions, and that antibody alone was insufficient to confer protection. The trial was successful, because the U.S. Army investigators and SmithKline Beecham were committed in partnership to expend the time, money, and effort required to develop a successful first generation adjuvanted malaria vaccine. Without such long-term committement, development efforts will not likely succeed.

12. Summary and Conclusion

Interest in vaccine adjuvants is intense and growing, because many of the new subunit vaccine candidates lack sufficient immunogenicity to be clinically useful. In this chapter, I have emphasized modern vaccine adjuvants injected parenterally or administered orally or intranasally with licensed or experimental human vaccines in volunteers. The terms "adjuvant," "carrier," "vehicle," and "adjuvant formulation" are defined. Every adjuvant has a complex and often a multifactorial immunological mechanism, usually poorly understood in vivo. Adjuvant safety, including the real and theoretical risks of administering vaccine adjuvants to humans, is a critical component that can enhance or retard adjuvant development. In addition to the problem of safety, at least four other issues impede the orderly preclinical development of adjuvanted vaccines. These include inconsistent immunopotentiation by candidate adjuvants, the unreliability of reference aluminum adjuvants, marked variation in response to the same adjuvant by different animal models, and the inability to consistently predict protective efficacy by immunoassays.

In preclinical studies of adjuvants and vaccines, the same adjuvant can enhance, inhibit or have no effect at all. The more important determinants of immunogenicity include the nature and dose of the immunogen, the stability of the adjuvant formulation, the schedule and route of immunization, and the animal species and strain studied. In addition to immunologic enhancement without unacceptable side effects and successful protection against challenge, choice of adjuvant for a clinical trial may depend upon cost and commercial availability. Entering the clinical arena, the extensive regulatory and administrative framework required for the conduct of phase I–3 clinical trials are summarized. Finally, several adjuvants combined with one antigen and administered by a common protocol to animals and humans are discussed to illustrate the strength and weaknesses of comparative adjuvant trials. Because the choice of an adjuvant often depends upon expensive trial and error, and because of continuing concerns about adjuvant safety, future vaccine development will focus increasingly on unique synthetic antigen constructs and DNA vaccines in the hope of avoiding the need to administer extraneous chemical or biological adjuvants to humans and to shorten the time of preclinical and clinical development.

References

1. Ramon, G. (1925) Sur l'augmentation anormale de l'antitoxine chez les chevaux producteurs de serum antidipherique. *Bull. Soc. Cent. Med. Vet.* **101,** 227-234.
2. Spriggs, D. R. and Koff, W. C. (1991) *Topics in Vaccine Adjuvant Research*, CRC, Boco Raton, FL.
3. Stewart-Tull, D. E. S. (1989) Recommendations for the assessment of adjuvants (immunopotentiators) in *Immunological Adjuvants and Vaccines* (Gregoriadis, G., Allison, A. C., and Poste, G., eds.), Plenum, New York, pp. 213–226.
4. Powell, M. F. and Newman, M. J. (1995) *Vaccine Design: The Subunit and Adjuvant Approach*, Plenum, New York.
5. Edelman, R. (1980) Vaccine adjuvants. *Rev. Infect. Dis.* **2,** 370–383.
6. Gupta, R. K., Relyveld, E. H., Lindblad, E. B., Bizzini, B., Ben-Efraim, and Gupta C. K. (1993) Adjuvants—a balance between toxicity and adjuvanticity. *Vaccine* **11,** 293–306.
7. Cooper, P. D. (1994) The selective induction of different immune responses by vaccine adjuvants, in *Strategies in Vaccine Design* (Ada, G. L., ed.), Landes, Austin, TX, pp. 125–158.
8. Hunter, R. L. and Lal, A. A. (1994) Copolymer adjuvants in malaria vaccine development. *Am. J. Trop. Med. Hyg.* **50,** 52–58.
9. Gupta, R. K. and Siber, G. R. (1995) Adjuvants for human vaccines—current status, problems and future prospects. *Vaccine* **13,** 1263–1276.
10. Cox, J. C. and Coulter, A. R. (1997) Adjuvants—a classification and review of their modes of action. *Vaccine* **15,** 248–256.
11. Douglas, R. G., Jr. (1993) The children's vaccine initiative—will it work? *J. Infect. Dis.* **168,** 269–274.
12. Ramon, G. (1926) Procedes pour accroitre la production des antitoxines. *Ann. Inst. Pasteur* **40,** 1–10.
13. Lesourd, B. M., Vincent-Falquet, J. C., Deslandes, D., Musset, M., and Moulias, R. (1988) Influenza vaccination in the elderly: improved antibody response with Imuthiol (Na diethyldithiocarbamate) adjuvant therapy. *Int. J. Immunopharmacol.* **10,** 135–143.

14. Gravenstein, S., Duthie, E. H., Miller, B. A., Roecker, E., Drinka, P., Prathipati, K., and Ershler, W. B. (1989) Augmentation of influenza antibody response in elderly men by thymosin alpha one. A double-blind placebo-controlled clinical study. *J. Am. Geriatr. Soc.* **37,** 1–8.
15. Goodman, M. G. (1995) A new approach to vaccine adjuvants: Immunopotentiation by intracellular T-helper-like signals transmitted by loxoribine, in *Vaccine Design: The Subunit and Adjuvant Approach* (Powell, M. F. and Newman, M. J., eds.), Plenum, New York, pp. 581–610.
16. Lin, R., Tarr, P. E., and Jones, T. C. (1995) Present status of the use of cytokines as adjuvants with vaccines to protect against infectious diseases. *Clin. Infect. Dis.* **21,** 1439–1449.
17. Hess, G., Kreiter, F., Kosters, W., and Deusch, K. (1996) The effect of granulocyte-macrophage colony-stimulating factor (GM-CSF) on hepatitis B vaccination in haemodialysis patients. *J. Viral. Hepat.* **3,** 149–153.
18. Drabick, J. J., Tang, D. B., Moran, E. E., Trofa, A. F., Foster, J. S., and Zollinger, W. D. (1997) A randomized, placebo-controlled study of oral cimetidine as an immunopotentiator of parenteral immunization with a group B meningococcal vaccine. *Vaccine* **15,** 1144–1148.
19. Evans, T. G., Judd, M. E., Dowell, T., Poe, S., Daynes, R. A., and Araneo, B. A. (1996) The use of oral dehydroepiandrosterone sulfate as an adjuvant in tetanus and influenza vaccination of the elderly. *Vaccine* **14,** 1531–1537.
20. Edelman, R. and Tacket, C. O. (1990) Adjuvants. *Int. Rev. Immunol.* **7,** 51–66.
21. Ockenhouse, C. F., Sun, P. F., Lanar, D. E., Wellde, B. T., Hall, B. T., Kester, K., et al. (1998) Phase I/IIa safety, immunogenicity, and efficacy trial of NYVAC-Pf7, a pox-vectored, multiantigen, multistage vaccine candidate for Plasmodium falciparum malaria. *J. Infect. Dis.* **177,** 1664–1673.
22. Stover, C. K., Bansal, G. P., Hanson, M. S., Burlein, J. E., Palaszynski, S. R., Young, J. F., et al. (1993) Protective immunity elicited by recombinant bacille Calmette-Guerin (BCG) expressing outer surface protein A (OspA) lipoprotein: a candidate Lyme disease vaccine. *J. Exp. Med.* **178,** 197–209.
23. MacGregor, R. R., Boyer, J. D., Ugen, K. E., Lacy, K. E., Gluckman, S. J., Bagarazzi, M. L., et al. (1998) First human trial of a DNA-based vaccine for treatment of human immunodeficiency virus type 1 infection: safety and host response. *J. Infect. Dis.* **178,** 92–100.
24. Hoffman, S. L., Edelman, R., Bryan, J. P., Schneider, I., Davis, J., Sedegah, M., et al. (1994) Safety, immunogenicity, and efficacy of a malaria sporozoite vaccine administered with monophosphoryl lipid A, cell wall skeleton of mycobacteria, and squalane as adjuvant. *Am. J. Trop. Med. Hyg.* **51,** 603–612.
25. Fries, L. F., Gordon, D. M., Richards, R. L., Egan, J. E., Hollingdale, M. R., et al. (1992) Liposomal malaria vaccine in humans: a safe and potent adjuvant strategy. *Proc. Natl. Acad. Sci. USA* **89,** 358–362.
26. Lidgate, D. M. and Byars, N. E. (1995) Development of an emulsion-based muramyl dipeptide adjuvant formulation for vaccines, in *Vaccine Design: The*

Subunit and Adjuvant Approach (Powell, M. F. and Newman, M. J., eds.), Plenum, New York, pp. 313–324.

27. Wintsch, J., Chaignat, C. L., Braun, D. G., Jeannet, M., Stalder, H., Abrignani, S., et al. (1991) Safety and immunogenicity of a genetically engineered human immunodeficiency virus vaccine. *J. Infect. Dis.* **163,** 219–225.
28. Stoute, J. A., Slaoui, M., Heppner, D. G., Momin, P., Kester, K. E., Desmons, P., et al. (1997) A preliminary evaluation of a recombinant circumsporozoite protein vaccine against Plasmodium falciparum malaria. *N. Engl. J. Med.* **336,** 86–91.
29. Levine, M. M. and Dougan, G. (1998) Optimism over vaccines administered via mucosal surfaces. *Lancet* **351,** 1375–1376.
30. Tacket, C. O., Reid, R. H., Boedeker, E. C., Losonsky, G., Nataro, J. P., Bhagat, H., and Edelman, R. (1994) Enteral immunization and challenge of volunteers given enterotoxigenic E. coli CFA/II encapsulated in biodegradable microspheres. *Vaccine* **12,** 1270–1274.
31. Lowell, G. H. (1997) Proteosomes for improved nasal, oral, or infectable vaccines, in *New Generation Vaccines*, 2nd ed. (Levine, M. M., Woodrow, G. C., Kaper, J. B., and Cobon, G. S., eds.), Marcel Dekker, Inc., New York, NY, pp. 193–206.
32. Chaicumpa, W., Chongsa-nguan, M., Kalambaheti, T., Wilairatana, P., Srimanote, P., Makakunkijcharoen, Y., et al. (1998) Immunogenicity of liposome-associated and refined antigen oral cholera vaccines in Thai volunteers. *Vaccine* **16,** 678–684.
33. Moldoveanu, Z., Love-Homan, L., Huang, W. Q., and Krieg, A. M. (1998) CpG DNA, a novel immune enhancer for systemic and mucosal immunization with influenza virus. *Vaccine* **16,** 1216–1224.
34. Gould-Fogerite, S., Edghill-Smith, Y., Kheiri, M., Wang, Z., Das, K., Feketeova, E., Canki, M., and Mannino, R. J. (1994) Lipid matrix-based subunit vaccines: a structure-function approach to oral and parenteral immunization. *AIDS Res. Hum. Retroviruses 10 Suppl.* **2,** S99–103.
35. Cryz, S. J., Jr. and Gluck, R. (1998) Immunopotentiating reconstituted influenza virosomes as a novel antigen delivery system. *Dev. Biol. Stand.* **92,** 219–223.
36. Saldinger, P. F., Blum, A. L., and Corthesy-Theulaz, I. E. (1997) Perspectives of anti-H. pylori vaccination. *J. Physiol. Pharmacol. 48 Suppl.* **4,** 59–65.
37. Glenn, G. M., Rao, M., Matyas, G. R., and Alving, C. R. (1998) Skin immunization made possible by cholera toxin [letter]. *Nature* **391,** 851.
38. Gonzalez, C., Hone, D., Noriega, F. R., Tacket, C. O., Davis, J. R., Losonsky, G. et al. (1994) Salmonella typhi vaccine strain CVD 908 expressing the circumsporozoite protein of Plasmodium falciparum: strain construction and safety and immunogenicity in humans. *J. Infect. Dis.* **169,** 927–931.
39. Edelman, R., Palmer, K., Russ, K. D., Secrest, H. P., Becker, J. A. Bodison, S. A., et al. (1998) Safety and immunogenicity of recombinant Bacille Calmette-Guerin (rBCG) expressing *Borrelia burgdorferi* outer surface protein A (OspA) lipoprotein in adult volunteers: A candidate Lyme disease Vaccine. *Vaccine*, **17,** 904–914.
40. Tacket, C. O., Losonsky, G., Lubeck, M. D., Davis, A. R., Mizutani, S., Horwith, G., et al. (1992) Initial safety and immunogenicity studies of an oral recombinant adenohepatitis B vaccine. *Vaccine* **10,** 673–676.

41. Tacket, C. O., Mason, H. S., Losonsky, G., Clements, J. D., Levine, M. M., and Arntzen, C. J. (1998) Immunogenicity in humans of a recombinant bacterial antigen delivered in a transgenic potato. *Nature* **4,** 607–609.
42. Krieg, A. M. (1996) An innate immune defense mechanism based on the recognition of CpG motifs in microbial DNA. *J. Lab. Clin. Med.* **128,** 128–133.
43. Newman, M. J. and Powell, M. F. (1995) Immunological and formulation design consideratins for subunit vaccines, in *Vaccine Design: The Subunit and Adjuvant Approach* (Powell, M. F. and Newman, M. J., eds.), Plenum, New York, pp. 1–42.
44. Newman, M. J., Wu, J. Y., Gardner, B. H., Munroe, K. J., Leombruno, D., Recchia, J., and Kensil, C. R. (1992) Saponin adjuvant induction of ovalbumin-specific CD8+ cytotoxic T lymphocyte responses. *J. Immunol.* **148,** 2357–2362.
45. Newman, M. J., Munroe, K. J., Anderson, C. A., Murphy, C. I., Panicali, D. L., Seals, J. R., et al. (1994) Induction of antigen-specific killer T lymphocyte responses using subunit SIVmac251 gag and env vaccines containing QS-21 saponin adjuvant. *AIDS Res. Hum. Retroviruses* **10,** 853–861.
46. Gupta, R. K. and Siber, G. R. (1994) Comparison of adjuvant activities of aluminium phosphate, calcium phosphate and stearyl tyrosine for tetanus toxoid. *Biologicals* **22,** 53–63.
47. Kensil, C. R., Newman, M. J., et al. (1993) The use of Stimulon adjuvant to boost vaccine response. *Vaccine Res.* **2,** 273–282 (Abstr.).
48. Hui, G. S., Chang, S. P., Gibson, H., Hashimoto, A., Hashiro, C., Barr, P. J., and Kotani, S. (1991) Influence of adjuvants on the antibody specificity to the Plasmodium falciparum major merozoite surface protein, gp195. *J. Immunol.* **147,** 3935–3941.
49. Kenney, J. S., Hughes, B. W., Masada, M. P., and Allison, A. C. (1989) Influence of adjuvants on the quantity, affinity, isotype and epitope specificity of murine antibodies. *J. Immunol. Methods* **121,** 157–166.
50. Tam, J. P. (1988) Synthetic peptide vaccine design: synthesis and properties of a high- density multiple antigenic peptide system. *Proc. Natl. Acad. Sci. USA* **85,** 5409–5413.
51. Nardin, E. H., Calvo-Calle, J. M., Oliveira, G. A., Clavijo, P., Nussenzweig, R., Simon, R., Zeng, W., and Rose, K. (1998) Plasmodium falciparum polyoximes: highly immunogenic synthetic vaccines constructed by chemoselective ligation of repeat B-cell epitopes and a universal T-cell epitope of CS protein. *Vaccine* **16,** 590–600.
52. Goldenthal, K. L., Cavagnaro, J. A., Alving, C. R., and Vogel, F. R. (1993) NCVDG working groups: Safety evaluation of vaccine adjuvants: National cooperative vaccine development meeting working group. *AIDS Res. Hum. Retrovirus* **9,** S47–S51.
53. Bussiere, J. L., McCormick, G. C., and Green, J. D. (1995) Preclinical safety assessment considerations in vaccine development, in *Vaccine Design: The Subunit and Adjuvant Approach* (Powell, M. F. and Newman, M. J., eds.), Plenum, New York, pp. 61–79.

54. Schultz, N., Oratz, R., Chen, D., Zeleniuch-Jacquotte, A., Abeles, G., and Bystryn, J. C. (1995) Effect of DETOX as an adjuvant for melanoma vaccine. *Vaccine* **13,** 503–508.
55. Keitel, W., Couch, R., Bond, N., Adair, S., Van Nest, G., and Dekker, C. (1993) Pilot evaluation of influenza virus vaccine (IVV) combined with adjuvant. *Vaccine* **11,** 909–913.
56. Brewer, M. A., Edwards, K. M., Palmer, P. S., and Hinson, H. P. (1994) Bacille Calmette-Guerin immunization in normal healthy adults. *J. Infect. Dis.* **170,** 476–479.
57. Kemp, E. B., Belshe, R. B., and Hoft, D. F. (1996) Immune responses stimulated by percutaneous and intradermal bacille Calmette-Guerin. *J. Infect. Dis.* **174,** 113–119.
58. Gordon, D. M., Duffy, P. E., Heppner, D. G., Lyon, J. A., Williams, J. S., Scheumann, D., et al. (1996) Phase I safety and immunogenicity testing of clinical lots of the synthetic Plasmodium falciparum vaccine SPf66 produced under good manufacturing procedure conditions in the United States. *Am. J. Trop. Med. Hyg.* **55,** 63–68.
59. Amador, R., Moreno, A., Murillo, L. A., Sierra, O., Saavedra, D., Rojas, M., et al. (1992) Safety and immunogenicity of the synthetic malaria vaccine SPf66 in a large field trial. *J. Infect. Dis.* **166,** 139–144.
60. Waters, R. V., Terrell, T. G., and Jones, G. H. (1986) Uveitis induction in the rabbit by muramyl dipeptides. *Infect. Immun.* **51,** 816–825.
61. Allison, A. C. and Byars, N. E. (1991) Immunological adjuvants: desirable properties and side-effects. *Mol. Immunol.* **28,** 279–284.
62. McElrath, M. J. (1994) Adjuvant effects on human immune responses in recipients of candidate HIV vaccines. IBC Conference, in *Novel Vaccine Strategies for Mucosal Immunization, Genetic Approaches and Adjuvants*, Rockville, MD, 24–26 (Abstr.).
63. Pearson, C. M. (1963) Experimental joint disease: Observations on adjuvant-induced arthritis. *J. Chron. Dis.* **16,** 863–874 (Abstract).
64. Kleinau, S., Erlandsson, H., Holmdahl, R., and Klareskog, L. (1991) Adjuvant oils induce arthritis in the DA rat. I. Characterization of the disease and evidence for an immunological involvement. *J. Autoimmun.* **4,** 871–880.
65. Murray, R., Cohen, P., and Hardegree, M. C. (1972) Mineral oil adjuvants: biological and chemical studies. *Ann. Allergy* **30,** 146–151.
66. Salk, J. and Salk, D. (1977) Control of influenza and poliomyelitis with killed virus vaccines. *Science* **195,** 834–847.
67. Stuart-Harris, C. H. (1969) Adjuvant influenza vaccines. *Bull. WHO* **41,** 617–621 (Abstract).
68. Beebe, G. W., Simon, A. H., and Vivona, S. (1972) Long-term mortality follow-up of Army recruits who received adjuvant influenza virus vaccine in 1951–1953. *Am. J. Epidemiol.* **95,** 337–346.

69. Page, W. F., Norman, J. E., and Benenson, A. S. (1993) Long-term follow-up of army recruits immunized with Freund's incomplete adjuvanted vaccine. *Vaccine Res.* **2,** 141–149.
70. Davenport, F. M. (1968) Seventeen years' experience with mineral oil adjuvant influenza virus vaccines. *Ann. Allergy* **26,** 288–292.
71. Keefer, M. C., Wolff, M., Gorse, G. J., Graham, B. S., Corey, L., Clements-Mann, M. L., et al. (1997) Safety profile of phase I and II preventive HIV type 1 envelope vaccination: experience of the NIAID AIDS Vaccine Evaluation Group. *AIDS Res. Hum. Retroviruses* **13,** 1163–1177.
72. Butler, N. R., Feng, S., Benson, P. F., et al. (1962) Response of infants to pertussis vaccine at one week and to poliomyelitis, diptheria, and tetanus vaccine at six months. *Lancet* **2,** 112–114 (Abstract).
73. Cvjetanovic, B. and Uemura, K. (1965) The present status of field and laboratory studies of typhoid and paratyphoid vaccines with special reference to studies sponsored by the World Health Organization. *Bull. WHO* **32,** 29–36 (Abstr.).
74. Woolridge, R. L., Grayston, J. T., Chang, I. A., et al. (1967) Long-term follow-up of the initial (1959–1960) trachoma vaccine field on Taiwan. *Am. J. Ophthalmol.* **63,** 1650–1653 (Abstract).
75. Kasel, J. A., Couch, R. B., and Douglas, R.G., Jr. (1971) Antigenicity of alum and aqueous adenovirus hexon antigen vaccines in man. *J. Immunol.* **107,** 916–919.
76. Davenport, F. M., Hennessy, A. V., and Askin, F. B. (1968) Lack of adjuvant effect of $AIPO_4$ on purified influenza virus haemagglutinins in man. *J. Immunol.* **100,** 1139–1140 (Abstr.).
77. Claesson, B. A., Trollfors, B., Lagergard, T., Taranger, J., Bryla, D., Otterman, G., et al. (1988) Clinical and immunologic responses to the capsular polysaccharide of Haemophilus influenzae type b alone or conjugated to tetanus toxoid in 18- to 23-month-old children. *J. Pediatr.* **112,** 695–702.
78. O'Hagan, D. T., Jeffery, H., and Davis, S. S. (1993) Long-term antibody responses in mice following subcutaneous immunization with ovalbumin entrapped in biodegradable microparticles. *Vaccine* **11,** 965–969.
79. Gupta, R. K., Rost, B. E., Relyveld, E., and Siber, G. R. (1995) Adjuvant properties of aluminum and calcium compounds, in *Vaccine Design: The Subunit and Adjuvant Approach* (Powell, M. F. and Newman, M. J., eds.), Plenum, New York: 229–248.
80. World Health Organization (1977) *Manual for the Production and Control of Vaccines—Tetanus Toxoid.* BLD/UNDP/77.2 Rev.1 ed.
81. Jensen, O. M. and Koch, C. (1988) On the effect of $AI(OH)_3$ as an immunological adjuvant. *Acta Pathol. Microbiol. Immun. Scand.* **96,** 257–264 (Abstract).
82. Bumford, R. (1989) Aluminum salts: prospectives in their use as adjuvants, in *Immunological Adjuvants and Vaccines* (Gregoriadis, G., Allison, A. C., and Poste, G., eds.), Plenum, New York, pp. 35–41.

83. Hardegree, M. C., Pittman, M., and Maloney, C. J. (1972) Influence of mouse strain on the assayed potency (unitage) of tetanus toxoid. *Appl. Microbiol.* **24,** 120–126.
84. Murphey-Corb, M., Ohkawa, S., Martin, L., et al. (1993) Comparative efficacy of a whole killed SIV vaccine in combination with various adjuvants, *Sixth Annu. Meet. Nat. Cooperative Vaccine Dev. Group for AIDS* (Abstract).
85. Tacket, C. O., Rennels, M. B., and Mattheis, M. J. (1997) Initial clinical evaluation of new vaccine candidates: phase 1 and 2 clinical trials of safety, immunogenicity, and preliminary efficacy, in *New Generation Vaccines* (Levine, M. M., Woodrow, G. C., Kaper, J. B., and Cobon, G. S., eds.), Marcel Dekker, New York, pp. 35–45.
86. U.S. Food and Drug Administration (1991) General Biological Products Standards, in *Anonymous Code of Federal Regulations*, Department of Health and Human Services, Bethesda, MD, pp. 43–53.
87. Davenport, L. W. (1995) Regulatory considerations in vaccine design, in *Vaccine Design: The Subunit and Adjuvant Approach* (Powell, M. F. and Newman, M. J., eds.), Plenum, New York, pp. 81–96.
88. Edelman, R. (1997) Adjuvants for the Future, in *New Generation Vaccines* (Levine, M. M., Woodrow, G. C., Kaper, J. B., and Cobon, G. S., eds.), Marcel Dekker, New York, pp. 173–192.
89. Hunsmann, G. (1995) Protection of macaques against simian immunodeficiency virus infection with inactivated vaccines: comparison of adjuvants, doses and challenge viruses. *Vaccine* **13,** 295–300.
90. Ballou, W. R., Hoffman, S. L., Sherwood, J. A., Hollingdale, M. R., Neva, F. A., Hockmeyer, W. T., et al. (1987) Safety and efficacy of a recombinant DNA Plasmodium falciparum sporozoite vaccine. *Lancet* **1,** 1277–1281.
91. Herrington, D. A., Clyde, D. F., Losonsky, G., Cortesia, M., Murphy, J. R., Davis, J., et al. (1987) Safety and immunogenicity in man of a synthetic peptide malaria vaccine against Plasmodium falciparum sporozoites. *Nature* **328,** 257–259.
92. Patarroyo, M. E., Amador, R., Clavijo, P., Moreno, A., Guzman, F., Romero, P., et al. (1988) A synthetic vaccine protects humans against challenge with asexual blood stages of Plasmodium falciparum malaria. *Nature* **332,** 158–161.
93. Alonso, P. L., Smith, T., Schellenberg, J. R., Masanja, H., Mwankusye, S., Urassa, H., et al. (1994) Randomised trial of efficacy of SPf66 vaccine against Plasmodium falciparum malaria in children in southern Tanzania. *Lancet* **344,** 1175–1181.
94. Fries, L. F., Gordon, D. M., Schneider, I., Beier, J. C., Long, G. W., Gross, M., et al. (1992) Safety, immunogenicity, and efficacy of a Plasmodium falciparum vaccine comprising a circumsporozoite protein repeat region peptide conjugated to Pseudomonas aeruginosa toxin A. *Infect. Immun.* **60,** 1834–1839.
95. Brown, A. E., Singharaj, P., Webster, H. K., Pipithkul, J., Gordon, D. M., Boslego, J. W., et al. (1994) Safety, immunogenicity and limited efficacy study of a recombinant Plasmodium falciparum circumsporozoite vaccine in Thai soldiers. *Vaccine* **12,** 102–108.

96. Gordon, D. M., McGovern, T. W., Krzych, U., Cohen, J. C., Schneider, I., LaChance, R., et al. (1995) Safety, immunogenicity, and efficacy of a recombinantly produced Plasmodium falciparum circumsporozoite protein-hepatitis B surface antigen subunit vaccine. *J. Infect. Dis.* **171,** 1576–1585.
97. Heppner, D. G., Gordon, D. M., Gross, M., Wellde, B., Leitner, W., Krzych, U., et al. (1996) Safety, immunogenicity, and efficacy of Plasmodium falciparum repeatless circumsporozoite protein vaccine encapsulated in liposomes. *J. Infect. Dis.* **174,** 361–366.

2

Harmful and Beneficial Activities of Immunological Adjuvants

Duncan E. S. Stewart-Tull

1. Introduction

There are no officially recognized regulations for the design and toxicity testing of adjuvants or adjuvant formulations; the former are also referred to as immunomodulators and immunopotentiators. At the "Immunological Adjuvants and Vaccines" meeting held in Greece in 1988, however, immunoadjuvant researchers discussed experimental toxicological tests that might be used to monitor new immunomodulators *(1)*. The usefulness of these tests for the range of immunomodulators and adjuvant formulations was examined over a 2-yr period and subsequently, at the next NATO meeting in 1990, further recommendations were made *(2)*. Although as yet, no final agreement has been reached and a variety of tests are still in use.

At the "Harmonization of regulatory procedures for Veterinary Biologicals" meeting in Ploufragan, Brittany, a number of scientists and administrators from the regulatory bodies of the United States of America and the European Community indicated that "adjuvants are too reactive for inclusion in vaccines" *(3)*. This viewpoint was challenged before discussions about new harmonized quality assurance, and quality control regulations were instigated, otherwise the development and release of new vaccines would be delayed. In addition, there has been a degree of lobbying against one or another immunomodulator in order to substantiate the efficacy claims for a particular substance or adjuvant formulation. Eventually, agreement will be reached among adjuvant researchers, vaccine producers, and licencing authorities in regard to the most suitable biological and toxicity tests for new immunomodulators or adjuvant

From: *Methods in Molecular Medicine, Vol. 42:*
Vaccine Adjuvants: Preparation Methods and Research Protocols
Edited by: D. T. O'Hagan © Humana Press, Inc., Totowa, NJ

formulations, but until then it would seem profitable to monitor the tests which are currently being appraised by adjuvant researchers. It should also be stressed that the battery of recommended tests may include some that would be specific for a particular group of immunomodulators; for example, the capacity of aluminum compounds to adsorb the vaccine antigen is an essential test.

In addition, comments expressed about the unsuitable and inadmissible use of adjuvants in vaccines contradict the *status quo*. Whole-cell vaccines of Gram-negative bacteria contain peptidoglycan and lipopolysaccharide (LPS), long established as efficient immunomodulators. Some 2.5 billion doses of BCG vaccine have been administered in the fight against tuberculosis and each dose contains approximately 3.0–5.0 mg of peptidoglycan, a good adjuvant. A course of three injections of the whole-cell pertussis vaccine would contain between 6.5–50.0 mg peptidoglycan and 6.0–35.0 mg of LPS ***(4)***. Would the critics really expect all whole-cell vaccines to be withdrawn irrespective of their efficacy because they contained an adjuvant? I suggest the answer would be No. Robbins ***(5)*** expressed the opinion that "any toxicity that we accept is a compromise." Such a compromise must become an accepted principle in the search for adjuvants suitable for use in human vaccines because one of their functions is to stimulate antigen-presenting cells (particularly dendritic cells and macrophages). It is doubtful whether this stimulation would occur if adjuvants were completely innocuous substances, lacking any cellular aggravation activity. This does not mean that an adjuvant should be designed to include low-level toxicity. The compromise adjuvant researchers seek is the design of adjuvant molecules with the insertion, substitution, or removal of chemical groups which will increase their immunopotentiating activity, while at the same time, reducing significantly their tissue reactivity, hence the array of MDP derivatives that the chemists have produced—of which very few have been shown to be acceptable.

An adjuvant or immunopotentiator should stimulate high antibody titres, but in the process it should have low toxicity and not induce harmful side effects after injection into either animals or human beings. The main function of an adjuvant is to stimulate antibody production against a range of antigens, even with small quantities of poorly antigenic substances, preferably in a small number of injections or administrations. These objectives would seem to be easy to achieve, but after much research the perfect adjuvant is still elusive to vaccinologists. Indeed, it is unlikely that such a universal adjuvant will be found as different vaccines will require different adjuvants. More than 100 adjuvants have been described ***(6)***, but many of these would not be routinely included in vaccines because of a variety of reasons, e.g., cost and the complex preparation of the injection mixture, and many are too reactive in toxicology tests.

The design of an adjuvant depends to a certain extent on the arm of the immune response one is attempting to enhance. But a high priority should be placed on the overall welfare of and possible stress caused to animals during the evaluation of a new prototype formulation to be included in the injection mixture. Furthermore, the nature of the adjuvant should be reflected in the route, protocols of injection, and the type of vaccine, e.g., "routine" preventative vaccines vs cancer vaccines.

2. Materials

2.1. Hemolysis Test

1. A New Zealand white (NZW) rabbit or equivalent.
2. Heparinized bleeding set, e.g., Vacutainer (Becton and Dickinson, Rutherford, NJ).
3. Sodium chloride (0.85% (w/v); Sigma, St. Louis, MO).
4. Saponin (Sigma).
5. Cyanmethemoglobin standard, Merck Ltd., Darmstadt-Mannheim, Germany, Cyanmethemoglobin standard for photometric determinations of hemoglobin, 1.0 mL in 200 mL distilled water. Cat. 36210P or Hemoglobin standard, Sigma, Cat. 525-A.
6. Hematocrit and bench centrifuge.
7. Phosphate buffer pH 7.5.
8. Drabkin's reagent: (Merck): this reagent is stable if stored in the dark.

Potassium hexacyanoferrate	200 mg
Potassium cyanide	50 mg
Potassium dihydrogen orthophosphate	140 mg
Colorless nonionic surfactant in distilled water, e.g., Nonidet P40	1.0 mL
Distilled water to 1 L	

9. Matburn blood cell suspension mixer (Matburn Surgical Equipment Ltd, Portsmouth, U.K.).
10. Spectrophotometer capable of reading from A540 nm to A592 nm with 1.0 cm lightpath cuvets.
11. Microhematocrit tubes (Volac; J. Poulten Ltd., Barking, Essex, U.K.).

2.2. Rabbit Pyrogenicity Test

1. NZW rabbits, 2–3 kg.
2. Pyrogen-free glassware, needles, and syringes, as well as pyrogen-free physiological saline.
3. Rectal thermometer.

2.3. Limulus Lysate Assay

1. Commercial *Limulus polyphemus* amoebocyte lysate (LAL) test kits, e.g., either Sigma E-Toxate, multiple test vial system sensitive to 0.005–0.5 endotoxin units (EU)/mL Cat. 210-2, or M.A. Bioproducts' LAL test system with a reagent which

will detect 0.25 ng/mL of FDA reference endotoxin with the addition of 1.0 ng/mL of *Escherichia coli* O 111 : B4. Sigma, Cat. 50-505U.
2. Pyrogen-free water for making dilutions of the standard, e.g., Endotoxin-free water Sigma Cat. 210-7.
3. All glassware must be pyrogen-free, autoclave at 121°C for 1 h followed by 3 h in the drying oven at 175°C or use commercially available pyrogen-free disposables.

2.4. Toxicity Assays

2.4.1. Cytoxicity Assay

1. Tissue-culture flasks (80 cm^2; Falcon, Los Angeles, CA) and tissue-culture plates, 24-well, Greiner.
2. Tissue-culture cell lines (European Collection of Cell cultures).
3. Minimal essential medium, Eagles' (Cat. 32360-026), fetal bovine serum (Cat. 10084-069), L-glutamine 200 m*M* (Cat. 25030-024), Fungizone (Cat. 152-018), penicillin/streptomycin (Cat. 15140-114), trypsin-EDTA (x1, Cat. 45300-019), all from Gibco, Gaithersburg, MD.
4. MEM nonessential amino acids (100x; Cat. 11140-035, Gibco) and Insulin-transferrin-selenium-G.
5. Supplement (Cat. 41400-045; Gibco) are required for the CaCO-2 cell-line growth.
6. Incubator (37°C and 5% CO_2).
7. Phosphate buffered physiological saline (BDH Merck).
8. Dialysis tubing (Medicell Int. Ltd.).
9. Millipore filters 0.22-µm pore size.
10. MTT, (3-[4,5-dimethylthiazol-2-yl] -2,5-diphenyltetrazolium bromide, thiazolyl blue) Sigma Cat. M2128).
11. DMSO (dimethyl sulfoxide; Sigma, Cat. D5879).
12. Triton-X 100 (t-octylphenoxy polyethoxy-ethanol) Sigma Cat. T9284.

2.4.2. Single and Multiple Dose and Systemic Toxicity Tests

1. Adjuvant in physiological saline as polar solvent.
2. Adjuvant in sesame oil (Sigma) as nonpolar solvent.
3. Needles and syringes.
4. Two mammalian species, e.g., rabbits and mice.

2.5. Induction of Allergy to Food Proteins

1. Ovalbumin and lactalbumin (Sigma).
2. Gelatin capsules.
3. Ascorbic acid.
4. Physiological saline.
5. 1.0 mL syringes.
6. Evans blue dye.
7. ELISA plates, coating buffer, washing buffer, peroxidase-labeled secondary antibody, substrate and reader.

3. Methods

3.1. Hemolysis Test

At very low concentrations, adjuvants should not be hemolytic. This is particularly relevant for the crude, triterpenoid plant saponins, which reportedly destroy erythrocytes if injected intravenously, although this effect may be owing to contaminatory substances *(7)*. The immune stimulating complexes (ISCOMs; see Chapter 14) contain a saponin, which is also used to produce the positive 100% lysis of erythrocytes in the method below. It is often stated that such complexes cannot be used in vaccines because of the hemolytic properties of this component, however, no such drastic hemolysis has been detected in the numerous successful studies with ISCOM vaccines in animals. Nevertheless, it is wise to check for the hemolytic activity of a new adjuvant compound either separately, or chemically conjugated to antigen, or in combination with an antigen in the final vaccine formulation. It is obviously very important to check new adjuvant preparations for hemolytic activity against erythrocytes from different sources and species, for example, if the vaccine is to be used in sheep, then a sheep hemolysis assay would be essential.

This procedure is based on the British Standard 5736: Part 11: *(8)*.

1. Bleed (10.0 mL) a NZW rabbit from the ear vein into a heparinized tube. Centrifuge at 2000*g* for 10 min and wash the cells twice in physiological saline. Resuspend the packed cells in a small quantity of saline and determine the percentage of erythrocytes in the suspension by the haematocrit method. Dilute an aliquot to 2.0% for use.
2. Tests and controls are set up as shown :

	Test	Test	Positive control	Negative control
Tube	1	2	3	4
Heparinized blood	2.0 mL	2.0 mL	2.0 mL	2.0 mL
Adjuvant in sterile physiological saline	0.1 mL	0.1 mL	—	—
Sterile physiological saline	—	—	0.1 mL	0.1 mL
White saponin 125 mg in sterile physiological saline	—	—	0.1 mL	—

3. Incubate the tubes at 37°C ± 2°C on a Matburn cell suspension mixer for 4 h. Centrifuge the tubes at 2000*g* for 10 min and determine the percentage hemolysis in each tube. This can be done by measurement of the A_{540nm} or more accurately by measurement of the hemoglobin concentration in the supernatant fluid by the cyanmethemoglobin conversion method.
4. Measurement of the total hemoglobin in blood as cyanmethemoglobin
   a. Spectrophotometric measurement at A_{540nm} in 1.0 cm-pathway cuvets. Add 20 µL of the positive or negative controls or test adjuvant samples to 4.0 mL

Drabkin's reagent and mix. Measure the A_{540nm} of these mixtures and the reference cyanmethemoglobin solution against a distilled water blank.

The hemoglobin concentration is calculated from:

$$\text{Hemoglobin concentration (g L}^{-1}) = \frac{A_{540}\text{ of test blood}}{A_{540}\text{ of reference cyanmethemoglobin}} \times \frac{200C}{1000}$$

where C = concentration of cyanmethemoglobin in the reference solution, expressed in mg/L.

b. Lyse freshly obtained heparinized blood from the NZW rabbit with distilled water. Measure the hemoglobin concentration by the cyanmethemoglobin conversion method described above. Prepare a series of reference hemoglobin solutions from 0.05 g/L to 0.75 g/L by diluting the lysed blood stock solution with a phosphate buffer, pH 7.5. Measure the A_{560nm}, A_{576nm}, and A_{592nm} against a distilled water blank with 1.0-cm path length. Measure test samples at the same wavelengths.
   i. Calculate the function for each reference hemoglobin solution from $2y - (x + z)$

   $$\text{i.e., } 2(A_{576nm}\text{ value}) - (A_{560nm}\text{ value} + A_{592nm}\text{ value})$$

   ii. Plot the values from $2y - (x + y)$ against the hemoglobin concentration.
   iii. Repeat with each of the test samples and read the hemoglobin concentrations off the graph. Express the results in g/L and calculate the percentage hemolysis by comparison with the reference.

Calculate and record the percentage hemolysis by:

$$\%\text{ hemolysis} = \frac{\text{Test hemoglobin concentration}}{\text{Total hemoglobin concentration in positive control}} \times 100$$

Tube	1	2	3	4
% Hemolysis				

The test is invalid if either the % hemolysis for the negative control is >5.0 or the % hemolysis for the positive control is <1.0 or >20.0. Hemolytic activity in the final adjuvanted vaccine formulation would preclude its general use.

3.2. Pyrogenicity Tests

*3.2.1. Rabbit Pyrogenicity Test **(9,10)***

The pyrogen test is designed to limit to an acceptable level the risks of febrile reactions that might occur after the injection of a product containing adjuvant. This method is a modification of the British Standard 5736: Part 5: ***(10)***. All glassware, solutions for washing or rinsing apparatus and diluents must be pyrogen-free, either heat at 250°C for not less than 30 min or use Toxaclean (Sigma) in washing solutions as applicable before use.

1. The adjuvant should be dissolved/suspended in pyrogen-free physiological saline and warmed to 38.5 ± 1.0°C.
2. Rabbits should be housed at a temperature of 20–23°C. Before use in a pyrogen test the rabbits should be sham-tested with an injection of 10.0 mL/kg physiological saline into a marginal ear vein 7 d before use. Withhold food from the rabbits the night before any test and until the completion of the test. Weigh the rabbits and record their temperature, with an accurate thermocouple or thermistor probe thermometer (+ 0.1°C) inserted into the rectum 50–75 mm, at 30-min intervals, beginning 90 min before injection of the saline solution, and at 30 min intervals for 3 h after injection. Exclude rabbits before the injection of the test adjuvant solution/suspension if:
   a. the difference between any two consecutive readings is >0.2°C.
   b. the range of temperature readings exceeds 0.4°C.
   c. the initial temperature is not in the range 38.0–39.8°C.
3. This procedure is repeated with each dose of adjuvant. Although it is more time-consuming, from the point of view of animal welfare it is reasonable to proceed with one animal at a time for each dose of adjuvant. Inject 10 ml/kg of the adjuvant preparation into the marginal vein of one ear of rabbit 1 within a period of 4.0 min. Record the temperature at 30-min intervals for 3 h after injection. If rabbit 1 passes the test, repeat with rabbits 2 and 3.
4. The adjuvant solution/suspension is deemed to be nonpyrogenic if either no rabbit showed an increase of 0.6°C above its respective control temperature before the injection of the adjuvant, or the sum of the three individual maximum temperature increases of rabbits 1–3 does not exceed 1.4°C.
5. If neither of the above criteria are met, it has been suggested that the test should be repeated with 5 other rabbits, although if there is excessive fever it may be deemed politic to reject the new adjuvant and save the needless use of animals. If the test is carried out, the adjuvant solution/ suspension is deemed to be nonpyrogenic if either 3 of the 8 do not show an average increase of 0.6°C, or the sum of the eight individual maximum temperature increases of the rabbits 1–8 does not exceed 3.7°C.

3.2.2. Limulus polyphemus Amoebocyte Lysate (LAL) Assay of Diluents and Adjuvants

The LAL assay for endotoxin, reviewed by McCartney and Wardlaw ***(11)***, is very sensitive and can detect as little as 0.1 ng/mL endotoxin activity. Nonspecificity may be a result of contaminatory endotoxin, so it is very important to ensure that all equipment and glassware used in the assay are endotoxin-free. The LAL assay was adopted by the U.S. Food and Drug Administration ***(12)*** for routine testing of biological products and medical devices, but as yet has not been accepted as an alternative for the rabbit pyrogenicity test by the

European Pharmacopoeia. One way forward would be to use the rabbit pyrogenicity test and the LAL assays in tandem during the development phase of a new vaccine containing an adjuvant and show negative results. Subsequently, it might be possible to persuade authorities to accept the LAL assay for routine batch-testing during manufacture of a new vaccine (*see* **Note 1**).

1. The precise procedure for this assay, which should include a series of control endotoxin dilutions from 4–0.005 ng/mL, is described by the manufacturer, but it is important that a minimum of 4 tests are set up for each sample.
2. A positive result is seen where a solid gel is formed in the test tubes and a negative result is where there is no solidification of the clottable protein extracted from the circulating amoebocytes of *L. polyphemus*.

3.3. Measurement of the Toxicity of Adjuvants

3.3.1. Cytotoxicity Assay in Cultured Monolayers of Human or Animal Cell Lines

This type of assay has the great merit of reducing the number of animals which must be used to comply with standardized toxicity tests. The MTT assay ***(13)*** was adapted for determining cell survival and proliferation by a number of workers ***(14–16)*** with different cell types and toxins.The assay compares favorably with other similar systems ***(17)***, is less time-consuming and objective than microscopic examination of cells, and eliminates the risks associated with assays involving radioisotope release. As examples, the protocols for three different cell lines have been described, but these are not exclusive.

1. Tissue culture cells and growth conditions. The cells should be checked for the absence of virus contamination. This is confirmed by electron microscopy and for the presence of contaminating mycoplasmas by a specific staining technique before use. Human colon adenocarcinoma (CaCO-2) cells are grown in Eagle's MEM medium with Earle's salts and 25 m*M* HEPES (Gibco) in 80-cm^2 tissue-culture flasks (Falcon). Non-essential amino acids (1.0% w/v), glutamine (2 mmol/L), 100 µg/mL penicillin/streptomycin, 1.0% v/v of growth promoter, insulin-transferrin-selenium, and 10% v/v fetal calf serum are added and the cells are incubated at 37°C in 5.0% carbon dioxide atmosphere. The cells are routinely split 1 in 5 by rinsing with 5.0 mL sterile PBS followed by 2.0 mL of 0.25% w/v trypsin/EDTA. A confluent monolayer of CaCO-2 cells in an 80.0-cm^2 flask is obtained usually within 5–7 d, with regular changes of medium. A cell suspension of cells prepared by trypsinization is used to inoculate wells in a 24-well plate.

   African green monkey kidney (VERO) or HeLa cells, are grown in Eagle's MEM medium (Gibco) containing 100 µg/mL penicillin/streptomycin and 5.0% v/v fetal calf serum. The cells are incubated at 37°C in an atmosphere of 5% CO_2. VERO and HeLa cells are routinely split in the same manner as the CaCO-2 cells.

2. HeLa or VERO cells are harvested with trypsin/EDTA and resuspended in growth medium to a density of 5×10^4 cells/mL. Each well of a flat-bottomed 24-well plate is loaded with 200 μL of the cell suspension and incubated at 37°C overnight. The growth medium (100 μL) is discarded and 100 μL of twofold dilutions of the adjuvant in tissue-culture medium is added to each well: duplicate wells of each dilution are set up. Cells with PBS only or 1.0% v/v Triton X-100 in PBS serve as the 100% and 0% live controls, respectively. After 24 h incubation at 37°C, 20 μL of MTT solution (5 mg/mL 3-[4,5-dimethylthiazol-2-yl]-2, 5-diphenyltetrazolium bromide (Sigma) in PBS, filter-sterilized are added to each well and incubation continued for 4 h. After emptying the wells the resultant formazan crystals are solubilized by the addition to each well of 100 μL 0.4 mol/L HCl in dimethyl sulphoxide v/v (DMSO; Sigma) and the absorbance measured at 540 nm in the Anthos 2001 plate reader. The percentage of cell deaths, adopted to take account of the variable growth of the cells, was calculated with the formula:

$$1 - \frac{[A_{540nm}\text{ test} - A_{540nm}\text{Triton X +ve Control}]}{[A_{540nm}\text{ PBS –ve control} - A_{540nm}\text{Triton X +ve Control}]} \times 100$$

3.3.2. Intracutaneous Toxicity Test

This procedure assesses any skin irritation at the site of injection and is based on the British Standard 5736: Part 7 ***(18)***. This test may be relevant with some adjuvants, which are to be included in vaccines injected by the intradermal or subcutaneous routes. For example, Kensil et al. ***(19)*** fractionated Quil A from *Quillaja saponaria*, the South American soap tree, and one preparation QS-7 was nontoxic at an intradermal dose of 500 μg whereas QS-18 was lethal at a dose of 25.0 μg. The latter preparation would not be acceptable either as a saponin adjuvant nor as part of any other adjuvant formulation. This type of test may involve single-dose toxicity or repeated dose toxicity reactions of the adjuvant formulation. The test is usually done by intraperitoneal (ip) or subcutaneous (sc) injection into two mammalian species, but the number of animals in the test groups is being questioned and some authorities may well invoke the 3 Rs, namely replacement, reduction, and refinement for the sake of animal welfare.

3.3.2.1. Single-Dose Toxicity Test

This is a qualitative and quantitative study of the possible toxic reactions, which may result from a single administration of the active substance, in this instance the adjuvant, in an acute toxicity test. As with other tests, it is important to use the adjuvant alone or in the injectable form. The test should be done in two mammalian species, with equal numbers of males and females, if a veterinary product the intended animal should be included. There should be at least two routes of administration, for example by ip and sc injection. After injection, the animals should be examined at regular intervals, at least three times daily, for not less than 7 d, and any animal with obvious signs of ill health or in a moribund state should be killed.

3.3.2.2. Repeated-Dose Toxicity Test

This is intended to monitor the effect of repeated administration of vaccines containing an adjuvant component. It is the responsibility of the investigator to give valid reasons for the extent and duration of the trials and the dosages chosen. However, the maximum dose should be selected so as to indicate potential harmful effects and lower doses will enable the animal's tolerance to the new adjuvant. The repeated-dose toxicity test should be done in two mammalian species (1 nonrodent).

Animals that are mentioned in European rules governing medicinal products *(28)* for use in these two tests are: mouse (*Mus musculus*), rat (*Rattus norvegicus*), guinea-pig (*Cavia porcellus*), golden hamster (*Mesocricetus auratus*), rabbit (*Oryctolagus cuniculus*), nonhuman primates, dog (*Canis familiaris*), cat (*Felis catus*), quail (*Coturnix coturnix*).

Evaluation of the adjuvant may be done by a variety of means: monitoring the behavior and weight gain of the animals, hematological, and physiological tests. If an animal dies, an autopsy and histological examination of tissues, including the sites of injection, should be done.

1. The adjuvant is dissolved/suspended in either a polar solvent, sterile physiological saline, or a nonpolar solvent, sesame oil (Ph. Eur), usually heated at 180°C for 60 min.
2. Preparation of animals. The fur is clipped on the back of each animal, e.g., rabbits, before injection.
3. Rabbit 1. (a) inject four sites on the left-hand side of the body with 0.1 mL of the test mixture subcutaneously or (b) inject four sites on the right-hand side with 0.01 mL intradermally with: (i) adjuvant in polar solvent; (ii) polar solvent alone; (iii) adjuvant in nonpolar solvent; iv) nonpolar solvent alone. The injection sites are examined for 5 d and the size of any skin reactions measured with precision calipers, for example, Mecanic in nylon-asbestos (Camlab, U.K.).
4. Rabbits 2, 3, and 4 should only be injected if the rabbit 1 test is negative.
5. The injection sites are examined for erythema (redness at the site of injection), eschar (scab formation at the site of injection), or edema (swelling at the injection site) (**Table 1**).

3.3.3. Systemic Toxicity Test

The aim of this procedure is to measure undesirable effect(s) at sites distant from the injection site, which may become apparent after the administration of

Table 1
Classification System for Skin Reactions

Reaction	Numerical grading
Erythema and eschar formation:	
No erythema	0
Very slight erythema	1
Well-defined erythema	2
Moderate to severe erythema	3
Severe erythema (beet-redness) to slight eschar formation	4
Edema formation:	
No edema	0
Very slight edema	1
Well-defined edema (edges of area well defined by definite raising)	2
Moderate edema (raised approximately 1 mm)	3
Severe edema (raised more than 1 mm and extending beyond exposure area)	4

NOTE: Other adverse changes at the skin sites should be recorded and reported.

the adjuvant alone or the adjuvant formulation. The adjuvant is injected intraperitoneally in polar or nonpolar diluents or intravenously in a nonpolar solvent with appropriate controls. These are tests which the regulatory bodies may require with groups of five mice, but there may be moves to reduce the number of animals to be tested. It is feasible that these tests could eventually be phased out when there are sufficient experimental results accumulated to allow the validation of alternative toxicity tests. The method is based on British Standard 5736: Part 3 ***(20)***.

1. Groups of five weanling mice, 3–4-wk old are weighed and injected, either intraperitoneally with 0.5-mL volumes of graded doses of the adjuvant mixtures:
   Group 1. Adjuvant in sesame oil
   Group 2. Sesame oil alone
   Group 3. Adjuvant in physiological saline
   Group 4. Physiological saline alone

   Or, intravenously with 1.0 mL of:
   Group 5. Adjuvant in physiological saline
   Group 6. Physiological saline alone
2. The animals are observed for 14 d, frequently during the 4 h immediately following injection and at least three times a day thereafter.
3. Record any visible signs of reaction after injection of the adjuvant preparation, for example, time of onset after injection, their duration, and intensity. Weigh all

the animals daily for 7 d, refer to the "weight-gain test" below, and kill all surviving animals and record the appearance of the animals. Record any deaths if they occur on the respective day after injection. Postmortem all animals at the end of the experiment and record the appearance of organs and the histological examination of tissues of interest including: heart, lungs, gastrointestinal tract, liver, spleen, kidneys, and gonads. The report could be produced in the format shown in **Table 2**.

3.3.4. Mouse Weight-Gain Test

The 7-d mouse weight-gain test is still a standard and reliable method. After injection of a substance containing endotoxin, the animal may show a decrease in weight during 24 h if endotoxin is present *(21)*. If this is followed by a steady increase in the animal's weight over 7 d, it is assumed that the product is acceptable. If, on the other hand, the product is highly toxic the animal may steadily continue to lose weight or in extreme cases become moribund and is killed. The tests in **Subheading 3.3.2.** and **3.3.3.** may provide evidence of unacceptable levels of toxicity in which case it may be unnecessary to proceed with a weight-gain test as the adjuvant is probably too reactive.

The protocols for these laboratory assays should not be regarded as alternatives to statutory tests required for licensed medical or veterinary products, however, they will show whether financial investment in a new immunopotentiator or adjuvant formulation is warranted. Invariably, if a new adjuvant formulation gives a positive reaction in one of the tests described above, it is highly unlikely that the preparation will be suitable for routine vaccine use (*see* **Note 2**).

3.4. Induction of Allergy to Nonvaccine or Food Proteins

This is a particularly important test when examining the suitability of an adjuvant for inclusion in an oral vaccine, as there could be a reaction to food proteins *(23)*. With the interest in the oral route as a means of stimulating mucosal immunity, there is a possibility that an adjuvant could induce an allergic response to dietary proteins. In this study, both lactalbumin and gluten failed to elicit an IgE response in the presence of the original Freund's Complete or Incomplete Adjuvants (FCA or FIA) in HAM1/CR mice or Dunkin Hartley guinea pigs. On the other hand, the guinea pigs showed increased IgE production after oral administration of ovalbumin or soy bean protein, both unusual proteins in their normal pellet diet. Such tests are valid only if all of the previous toxicity tests are negative.

1. Groups of mice or guinea pigs are fed freely with moistened ovalbumin or lactalbumin as the main food supply for 24 h. This does not affect their normal weight gain or health. Subsequently, the mice are dosed orally with 0.2 mL of the

Table 2
Style of Report for the Toxicity Tests

	Mouse groups					
	1	2	3	4	5	6
Weight (g) at the start of the test						
Weight (g) at the end of the test						
Difference in weight (g)						
Deaths						
Autopsy report						
Histology report						
Assessment. P = Pass; F = Fail						

adjuvanted formulation or with physiological saline, as the control, containing 2.0 mg of the test protein. The dose in guinea pigs is 0.3 mL of adjuvanted formulation, administered in a gelatin capsule, whereas the saline is delivered from a syringe without a needle at the back of the oral cavity.

2. All animals are fed on the protein diet for a further 24 h after adjuvant dosing and then returned to their normal pellet diet and water. The guinea pigs are also given ascorbic acid to prevent vitamin C deficiency. All animals were bled out on day 21.
3. Passive cutaneous anaphylaxis (PCA) reactions are measured in hairless mice, *hrhr*, injected intradermally with 0.05 mL of serum diluted 1 in 2 at four sites on the dorsal surface. For IgG PCA tests, the sera are heated for 2 h at 56°C to inactivate IgE. After 2 h for IgG and 48 h for IgE, 1.0 mg of the respective protein in 0.2 mL saline containing 0.5% (w/v) Evans Blue dye is injected into the caudal vein, and after 30 min the areas of blueing on the skin are measured. The hair is clipped from the dorsal surface of the guinea pig, injected with 0.1 mL of the serum and after 4 h for IgG and 12 d for IgE injected with 0.1 mL saline containing 1.0% dye and 1.0 mg of the respective protein. The zones of blueing are measured after 2 h, intensively staining zones of >0.5 cm^2 are indicative of a positive reaction, although the positive zones appear more diffuse with the IgE response in the guinea pig.
4. The sera may also be examined for the presence of antibodies by a standard ELISA.

3.5. Standard Adjuvants and Antigens, Routes, and Volumes of Injection Mixtures for Use with New Adjuvant Formulations in Tests to Measure the Stimulation of Humoral and Cell-Mediated Responses

3.5.1. Standard Adjuvants

Those recommended were Alhydrogel and the FCA produced by the Statens Serum Institute, Copenhagen *(1)*. A suitable alternative for the latter is a "Non-

Ulcerative Freund's Complete Adjuvant (NUFCA)" which contains BCG vaccine BP, BNF intradermal (*see* **Note 3**). The BCG vaccine for sc injection should not be used as this will cause local ulceration. The id BCG vaccine is reconstituted according to the manufacturer's instructions and 0.1 mL is added to 0.9 mL of the aqueous phase-containing antigen. Note that this is a major difference between FCA and NUFCA as the *Mycobacterium tuberculosis* in FCA was suspended in the oil phase. The aqueous phase is emulsified with the oil phase before use. The manufacturers indicate that this NUFCA can be administered by id, im, or sc routes and agree with the WHO *(22)* that the im route produces fewer adverse reactions and creates a longer-lived slow-release depot which tends to provide a better immune response.

3.5.2. Standard Antigens

For the comparative biological testing of immunomodulators, the antigens chosen were ovalbumin (Ovalbumin,grade V crystallized and lyophilized, Sigma), and influenza H3N2 type A hemagglutinin *(1)*, however, it was pointed out that the latter antigen is an unsuitable standard for guinea pigs *(2)* (*see* **Note 5**).

3.5.3. Animals for Standard Antibody Production Tests

The guinea pig was the animal of choice for biological tests. In regard to mice, the influence of the animal's genetic background and MHC haplotype must also be considered. For this reason, animals with either similar genetic background and variable H-2 haplotype (e.g., C3H H-2^k and C3H.B10 H-2^b) or variable genetic background and similar H-2 haplotype (e.g., Balb/c H-2^d and DBA/c H-2^d) should be included in comparative tests.

3.5.4. Route of Injection

In most instances, researchers have their own preferences in regard to the site of injection of an adjuvant-formulated, experimental vaccine, however, consideration should be given to whether the vaccine is for human or veterinary use. It is doubtful whether patients would be willing to accept ip or iv injections as a routine vaccination procedure. Consequently, it is advisable to give the injections either subcutaneously or intramuscularly. Similarly, in no circumtances should an oil or alum-adjuvanted veterinary vaccine be injected intravenously nor booster injections administered iv or ip as there is a danger of inducing anaphylactic shock in the animals. Intraperitoneal injection of adjuvanted mixtures into some animals may result in decreased weight gain over 7 d. This inflammation may resolve itself after 7 d, but later postmortem

Table 3
Some Recommended Routes and Volumes for Injection Doses

Species	Maximum volume per injection site	Injection Sites: Primary	Injection Sites: Secondary
Mice or hamsters	50 µL	sc; im	sc; im
	200 µL		oral
Guinea pigs or rats	200 µL	sc; im. into one hindlimb	sc; im into one hindlimb
	300 µL		oral
Rabbit	250 µL (if in multiple sites <25 µL/site*)	sc; im. into one thigh muscle; id*	sc; im into one thigh muscle; id*
Large animal	500 µL (if in multiple sites <250 µL/site*)	sc; im into one hindlimb; id*	sc; im into one hindlimb; id*
Chicken	250 µL	sc; im	sc; im

sc: subcutaneous; im: intramuscular.
* If the intradermal (id) multiple injection site schedule is used.

examination may reveal macroscopic evidence of such a response. There may be specific tests where there is a requirement for another route, for example, id injections.

3.5.5. Volume of Injection Mixture

For animals the maximum volumes per site of injection are shown in **Table 3**. These dosages are based on the use of an adjuvanted vaccine which has already been shown to be nontoxic and nonpyrogenic.

3.5.6. Dose of Adjuvant

The upper limit of adjuvant per dose may be dictated by the results obtained in the toxicity and pyrogenicity tests, although it may be preferable for economic reasons to determine a lower dose at which an adjuvant response is obtained. In general however, the weight in the injection mixture should not exceed 25 µg for a mouse and 200 µg for guinea pigs, rats, or rabbits. If the dose is to be spread among multiple injection sites in larger animals, the volume should be not more than 250 µL per site and preferably as little as 25 µL. If a new adjuvant is being developed for veterinary use, it is important that, if possible, the animal species ear-marked for the vaccine is tested during the development phase.

3.6. Discussion

Manufacturers are expected to provide safety data sheets for their products and these will confirm the lack of toxicity of the product (*see* **Note 4**), but the addition of the vaccine candidate antigen may also alter the overall reactivity of the complete vaccine. Therefore, it is unwise to rely completely on manufacturer's specifications alone. Before evaluating the possible toxicity of a new adjuvant formulation, it is assumed that the investigator will have checked for either the innate toxicity of the antigen preparation, e.g., for lipopolysaccharide (endotoxin), or for chemicals used in antigen preparation, e.g., formaldehyde, glutaraldehyde, sodium azide. The inoculation mixture should be prepared aseptically to minimize contamination with endotoxins. In addition, the immunogen itself may have innate adjuvant activity and this should be checked before preparing complex adjuvant formulations. Conjugation of the immunogen to a carrier may impart innate adjuvant activity (*see* **Note 5**).

Because of necessity, many of these tests require the use of living animals to obtain standard values for the various tests, however, some attempts could be made to extrapolate from data in published records of adjuvant research. It does appear that the criteria required for animal vaccines are not applicable to human vaccines. In the Rules Governing Medicinal Products in the European Community (Volume 5) under veterinary medicinal products it states "it is recognized that for veterinary medicinal products a degree of toxicity and hazard for the animal are acceptable, provided that such toxicity has no consequences for man." (*See* **Note 4**.) Although much effort has gone into the development of alternative toxicological tests to recommended animal tests it is important to remember that the mammalian system is a complex series of interrelated physiological reactions, which are impossible to mimic in the test tube. Therefore, it is doubtful whether it will be possible to eliminate completely all use of experimental animals. It is more likely that in vitro tests could be developed to eliminate highly toxic test substances before animal tests must be considered. The debate will continue about the tests required to ensure that adjuvants, (immunopotentiators or immunomodulators) will be safe for use as vaccine additives in human vaccines.

4. Notes

1. Limulus assay. This requires very careful preparation and experience in reading the tests, therefore it is wise to run the tests with more than one person to check any differences from one operator to another. It should be borne in mind that false-positive results can be produced by substances other than endotoxin, lipopolysaccharide of Gram-negative bacteria.

2. Creatine kinase assay. The creatine kinase (CK) assay is measured in the serum of the test animal 3 d after the injection of the adjuvant. The test is not difficult to do as there is a standardized kit available from Sigma, Creatine kinase diagnostic kit, Cat. 520 or 520-C, but there are difficulties in regulating the standard values for each animal species. In our laboratory, a narrow range of CK values was not obtained with the guinea pig and one suggestion was that pain following injection or the mere handling of timid animals could lead to elevation of their normal CK levels for a period of time.
3. Freund's Complete Adjuvant. It is now time to commit to history FCA. Few laboratories are in a position to make the original FCA because it was formulated with heat-killed, whole cells of *Mycobacterium tuberculosis* in a mineral oil manufactured before 1969, the antigen in the aqueous phase and both of these emulsified with mannide monooleate ***(24)***. Today, adjuvant immunologists retain the use of FCA manufactured by the State Serum Institute in Copenhagen as a "gold" standard against which new adjuvants are compared. There may also be specific examples where FCA is required to stimulate a cell-mediated immune response but in general it is unnecessary to produce routine antisera with this material.

   There are some modern formulations that can achieve the same effect. A ready-to-use preparation at a ratio of 70 parts Montanide ISA 720 to 30 parts aqueous phase-containing antigen did not cause adverse reactions in human volunteers (Montanide ISA 720. Seppic, Paris, France). Similarly, NUFCA antigen in saline plus the BCG vaccine (BCG vaccine prepared by Evans Medical for intradermal use from John Bell & Croydon, 52-54 Wigmore Street, London, W1H 0AU, UK) in oil that conforms to the United States and EC Pharmacopoeias and comply with FDA regulations 21 CFR 172.878 and 178.3620a (Guildhay Ltd., 6, Riverside Business Centre, Walnut Tree Close, Guildford, Surrey, GU1 4UG, UK) may work just as well.
4. Mineral oil adjuvants. Reference to adverse effects of mineral oils from the petroleum industry in experiments completed prior to the late 1960s should not be seen as relevant to current experimental results. During earlier studies with FCA and FIA, the mineral oil produced by the acid treatment or oleum method was obtained as an intermediate stage in the refining process with an estimate of the hydrocarbon chain length but with no quality control. Published reports that oil emulsions can never be used in human vaccines ignore the fact that an oil-adjuvanted influenza vaccine was administered to many American servicemen more than 50 years ago. Surveillance of these vaccinees showed no evidence of increased disease states when compared to the incidences in the normal population ***(25)***.

   Since the 1970s, white mineral oil has been produced by the single or double hydrogenation procedure and far superior grades of oil have been obtained. A number of oils and emulsifiers are available now which lack the adverse effects of old crude mineral oils and conform to the requirements of the US and EC

Pharmacopoeias and comply with the FDA regulations 21 CFR 172.878 and 178.3620a. Manufacturers safety data sheets should provide QA data with new oils, e.g., mass spectrometer and gas liquid chromatography analyses,which may be used in adjuvanted vaccine oil formulations *(26)*. Many adverse reactions attributed to oil-adjuvanted vaccines were caused by the poor quality control of the original oils obtained from the petroleum industry. Unacceptable footpad reactions were obtained with mineral oils containing short-chain hydro-carbons (C_8-C_{12}), but medium-chain length hydrocarbons (C_{16}-C_{18}) showed minimal toxicity. The toxicity test must be relevant to the use of oils in vaccines: a 90-d feeding study does not necessarily equate with either oral administration or a parenteral injection of a vaccine dose containing ~0.5 mL oil *(24)*.

The induction of adjuvant arthritis test in Lewis rats was mainly required for oils produced prior to 1970 which were commonly used in experimental vaccines *(27)*. It is doubtful if it is required as a routine test for adjuvants, but may prove useful in some QA/QC procedures for selective adjuvants.

5. Sometimes an antigen alone or conjugated to another molecule will possess innate adjuvanticity *(2)*, therefore the addition of another separate adjuvant to the new vaccine may lead to a depression of the antibody response. Therefore, it is advisable to test whether the antigen requires the presence of an adjuvant. This can be done by testing the antigen as an adjuvant with the standard antigen ovalbumin. If the antibody response is greater than that obtained with ovalbumin in saline alone, it is reasonable to assume that the antigen has innate adjuvanticity.

References

1. Stewart-Tull, D. E. S. (1989) Recommendations for the assessment of adjuvants (immuno-potentiators), in *Immunological Adjuvants and Vaccines* (Gregoriadis, G., Allison, A. C., and Poste, G., eds.), Plenum, New York, pp. 213–226.
2. Stewart-Tull, D. E. S. (1991) The assessment and use of adjuvants, in *Vaccines* (Gregoriadis, G., Allison, A. C., and Poste, G., eds.), Plenum, New York, pp. 85–92.
3. Stewart-Tull, D. E. S. and Brown, F. (1993) First steps towards an international harmonization of veterinary biologicals. *Vaccine* **11,** 692–695.
4. Stewart-Tull, D. E. S. (1985) Immunopotentiating activity of peptidoglycan and surface polymers, in *Immunology of the Bacterial Cell Envelope* (Stewart-Tull, D. E. S. and Davies, M., eds.), Wiley, Chichester, pp. 47–89.
5. Robbins, J. (1980) in *New Developments with Human and Veterinary Vaccines* (Mizrahi, A., et al.) A R Liss, New York, pp. 393–394.
6. Vogel, F. R. and Powell, M. F. (1995) A compendium of vaccine adjuvants and excipients, in *Vaccine Design. The subunit and adjuvant approach* (Powell, M. F. and Newman, M. J., eds.), Plenum, New York, pp. 141–227.
7. Campbell, J. B. (1995) Saponins, in *The Theory and Practical Application of Adjuvants* (Stewart-Tull, D. E. S., ed.), Wiley, Chichester, pp. 95–127.
8. British Standards Institution (1990) Evaluation of medical devices for biological hazards Part 11. Method of test for haemolysis, British Standard 5736. British Standards Inst., 2, Park Street, London, W1A 2BS, England.

9. Wolff, S. M., Rubenstein, M., Mulholland, J. H., and Alling, D. W. (1965) Comparison of hematologic and febrile response to endotoxin in man. *Blood* **26,** 190–201.
10. British Standards Institution (1990) Evaluation of medical devices for biological hazards, Part 5. Method of test for systemic toxicity; assessment of pyrogenicity in rabbits of extracts from medical devices, British Standard 5736, 5, British Standards Inst., 2, Park Street, London, W1A 2BS. England, pp. 1–3.
11. Wardlaw, A. C. and McCartney, A. C. (1985) Endotoxic activities of lipopolysaccharides, in *Immunology of the bacterial cell envelope* (Stewart-Tull, D. E. S. and Davies, M., eds.), Wiley, Chichester, pp. 203–238.
12. Federal Register (1977) **42,** No. 213, 57749.
13. Mosmann, T. (1983) Rapid colorimetric assay for cellular growth and survival: application to proliferation and cytotoxicity assays. *J. Immunolog. Meth.* **65,** 55–63.
14. Vega, M. V., Maheswaran, S. K., Leininger, J. R., and Ames, T. R. (1987) Adaptation of a colorimetric microtitration assay for quantifying *Pasteurella haemolytica* A1 leucotoxin and anti-leukotoxin. *Am. J. Vet. Res.* **48,** 1559–1564.
15. Craig, F. F., Dalgleish, R., Sutherland, A. D., Parton, R., Coote, J. G., Gibbs H. A., and Freer, J. H. (1990) A colourimetric, microplate assay for the leucotoxin of Pasteurella haemolytica. *Vet. Microbiol.* **22,** 309–317.
16. Ferrari, M., Fornasiero, M. C., and Isetta, A. M. (1990) MTT colorimetric assay for testing macrophage cytotoxicity activity in vitro. *J. Immunolog. Meth.* **131,** 165–172.
17. Borefreund, E., Babich, H., and Martin-Alguacil, N. (1988) Comparisons of two in vitro cytotoxicity assays—the neutral red (NR) and tetrazolium MTT tests. *Toxicol. in Vitro* **2,** 1–6.
18. British Standards Institution (1983) Evaluation of medical devices for biological hazards. Part 7. Method of test for skin irritation of extracts from medical devices. British Standard 5736, 7. British Standards Inst., 2, Park Street, London, W1A 2BS, England, pp. 1–3.
19. Kensil, C. R., Patel, U., Lennick, M., and Marciani, D. (1991) Structure and characterization of saponins with adjuvant activity from Quillaja saponaria Molina cortex. *J. Immunol.* **146,** 431–437.
20. British Standards Institution (1983) Evaluation of medical devices for biological hazards. Part 3. Method of test for systemic toxicity; assessment of acute toxicity of extracts from medical devices. British Standard 5736, 3, British Standards Inst., 2, Park Street, London, W1A 2BS, England, pp. 1–2.
21. Christodoulides, M., Sidey, F. M., Parton, R., and Stewart-Tull, D. E. S. (1987) Acellular pertussis vaccine prepared by a simple extraction and toxoiding procedure. *Vaccine* **5,** 199–207.
22. World Health Organization (1976) Immunological adjuvants. *Tech. Rep. Ser.* **595,** 3.
23. Stewart-Tull, D. E. S. and Jones, A. C. (1992) Adjuvants should not induce allergic reactions to protein antigens. *FEMS Lett.* **100,** 489–496.

24. Stewart-Tull, D. E. S. (1995) Freund-type mineral oil adjuvant emulsions, in *The Theory and Practical Application of Adjuvants* (Stewart-Tull, D. E. S., ed.), Wiley, Chichester, pp. 1–19.
25. Davenport, F. M. (1968) Seventeen years experience with mineral oil adjuvant influenza virus vaccines. *Ann. Allergy* **26,** 288–292.
26. Stewart-Tull, D. E. S., Shimono T., Kotani S., and Knights, B. A. (1976) Immunosuppressive effect in mycobacterial adjuvant emulsions of mineral oils containing low molecular weight hydrocarbons. *Int. Arch. Allergy Appl. Immunol.* **52,** 118–128.
27. Pearson, C. M. (1956) Development of arthritis, periarthritis and periostitis in rats given adjuvant. *Proc. Soc. Exp. Biol. Med.* **91,** 95–101.
28. European Community (1989) The rules governing medicinal products in the European Community, Vol. III, Guidelines on the quality, safety, and efficacy of medicinal products for human use. CB-55-89-293-EN-C.

3

Freund's Adjuvants

Erik B. Lindblad

1. Introduction

Freund's adjuvants are water-in-mineral oil emulsions (W/O emulsions) without heat-killed mycobacteria added (Freund's incomplete adjuvant) or with heat-killed mycobacteria added (Freund's complete adjuvant). Freund's adjuvants are, in a way, historic adjuvants and for many researchers the first and most obvious association to the word *adjuvant* at all. The adjuvants have been used extensively in experimental immunology owing to their high efficacy, and Freund's incomplete adjuvant has been used for decades in practical veterinary vaccination. Vaccination of humans with Freund's incomplete adjuvant was undertaken in the 1950s and was stopped because of adverse reactions in the mid-1960s.

Every author who is to write about Freund's adjuvants faces the problem that data on the use of the adjuvant have been compiled over a timespan of more than 40 years. During this time, the composition of the oils used in the formulation has changed several times. Accordingly, the composition of the adjuvants also changed. Further, some commercial suppliers of Freund's complete adjuvant have chosen to substitute the original *Mycobacterium tuberculosis* with other mycobacteria.

One should bear this in mind when, over the years, differing results from the use of Freund's adjuvants have been described. In order to give the reader a basic understanding of Freund's adjuvants, it therefore seems inevitable to put some emphasis on historical aspects. It should further be underlined that the Freund's adjuvants discussed in this chapter are the *classical* Freund's adjuvants. The French company SEPPIC has developed an oil that is better tolerated than the traditional mineral oils used in Freund's adjuvants. This product,

From: *Methods in Molecular Medicine, Vol. 42: Vaccine Adjuvants: Preparation Methods and Research Protocols*
Edited by: D. T. O'Hagan © Humana Press, Inc., Totowa, NJ

Table 1
Side Effects in Laboratory Animals Historically Attributed to the Use of Freund's Adjuvants

Freund's Complete Adjuvant	Sterile abscesses
	Granulomas
	Muscle indurations
	Plasma cell neoplasia in BALB/c mice
	Ascites in BALB/c mice
	Amyloidosis
	Adjuvant arthritis in Lewis rats
	Experimental allergic encephalomyelitis in guinea pigs
Freund's Incomplete Adjuvant	Sterile abscesses
	Granulomas
	Muscle indurations
	Plasma cell neoplasia in BALB/c mice
	Ascites in BALB/c mice

when used in a W/O adjuvant emulsion, is referred to as Montanide ISA (Incomplete Seppic adjuvant). Discussion of this formulation has not been included in this chapter.

1.1. Historical Background

The first evidence of the use of oil emulsions as adjuvants in vaccine formulations dates back to 1916. At that time, Le Moignic and Pinoy immunized mice with heat-inactivated *Salmonella typhimurium* in an emulsion of water and vaselin oil, using lanolin as an emulsifier *(1)*. The oil emulsions as adjuvants, however, did not receive much attention before Jules Freund and coworkers *(2,3)* decades later combined a paraffin (mineral) oil emulsion and heat-killed mycobacteria to produce an extremely potent adjuvant, Freund's complete adjuvant (FCA).

Until then, adjuvants in general had been characterized mainly by their ability to raise high antitoxin titres. In contrast, FCA proved to be a highly efficient stimulator of cell-mediated immunity in addition to its ability to augment the humoral immune response. FCA, however, had a profile of adverse side-effects (**Table 1**), severe enough to restrict its use to experimental immunology in laboratory animals. A modified version of FCA is known as Freund's incomplete adjuvant (FIA). In this formulation the antigen is administered in a similar water-in-oil (W/O) emulsion, but without mycobacterial components. With FIA, an excellent stimulation of the humoral immune response was still

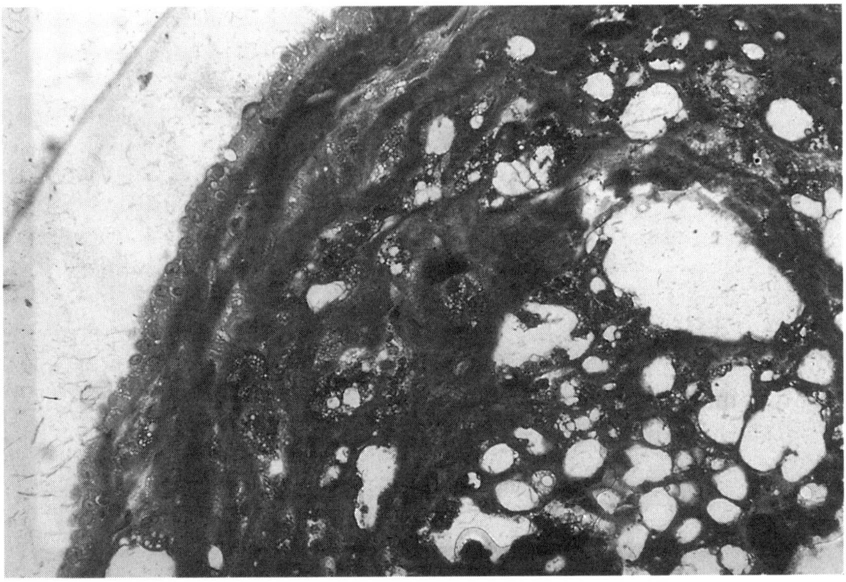

Fig. 1. Adjuvant granuloma in BALB/c mouse induced by FIA. Cross-section shows stratified layers of cells surrounding circular vacuoles, where the oil depot resided. (Preparation and photo, Jens Blom and E. B. Lindblad.)

achieved, but it is not efficient in stimulating delayed-type reactions *(4)*. Further, although less reactogenic than FCA, e.g., granuloma formation is commonly seen following use of FIA (**Fig. 1**).

FIA has been included in veterinary, as well as human, vaccines. The veterinary vaccines included vaccines against foot-and-mouth disease *(5)*, equine influenza virus *(6)*, hog cholera *(7)*, rabies *(8)*, parainfluenza 3 *(9)*, Newcastle disease *(10)*, and infectious canine hepatitis *(11)*. In cattle, FIA was inefficient in combination with herpesvirus *(12)*. In humans, FIA was used for a period of about two decades, particularly with vaccines against influenza virus *(13)*, tetanus toxoid *(14)*, and killed polio-myelitis virus *(15)*, whereas it failed to increase vaccine efficacy when used with adenovirus *(16)* and trachoma *(17)*.

In Britain alone, approximately 900,000 doses of a mineral oil-adjuvanted influenza vaccine were administered to humans in the early 1960s. The most frequent side-effects recorded after the use of FIA-adjuvanted vaccines in patients were cystic swellings and muscle indurations. Indurations could persist for up to 1 yr after injection. Histological examination of the indurated loci showed oil granulomas with central vacuoles where the oil was assumed to have resided. The vacuoles were surrounded by epitheloid and fibroblast cells

Table 2
Examples of Light Mineral Oils Used in Oil Adjuvants

Drakeol 6VR	(source: PenReCo)
Bayol F	(source: ESSO)
Marcol 52	(source: ESSO)
Marcol 82	(source: ESSO)
MedicWay M7	(source: Statoil)

with scattered plasma cells. All together, more than 500,000 humans have been vaccinated with FIA adjuvanted vaccines. However, in the mid-1960s, the use of FIA in human vaccination was discontinued because of concerns about the safety of the adjuvant.

1.2. Composition of Mineral Oil Adjuvants

As mentioned, the classical Freund's incomplete adjuvant consists of a mixture of mineral oil and emulsifier in a ratio of 85% v/v oil and 15% v/v emulsifier. This mixture will then be mixed with an equal volume of aqueous solution of antigen and subsequently emulsified prior to use. Ratios of 90% oil and 10% emulsifier have also been described. Both components will be discussed below.

1.2.1. The Mineral Oil Component

The oil component of mineral oil adjuvants is normally light mineral oil of a highly purified quality. Some examples are given in **Table 2**.

Crude oils contain (a) paraffins (alkanes, saturated noncyclic hydrocarbon chains); (b) olefins (alkenes, unsaturated, noncyclic hydrocarbon chains); (c) cycloparaffins (cycloalkanes, naphtenes, saturated cyclic hydrocarbon rings); and (d) aromatic hydrocarbons (cyclic compounds with resonating double bonds) ***(18)***. Through refining of the oil for use in adjuvants, a so-called "white mineral oil" is obtained by sulfonation to remove aromatic hydrocarbons. Unsaturated and other reactive hydrocarbons, as well as sulfur and nitrogen derivatives and volatiles, are also removed. Further refining may take place through filtration and extraction with alcohol.

Several pharmacopeias contain a set of specifications for the mineral oil "petrolatum" or *paraffinum liquidum* intented for general pharmaceutical use, e.g., as a laxative. However, following the work of Friedewald ***(19)***, Henle and Henle ***(20)***, and Salk ***(21,22)*** leading to a mineral oil-influenza vaccine for humans in the mid-1940s and early 1950s, a special set of requirements was set up for acceptance of the mineral oil preparation for adjuvants. This so-called *Tentative Draft, Minimum Requirements for Influenza Vaccines Emulsified in Mineral Oil* was prepared by The National Institutes of Health, USA, in 1956

Table 3
Chemical Specifications
For Refined Arlacel A (Ref. *26*)

Saponification number	164–172
Iodine number	70–74
Hydroxyl number	90–100
Acid number (max.)	1.0
Viscosity (25°C)	300–350 cp
Color, Hess-Ives scale (max.)	45 units

(23). These requirements will not be described in details here. They contain a set of basic physicochemical requirements regarding refractive index, viscosity, specific gravity, etc., but beside these, there was a requirement for absence of unsaturated hydrocarbons. The aim of these specifications was to exclude the presence of reactive groups, because, e.g., polycyclic aromatic hydrocarbons may be carcinogenic *(24)*.

1.2.2. The Emulsifier

The emulsifier used in Freund's complete and incomplete adjuvant to form the W/O emulsion is mannide monooleate, an ester consisting of mannitol as the hydrophilic residue and oleic acid, a C_{18} fatty acid, as the hydrophobic residue. Arlacel A is a tradename for mannide monooleate.

The initial finding that mannide monooleate was suitable for emulsifying aqueous antigen preparations in mineral oil was done by Jules Freund *(25)*. In his earlier work, he used commercially available lanolin-like substances, such as Aquaphor™ and Falba™. Mannide monooleate preparations, when intended for use in adjuvants, should be refined to remove toxic substances and free oleic acid.

Berlin *(26)* devised a set of requirements that should be met chemically (**Table 3**) and in terms of toxicity testing. These imply that young mice injected ip with 0.25 mL Arlacel A should not suffer from transient weight loss. The difference in weight gain between young mice injected ip with an acceptable preparation of Arlacel A and a control group receiving saline should be less that 10.5%. Further, the preparation should not induce chemical peritonitis. A set of standards for testing skin erythemas and skin thickening in guinea pigs following intracutaneous injection of Arlacel A was also devised.

1.3. The Mechanism of Action of Mineral Oil Adjuvants

Traditionally, the *modus operandi* of the mineral oil emulsions is associated with at least three different mechanisms: (1) The establishment of a repository antigen-containing locus at the site of injection allowing a gradual and continous release of the antigen; (2) provision of a vehicle capable of transporting emulsified antigen through the lymphatic system to distant sites (e.g., draining lymphnodes and the spleen) creating additional foci of antibody formation; and (3) interaction with mononuclear cells, such as phagocytic cells, antigen presenting cells, etc.

The effect of the gradual release of antigen from the W/O emulsion upon injection and the significance of possible alternative mechanisms was elucidated by the work of Herbert *(27)*. Here, the antibody production after injection of a single dose of antigen-containing mineral oil emulsion was compared to a regimen in which small amounts of the same antigen in saline were injected daily over a period of 50 d to parallel the gradual release. The antibody response in the group that received the oil emulsion remained elevated after day 50, whereas the response of the other group soon declined. Possible differences in isotypic profiles were not determined. On the other hand, when rabbits were immunized intracutaneously with killed typhoid bacilli in a W/O emulsion, excision of the injection site as early as 30 min following injection did not prevent antibody formation *(3)*.

Wilner et al. pioneered an important line of work that allowed evaluation of the relative importance of the various groups of organic hydrocarbons normally found in refined mineral oil, including branched, as well as unbranched, and saturated hydrocarbons *(28)*. Stewart-Tull and coworkers substituted the mineral oil with pure, straight-chain hydrocarbons *(29)* of various chain lengths, and found that fully saturated hydrocarbons of C-16 to C-19 were the most effective in adjuvant preparations. Earlier work by Shaw et al. *(30)* showed that short-chain straight hydrocarbons of C-6 to C-13 induced a local inflammatory reaction, but were not particularly effective as adjuvants. Long-chained hydrocarbons of C-22 and C-24 were solid at body temperature and, hence, unsuited for the purpose. In contrast, Shaw et al. obtained good results with saturated straight-chain hydrocarbons of C-15 to C-20 *(30)*. These authors suggested that the retention of the antigen within the oil emulsion depended upon the hydrocarbon chain length. Longer hydrocarbon chains retained the antigen for a longer period of time. The neccessity of using an oil that was not readily cleared or metabolized from the body has been emphasized as a prerequisite for a continous stimulus *(31)*.

This point of view may seem to be supported indirectly by the observations of Herbert *(27)*. For a long time, the mineral oil was considered nonmetabolizable. However, although no specific metabolic pathways for catabolism of saturated hydrocarbons have been described, the work of Stetten *(32)* and of Bollinger *(33,34)* strongly indicates that mineral oil adjuvants are indeed, to a certain extent, metabolized.

1.4. Metabolic Degradation of Mineral Oil Adjuvants

Much of the understanding of the metabolic fate of mineral oil adjuvants was provided by the work of James Bollinger. Bollinger studied the clearing of mineral oil *(33)*, as well as mannide monooleate *(34)*, in rats and monkeys by use of ^{14}C-labeled tracers.

1.4.1. The Mineral Oil

To study the clearing of mineral oil he injected ^{14}C-labeled hexadecane in an emulsion with unlabeled mannide monooleate im and sc in the thigh of the animals. One week after injection 85–98% of the radioactivity remained at the site of injection. After 1 mo 65–75%; after 3 mo 55–65%; and after 10 mo approx 30% of the labeled oil could still be found at the injection site. Thin-layer chromatography separation was undertaken to tell in which type of lipid the radioactivity was found. It was clearly shown that after 10 mo, the radioactivity at *the injection site* was still found in the hydrocarbon fraction. Samples from the major organs showed that there was an increasing level of radioactivity in the liver that peaked after 1 wk to 1 mo. After 10 mo, the level was back to normal. This was accompanied by a slightly later, but analogous rise-and-fall pattern in the radioactivity of the depot fat. No other organs achieved high levels of radioactivity. In the liver, the radioactivity after 1 mo was predominantly found in triglycerides, sterol esters, and free sterols, whereas in the depot fat, it was primarily found in triglycerides and free fatty acids. After 3 mo, practically all the radioactivity of the depot fat was found in triglycerides, whereas most of the radioactivity at that time in the liver was found as phospholipids *(33)*.

1.4.2. The Emulsifier

To investigate the metabolic fate of mannide monooleate, either the mannitol or the oleic acid was labeled with ^{14}C and subsequently incorporated into a FIA preparation *(34)*. The clearing from the injection site of the emulsifier took place significantly faster than was the case with the mineral oil. After 1 wk, approx only 50% of the radioactivity could be found at the injection site. The ^{14}C-mannide monooleate containing inoculum lost about 40% of its *in situ* radioactivity in about 2 d. The clearing rate was, in this case, faster than when ^{14}C-oleate mannide was incorporated. When the oleate was labeled, a similar rise-and-fall pattern of the radioactivity in the liver and depot fat, as was seen with ^{14}C-hexadecane *(33)*, could be found. This was not the case when the mannitol had been labeled. In that case, radioactivity in the inguinal lymph nodes was seen and a significant amount of radioactivity was excreted with the urine *(34)*.

In conclusion, the general picture was that upon injection of a mineral oil emulsion, the emulsifier tended to leave the inoculum depot faster than the oil itself, giving lead to a coalesced oil depot. Bollinger, however, emphasized that the preparation of mannide monooleate had a high content of free mannitol and oleic acid due to incomplete esterification. This could account for the rapid clearing of mannitol from the injection site. The transport of the mannitol appears to take place through the lymphatics. The lipids, i.e., both the oleic acid and the hydrocarbons of the mineral oil (which is very slowly transported away from the inoculum) can be metabolized in the liver and may end up in the depot fat as triglycerides. The mannitol is excreted with the urine *(34)*.

1.5. Reaction Profile of Freund's Adjuvants

Freund's adjuvants are used in priming immunizations. In boosters, FIA can be used with antigen or antigen alone can be administered in saline. Interestingly, it was shown by Paraf and coworkers in mouse studies, that injection of human serum albumin in saline prior to a stimulating injection of HSA in FCA, could completely suppress the antibody reponse *(35)*. In rabbits, injection of HSA with Freund's adjuvant was able to elicit a significant antibody response in the newborn individual, which is normally regarded as immunologically immature and unable to respond *(35)*.

In general, both FIA and FCA are indeed very efficient in raising high antibody titres. FCA with its mycobacterial components is able to skew a humoral immune response toward the Th1 profile with pronounced IgG2a stimulation with high titres in mice. The antibody profile, however, is not entirely limited to IgG2a; other subclasses are seen as well. This ability to stimulate Th1 immunity is further sustained by a number of studies where FCA has been tested alone or in comparison with aluminium hydroxide, which is well documented *(36,37)* as a Th2 adjuvant.

This model of investigating FCA vs aluminium hydroxide adjuvant is suited to illustrate the dichotomy of the immune response in terms of Th1 and Th2 immunity and its modulation. Uede and coworkers *(38)* isolated 13kDa IgE binding factors from the spleen cells of rats immunized with keyhole limpet hemocyanin (KLH) and $Al(OH)_3$. This factor selectively potentiated the IgE response, whereas factors from KLH-FCA primed spleen cells supressed it. Further studies showed *(39)* that KLH-alum primed T cells formed "inducers" of IgE binding factors and glycosylation-enhancing factors, and together these factors stimulated unprimed $Fc\gamma R^+$ T cells to form IgE potentiating factors. KLH-FCA primed T cells formed inducing factors and glycosylation *inhibiting* factors and these two lymphokines collectively stimulated $Fc\gamma R^+$ T-cells to form IgE suppresive factors *(39)*.

Smith and Butchko ***(40)*** demonstrated a suppression of the IgE response in mice following immunization with FCA. Freund's adjuvant, both complete and incomplete, has been shown to induce cytotoxic T lymphocytes (CTL), but there is no simple, clear-cut reaction pattern. Early studies ***(41)*** had shown that FCA was unable to elicit CTL in C57BL/6 mice when used as an adjuvant with allogeneic P815 cells. However, Ke et al. demonstrated $CD8^+$, class I MHC restricted ovalbumin-specific CTL in mice following priming with ovalbumin emulsified with FCA. These CTL produced TNF-α and interferon-γ upon activation and they were confirmed to recognize the $OVA_{257\text{-}264}$ epitope ***(42)***.

Kuzu and coworkers found ***(43)*** that priming BALB/c mice using influenza A virus nucleoprotein (NP) peptide with FCA, followed by a single boost of NP with FIA was superior to no boosts or two boosts in raising a CTL response.

Strong CTL reponses against peptides representing poorly immunogenic malaria CTL epitopes were elicited when mixing with peptides representing defined T-helper epitopes and injected with FIA. Preinjection of FIA alone also had a stimulatory effect ***(44)***. In contrast, virus-like particles (VLP) from HIV-1, which are noninfectious constructs, gave significant responses of $CD8^+$, class I MHC restricted CTL in BALB/c mice when injected alone, whereas injection together with FIA drastically reduced the CTL reponse ***(45)***.

It is apparent that the data on the ability of Freund's adjuvants in eliciting CTL reponses do not call for generalizations. There may be many explanations for this, but a better identification of specific CTL epitopes on the antigen in question will be valuable.

2. Materials

2.1. Preparation of the Emulsion

1. Sterilized Wassermann (or Vidal or Eppendorf) test tubes.
2. Sterility filters (0.22 µm) to be mounted with Luer locks on syringes.
3. Freund's complete or incomplete adjuvant, sterilized.
4. Antigen.
5. Saline or PBS for preparation of the antigen solution.
6. Sterile pipets.
7. A 21-gage double-hubbed transfer needle inserted between two (preferably glass) syringes (all sterilized).
8. Syringes (preferably glass) and needles for injection (*see* **Notes 1** and **7**).

2.2. The Trypan Blue Test

1. All the above plus Trypan blue.
2. A microscope and glass slides.

2.3. The Droplet Test

1. A beaker or Petri dish.
2. A syringe equipped with a needle.
3. Cold water.

3. Methods

3.1. Preparation of the Emulsion

1. Decide the volume of a single-dose inoculum (if immunizing mice the total volume of the inoculum should not exceed 100 µL).
2. Decide the required amount of antigen in a single inoculum dose.
3. Prepare an aqueous solution of the protein antigen in a Wassermann test tube in such a concentration that the required amount of antigen in a single inoculum is contained in half the total volume of the inoculum. Pass the solution through a sterility filter (0.22 µm) equipped with a Luer lock and collect in a sterile test tube.
4. Pipet into a sterile test tube a volume corresponding to the number of doses to be prepared and allow a surplus of the antigen solution equaling a volume no less than 200 µL.
5. Add a similar volume of sterilized Freund's adjuvant to the test tube and close it. You will now end up with enough mixture to immunize the required number of animals and a further surplus of 400 µL to assure that there will be no shortage of mixture because of adherence to the glass surface.
6. The final emulsion can be prepared by repeated passage of the oil/water + antigen mixture through a 21-gage double-hubbed transfer needle inserted between two (preferably glass) syringes each holding a volume no less than 50% higher than the volume of the mixture. The mixture should be aspirated into one of the syringes and the air should be expelled prior to applying the transfer needle and the second syringe. Press the mixture from the one syringe to the other and continue doing so. Along with the repeated alternate expulsions/passages, the emulsion becomes gradually thicker and it turns milky in appearance (*see* **Note 1**).

It is difficult to give a definite recommendation as to how many passages are required, because it would depend upon the shear rate and the pressure applied to the piston of the syringes.

3.2. The Trypan Blue Test

The preparation of an emulsion can be checked by adding Trypan blue to the aqueous phase prior to emulsification. After the emulsification, the blue staining will be visible in light microscopy. In a W/O emulsion, the blue color will be seen in the antigen-containing water droplets. In a O/W emulsion, the blue staining will be seen in the water phase outside the (oil) droplets.

1. Prepare a 1–10% solution of Trypan blue and filter it through a sterility filter equipped with a Luer lock mounted on a syringe. Add filtered Trypan blue soln dropwise to the aqueous antigen solution under stirring.

2. Prepare the emulsion as described above taking any added volume of Trypan blue soln into consideration. The emulsion should not be too thick for this test because the water droplets may then attain a size below the resolution of the light microscope.
3. Place a droplet of the emulsion on a glass slide for microscopy and apply a cover very carefully (*see* **Note 2**).

3.3. The Droplet Test

A simple test to check if you have prepared a W/O emulsion is to place carefully a drop of the emulsion in cold water in a shallow dish, e.g., a Petri dish. A W/O emulsion will then retain the integrity of the drop, whereas it is indicative of a O/W emulsion if the drop disperses on the water surface ***(46)***.

4. Notes

1. Preparation of the emulsion: The syringes should preferably be glass syringes instead of plastic, because the rubber-tipped plungers in plastic syringes are not compatible with the paraffin oil. In case air is not excluded during the emulsification, minute air bubbles will be trapped within the emulsion. During injection, (because of compression and decompression of entrapped air) the syringe may then continue to inject emulsion from the needle after the finger pressure has been relieved ***(47)***. The consequence being a risk of overdosing the emulsion. Thick emulsions are normally more stable than thin emulsions.

   It is not possible to carry out fixation of the emulsions for electron microscopy using glutaraldehyde or formaldehyde, but there is evidence that fixation can be undertaken using osmium tetraoxide ***(46)***.
2. The Trypan blue test: The Trypan blue test requires light microscopy. The blue, stained water droplets in the W/O emulsions are readily recognizable in thin emulsions, because these have droplets of a size appropriate for light microscopy. However, in thick emulsions, the droplet size is smaller and the emulsion here may appear as a fine mesh, which cannot be resolved in the light microscope.
3. The droplet test: The water phase on which the droplet is to be placed should be cold.
4. General comments on emulsifiers: Arlacel A (mannide monooleate) is preferentially wetted by oil (low HLB-value). Because of this, more molecules of the emulsifyer can be accomodated at the oil–water interface if it is convex to the oil phase and consequently it favors a W/O emulsion ***(46)***.

   Alternative emulsifiers, such as Tween-80, may preferentially be wetted by the aqueous phase (having higher HLB values), giving lead to O/W instead of W/O emulsions.
5. General comments on mineral oil: It is recommended to obtain a GLC spectrometer analysis of the oil to document the hydrocarbon composistion. The following method is recommanded by Stewart-Tull ***(48)***. The analysis could be carried out using a 2.77-column packed with 3% OV-17 coated with Gas Chrom Q (obtainable from Phase Separations Ltd.). The oil samples are dissolved in ether, use approx 5 mg/mL. Inject an aliquot of 1–2 µL via a self-sealing septum into

Table 4
Recommended Maximum Volumes for Injection of Antigen/Mineral Oil Adjuvant Mixtures Per Site of Injection for Laboratory Animals

Species	Max. volume per site	Primary injection	Subsequent injections
Mice, hamsters	100 µL	sc	sc
Mice, hamsters	50 µL	im*	im
Guinea pigs	200 µL	sc; im	sc; im
Rats	200 µL	sc; im	sc; im
Rabbits	250 µL	sc; im	sc; im

* In the thigh

the GLC apparatus. The analyses are carried out initially for 16 min at 100°C followed by a temperature programming at 8°C/min until you reach 275°C. As reference compounds, use standard hydrocarbons of $nC_{11}H_{22}$, $nC_{18}H_{38}$, and $nC_{20}H_{42}$ ***(48)***.

6. The mycobacterial component: The mycobacterial component of the classical Freund's complete adjuvant was heat-killed *Mycobacterium tuberculosis* (0.5 mg/mL). The only commercially available preparation of FCA that still contains *M. tuberculosis* is prepared by Statens Seruminstitut (Copenhagen, Denmark). Other preparations may contain *M. butyricum* ***(49)***.

   FCA can be blended with FIA prior to emulsification in case a dilution of the mycobacterial content is desired. In FCA, the mycobacterial component will essentially be found in the oil phase ***(46)***.
7. Injection of Freund's adjuvant: Injections should be undertaken intramuscularly or subcutaneously using sterile needles after having disinfected the skin of the animal with 70% ethanol. It is recommendable to use glass syringes, since injection of emulsions requires a higher pressure than nonemulsion vaccines. It is also recommended to heat the emulsion up to room temperature prior to injection. It eases the flow of the emulsion through the needle. Recommended injection volumes are given in **Table 4**.

   For animal ethics reasons, the use of FCA should be restricted and never used simply for raising an antibody response routinely. It should only be used when it is specifically and scientifically justified, such as for raising an immune response to weak antigens in cases where other options failed. Even in such cases, it should not be used more than once in an animal. If boosters need emulsion adjuvants these should be FIA and not FCA.

   Caution: Accidental selfinoculation of Freund's adjuvants may lead to severe local adverse reactions.

References

1. Le Moignic and Pinoy (1916) Les vaccins en emulsion dans les corps gras ou "lipo-vaccins." *Comptes Rendus de la Societe de Biologie* **79,** 201–203.

2. Freund, J., Casals, J., and Hosmer, E. P. (1937) Sensitization and antibody formation after injection of tubercle bacili and paraffin oil. *Proc. Soc. Exp. Biol. Med.* **37,** 509–513.
3. Freund, J. (1956) The mode of action of immunologic adjuvants, in *Adv. Tuberc. Res.* S. Karger, Basel, New York, pp. 130–148.
4. Raffel, S. (1948) The components of the tubercle bacillus responsible for the delayed type of "Infectious" allergy. *J. Infect. Dis.* **82,** 267–293.
5. McKercher, P. D. and Graves, J. H. (1977) A review of the current status of oil adjuvants in foot-and-mouth disease vaccines. *Dev. Biol. Stand.* **35,** 107–112.
6. Street, B. K. (1967) The use of an oil adjuvant equine influenza virus vaccine, in *Symp.series immunobiol. Standard.,* vol. 6, Karger, Basel, New York, pp. 241–250.
7. Ott, G. L., Yaillen, A. J., and Korschak, J. (1962) Adjuvant killed hog cholera vaccine. *Vet. Med.* **57,** 1060–1063.
8. Freund, J., Lipton, M. M., and Pisani, T. M. (1948) Immune response to rabies vaccine in water-in-oil emulsion. *Proc. Soc. Exp. Biol. Med.* **68,** 609–610.
9. McClelland, L., Hampil, B., Hamparian, V. V., Potash, L., Ketler, A., and Hilleman, M. R. (1961) Laboratory and field investigations of bovine myxovirus parainfluenza 3 virus and vaccine. II. Development and appraisal of potency of SF-4 (Shipping Fever) virus vaccine. *J. Immunol.* **87,** 134–138.
10. Eidson, C. S. (1982) Vaccination of breeder chickens and their progeny with a live or with an inactivated oil emulsion newcastle disease vaccine, in *Develop. Biol. Stand.* vol. 51, Karger, Basel, New York, pp. 191–205.
11. Fastier, L. B. and Hansen, N. F. (1964) An adjuvant vaccine against infectious canine hepatitis. *New Z. Vet. J.* **12,** 89–91.
12. Plowright, W., Herniman, K. A. J., Jessett, D. M., Kalunda, M., and Rampton, C. S. (1975) Immunization of cattle against the herpesvirus of malignant cattarrhal fever: failure of inactivated culture vaccines with adjuvant. *Res. Vet. Sci.* **19,** 159–166.
13. Salk, J. E., Bailey, M. L., and Laurent, A. M. (1952) The use of adjuvants in studies on influenza immunization II. Increased antibody formation in human subjects inoculated with influenza virus vaccine in a water-in-oil emulsion. *Amer. J. Hyg.* **55,** 439–456.
14. Pittman, M. (1967) Some remarks regarding the reaction provoking properties, in *Symp.series immunobiol. Standard.,* vol. 6, Karger, Basel, New York, pp. 101–102.
15. Salk, J. E., Benneth, B. L., Lewis, L. J., Ward, E. N., and Youngner, J. S. (1953) Studies in human subjects on active immunization against poliomyelitis. *J. Am. Med. Assoc.* **151,** 1081–1098.
16. Miller, L. F., Peckinpaugh, R. O., Arlander, T. R., Pierce, W. E., Edwards, E. A., DeBerry, P., et al. (1965) Epidemiology and prevention of acute respiratory disease in naval recruits. II. Effect of adjuvant and aqueous adenovirus vaccines in prevention of naval recruit respiratory disease. *Am. J. Publ. Health* **55,** 47–59.
17. Woolridge, R. L., Grayston, J. T., Chang, I. H., Cheng, K. H., Yang, C. Y., and Neave, C. (1967) Field trial of a monovalent and bivalent mineral oil adjuvant trachoma vaccine in Taiwan school children. *Am. J. Ophthalmol.* **63,** 1645s.

18. Cram, J. M. and Cram, D. J. (1978) Alkenes and alkynes, in *The Essence of Organic Chemistry,* Addison-Wesley, New York, pp. 77–97.
19. Friedewald, W. F. (1944) Adjuvants in immunization with influenza virus vaccines. *J. Exp. Med.* **80,** 477–491.
20. Henle, W. and Henle, G. (1945) Effect of adjuvants on vaccination of human beings against influenza. *Proc. Soc. Exp. Biol. N.Y.* **59,** 179–181.
21. Salk, J. E., Laurent, A. M., and Bailey, M. L. (1951) Direction of research on vaccination against influenza—new studies with immunologic adjuvants. *Am. J. Publ. Health* **41,** 669–677.
22. Salk, J. E. (1953) The use of adjuvants in studies on influenza immunization III. Degree of persistence of antibody in human subjects two years after vaccination. *J. Am. Med. Assoc.* **151,** 1169–1175.
23. Tentative draft, minimum requirements for influenza vaccines emulsified in mineral oil. National Inst. of Health, 1956, USA.
24. Dietz, W. A., King, W. H., Priestly, W., and Rehner, J. (1952) Properties of high boiling petroleum products. *Ind. Eng. Chem.* **44,** 1818–1827.
25. Freund, J., Thomson, K. J., Hough, H. B., Sommer, H. E., and Pisani, T. M. (1948) Antibody formation and sensitization with the aid of adjuvants. *J. Immunol.* **60,** 383–398.
26. Berlin, B. S. (1962) Tests for biological safety of Arlacel A. *Ann. Allergy* **20,** 472–479.
27. Herbert, W. J. (1967) Some investigations into the mode of action of the water-in-mineral-oil emulsion antigen adjuvants. *Symp. Series Immunobiol. Standard.,* vol. 6, Karger, Basel, New York, pp. 213–220.
28. Wilner, B. I., Evers, M. A., Troutman, H. D., Trader, F. W., and McLean, I. W. (1963) Vaccine potentiation by emulsification with pure hydrocarbon compounds. *J. Immunol.* **91,** 210–229.
29. Stewart-Tull, D. E. S., Shimono, T., Kotani, S., and Knights, B. A. (1976) Immunosuppressive effect in mycobacterial adjuvant emulsions of mineral oils containing low molecular weight hydrocarbons. *Int. Archs Allergy Appl. Immun.* **52,** 118–128.
30. Shaw, C., Alvord, E. C., and Kies, M. W. (1964) Straight chain hydrocarbons as substitutes for the oil in Freund's adjuvants in the production of experimental "allergic" encephalomyelitis in the guinea pig. *J. Immunol.* **92,** 24–27.
31. Freund, J. (1951) The effect of paraffin oil and mycobacteria on antibody formation and sensitization. A review. *Am. J. Clin. Pathol.* **21,** 645–656.
32. Stetten, D. (1943) Metabolism of paraffin. *J. Biol. Chem.* **147,** 327–332.
33. Bollinger, J. N. (1970) Metabolic fate of mineral oil adjuvants using ^{14}C-labeled tracers I: mineral oil. *J. Pharm. Sci.* **59,** 1084–1088.
34. Bollinger, J. N. (1970) Metabolic fate of mineral oil adjuvants using ^{14}C-labeled tracers II: mannide monooleate. *J. Pharm. Sci.* **59,** 1088–1092.
35. Jollès, P. and Paraf, A. (1973) Biological activty of adjuvants, in *Chemical and Biological Basis of Adjuvants* (Kleinzeller, Springer, and Wittmann, eds.), *Molecular Biol. Biochem. and Biophys.* **13,** 53–77.

36. Grun, J. L. and Maurer, P. H. (1989) Different T-helper cell subsets elicited in mice utilizing two different adjuvant vehicles: the role of endogenous interleukin-1 in proliferative responses. *Cell. Immunol.* **121,** 134–145.
37. Lindblad, E. B., Elhay, M. E., Silva, R., Appelberg, R., and Andersen, P. (1997) Adjuvant modulation of the immune responses to tuberculosis subunit vaccines. *Infect. Immun.* **65,** 623–629.
38. Uede, T., Huff, T. F., and Ishizaka, K. (1982) Formation of IgE binding factors by rat T lymphocytes. V.: effect of adjuvant for the priming immunization on the nature of IgE binding factors formed by antigenic stimulation. *J. Immunol.* **129,** 1384–1390.
39. Uede, T. and Ishizaka, K. (1982) Formation of IgE binding factors by rat T lymphocytes. VI.: cellular mechanisms for the formation of IgE-potentiating factor and IgE-suppressive factor by antigenic stimulation of antigen primed spleen cells. *J. Immunol.* **129,** 1391–1397.
40. Smith, W. G. and Butchko, G. M. (1986) Regulation of in vivo IgE biosynthesis in mice with complete freund's adjuvant. *Int. Archs. Allergy Appl. Immun.* **79,** 337–342.
41. Reinisch, C. L., Gleiner, N. A., and Schlossman, S. F. (1976) Adjuvant regulation of T cell function *J. Immunol.* **116,** 710–715.
42. Ke, Y., Li, Y., and Kapp, J. A. (1995) Ovalbumin injected with complete Freund's adjuvant stimulates cytotoxic responses. *Eur. J. Immunol.* **25,** 549–553.
43. Kuzu, H., Kuzu, Y., Zaghouani, H., and Bona, C. (1993) In vivo priming effect during various stages of ontogeny of an influenza A virus nucleoprotein peptide. *Eur. J. Immunol.* **23,** 1397–1400.
44. Valmori, D., Romero, J. F., Men, Y., Maryanski, J. L., Romero, P., and Corradin, G. (1994) Induction of a cytotoxic T cell response by co-injection of a T helper peptide and a cytotoxic T lymphocyte peptide in incomplete Freund's adjuvant (IFA): further enhancement by preinjection of IFA alone. *Eur. J. Immunol.* **24,** 1458–1462.
45. Wagner, R., Deml, L., Schirmbeck, R., Niedrig, M., Reimann, J., and Wolf, H. (1996) Construction, expression and immunogenicity of chimeric HIV-1 virus-like particles. *Virology* **220,** 128–140.
46. Dvorak, A. M. and Dvorak, H. F. (1974) Structure of Freund's complete and incomplete adjuvants. *Immunology* **27,** 99–114.
47. Chase, M. W. (1967) Production of antiserum, in *Methods in Immunology and Immunochemistry* (Williams, C. A. and Chase, M. W., eds.), vol. 1, Academic, New York, p. 197.
48. Stewart-Tull, D. E. S. (1996) The Use of Adjuvants in Experimental Medicine II. Water-in-Oil Emulsions, in *Methods in Molecular Medicine: Vaccine Protocols* (Robinson, A., Farrar, G., and Wiblin, C., eds.), Humana, Totowa, NJ.
49. Stewart-Tull, D. E. S. (1995) Freund-type mineral oil adjuvant emulsions, in *The Theory and Practical Application of Adjuvants* (Stewart-Tull, D. E. S., ed.), Wiley, New York, pp. 1–19.

4

Aluminum Compounds as Vaccine Adjuvants

Rajesh K. Gupta and Bradford E. Rost

1. Introduction

Aluminum compounds, including aluminum phosphate ($AlPO_4$), aluminum hydroxide ($Al(OH)_3$), and alum precipitated vaccines, historically referred to as protein aluminate, are currently the most commonly used adjuvants with human and veterinary vaccines ***(1–6)***. These adjuvants are often referred to as "alum" in the literature, which is misleading because (1) two most widely used adjuvants from this group, aluminum hydroxide and aluminum phosphate, have very different physical characteristics *(7)* and differ in their adjuvant properties *(3,6)*; and (2) alum, chemically potassium aluminum sulfate ($KAl(SO_4)_2.12H_2O$), has not been used as an adjuvant as such. Alum was originally used to partially purify protein antigens, mainly tetanus and diphtheria toxoids, by precipitating them in the presence of anions including phosphate, sulphate, and bicarbonate ions resulting in a mixture of compounds, mainly aluminum phosphate and aluminum hydroxide ***(4,8,9)***. The amounts of aluminum phosphate and aluminum hydroxide in the mixture depended upon the amount and nature of anions present in the reaction mixture and adjustment of pH of the final product with sodium hydroxide ***(3,4,6,10,11)***. Although alum-precipitated tetanus and diphtheria toxoids had been used for human immunization for many years, their use has declined considerably because of variability in production of alum precipitated toxoids ***(1,4,8,9,12)***.

Procedures described in this paper for making aluminum adjuvants and for adsorption of vaccines onto these adjuvants are for experimental purposes only. Before performing any clinical trials or studies in humans, the adjuvanted preparations, even for established vaccines, should be thoroughly evaluated for toxicology and other safety studies in animals as required by regulatory agencies or national control authorities. Any clinical trials using the adjuvanted preparations should be performed under protocols approved by these agencies.

From: *Methods in Molecular Medicine, Vol. 42: Vaccine Adjuvants: Preparation Methods and Research Protocols*
Edited by: D. T. O'Hagan © Humana Press, Inc., Totowa, NJ

Although there has been a search for alternate adjuvants, aluminum compounds will be continued to be used as adjuvants for human vaccines for many years owing to their good track record of safety, low cost, and adjuvanticity with a variety of antigens ***(1–4,6,7,9,11,12)***. Aluminum adjuvants have certain limitations, such as occasional induction of local reactions at the site of injection, augmentation of IgE antibody responses, ineffectiveness for some antigens, and inability to augment cell-mediated immune responses, especially cytotoxic T-cell responses ***(1–3,5,6,13)***. For diseases that can be prevented by induction of serum IgG antibodies, aluminum adjuvants formulated under optimal conditions are the adjuvants of choice.

Because aluminum compounds are the only adjuvants currently used routinely for human vaccines, these have become the benchmark or reference for evaluating new adjuvant formulations. It is very important to prepare optimal formulations of vaccines adsorbed onto aluminum adjuvants to correctly evaluate the new adjuvants. Two methods have commonly been used to prepare vaccines and toxoids with aluminum compounds—*in situ* precipitation of aluminum compounds in the presence of antigen (developed originally to purify toxoids by precipitation with alum), and adsorption of antigen onto preformed aluminum gel ***(3,4,6–9,14)***. Adsorption of antigens on aluminum adjuvants, either during *in situ* precipitation of aluminum adjuvants or onto preformed aluminum gels, depends upon physical and chemical characteristics of antigen, type of aluminum adjuvant and conditions of adsorption ***(3,4,6,7,11,12,14–16***, **Table 1**, *see* **Note 1**). These conditions are often overlooked and a poorly formulated aluminum adjuvant preparation does not exhibit optimal adjuvanticity. Further, characteristics of aluminum adjuvants, such as size of the gel particles, adsorption capacity, isoelectric point, and ratio of aluminum to phosphate, depend upon the conditions of making these gels, including order of adding reagents, speed at which the reagents are added and mixed, mixing speed, time taken to adjust pH, and scaling-up the production. Therefore, aluminum adjuvants have been described as difficult to manufacture in a physicochemically reproducible way, thus resulting in batch to batch variations ***(4,14,17)***. To minimize variations and to avoid nonreproducibility as a result of use of different preparations of aluminum compounds, a specific preparation (Alhydrogel®, aluminum hydroxide, from Superfos Biosector, Vedbaek, Denmark) was chosen as a scientific standard for evaluation of new adjuvant formulations ***(18)***. However, certain antigens do not adsorb onto Alhydrogel because of the same charge on the adjuvant and antigens ***(7,19)***. Therefore, selection of appropriate aluminum adjuvant to give an optimal adjuvant effect is very important (*see* **Note 1**).

Table 1
Factors Affecting Adsorption of Antigen Onto Aluminum Adjuvants

Factor	Optimal Conditions
Electrostatic forces Hydrophobic interactions Van der Waals forces Hydrogen bonding	Opposite charge on antigen and adjuvant
pH	6.0–7.5, at optimal pH adjuvant and antigen should have opposite charges
Temperature	4–25°C, depending upon the stability of antigen
Size of gel particles	<10 μm
Ionic strength of reaction mixture	Low, absence of phosphate ions for aluminum phosphate

2. Materials (*see* Note 2)

2.1. Alum-Precipitated Vaccines

1. 10% solution of sodium alum (Na_2SO_4. $Al_2(SO_4)_3.18H_2O$) is prepared in distilled water and is sterilized by autoclaving or by filtration through 0.2 μm filter.
2. 0.85% NaCl, sodium chloride solution (physiological saline) is prepared in distilled water and is sterilized by autoclaving or by filtration through 0.2 μm filter.
3 1% Thimerosal (Ethyl [2-mercaptobenzoato-S] mercury sodium salt) solution, prepared in distilled water, is a filter (0.2 μm) sterilized solution.

2.2. Aluminum Hydroxide

1. Aluminum chloride/sodium acetate solution. Final concentration of aluminum chloride ($AlCl_3$.$6H_2O$) and sodium acetate ($CH_3COONa.3H_2O$) is 0.0513*M* and 0.01*M*, respectively. Prepare 5X solution (0.257*M* aluminum chloride and 0.05*M* sodium acetate) by dissolving 62.05 g aluminum chloride ($AlCl_3$.$6H_2O$) and 6.8 g of sodium acetate ($CH_3COONa.3H_2O$) per liter of distilled water. Sterilize the solution either by autoclaving or by filtration (0.2 μm). If filter sterilization is used, filter membrane should be compatible with the solution. The pH of this solution is between 3 and 4. The sterile solution is stored at room temperature (20 to 30°C).
2. Sodium hydroxide solution. Final concentration of sodium hydroxide (NaOH) is 0.0513*M*. Prepare 5X solution (0.257*M*) by dissolving 10.25 g of sodium hydroxide per liter of distilled water. Sterilize the solution by heat or filter sterilization. As with other solutions, if filtration is used, test the compatibility of filter

membranes with the solution. The pH of the 5X concentrate solution is between 12 and 14. The sterile solution should be stored at room temperature (20 to 30°C).
3. 1% Thimerosal (described in **Subheading 2.1.**).
4. Sterile solutions of 5*N* NaOH and 5*N* acetic acid for pH adjustment.

2.3. Aluminum Phosphate

1. Aluminum chloride/sodium acetate solution. Final concentration of aluminum chloride ($AlCl_3 .6H_2O$) and sodium acetate ($CH_3COONa.3H_2O$) is 0.0328*M* and 0.01*M*, respectively. Prepare 5X solution (0.164*M* aluminum chloride and 0.05*M* sodium acetate) by dissolving 39.7 g $AlCl_3 .6H_2O$ and 6.8 g of $CH_3COONa.3H_2O$ per liter of distilled water. Sterilize the solution either by autoclaving or filter (0.2 µm) sterilization. If filter sterilization is used, filter membranc should be compatible with the solution. The pH of this solution is between 3 and 4. The sterile solution is stored at room temperature (20 to 30°C).
2. Disodium phosphate solution. Final concentration of disodium phosphate ($Na_2HPO_4.7H_2O$) is 0.0287M. Prepare 5X solution (0.144*M*) by dissolving 38.59 g of $Na_2HPO_4.7H_2O$ per liter of distilled water. Sterilize the solution by heat or filter sterilization. As with other solutions, if filtration is used, test the compatibility of filter membranes with the buffer solution. The pH of the 5X concentrate solution is between pH 8.5 and 9.5. The sterile solution should be stored at room temperature (20 to 30°C).
3. 1% thimerosal (described in **Subheading 2.1.**).
4. Sterile solutions of 5*N* NaOH and 5*N* acetic acid for pH adjustment.

2.4. Quantitation of Aluminum Adjuvants

1. 50% w/v sodium hydroxide (NaOH).
2. Acetate buffer. Dissolve 68 g sodium acetate and 38.5 g of ammonium acetate in approximately 200 mL distilled water. Add 125 mL glacial acetic acid and make the final volume to 500 mL. Buffer contains 1*M* sodium acetate, 1*M* ammonium acetate, and 4.35 *M* acetic acid.
3. 0.01*M* disodium ethylenediamine tetra acetate.
4. 0.01*M* Cuprous sulphate ($CuSO_4.5H_2O$).
5. Sulphuric acid, nitric acid.
6. Methyl orange indicator and pyridylazonaphthol indicator (0.1% solution in 95% ethanol).

3. Methods

3.1. Alum-Precipitated Vaccines

Alum-precipitated vaccines are prepared by *in situ* precipitation of vaccine antigens with potassium or sodium alum. These antigens are usually in culture medium, employed for growing the organisms, containing anions (phosphate, sulphate, and bicarbonate ions). This is the original method developed primarily for purifying tetanus and diphtheria toxoids ***(8,15,20)***. Alum-precipitated toxoids, prepared in this way, were more immunogenic than the soluble formulations and contained a mixture of aluminum compounds, mainly aluminum phosphate and aluminum hydroxide. This product was highly heterogeneous ***(4)*** and difficult to manufacture in a consistent and reproducible manner ***(8,9,12)***. In 1976, a World Health Organization report ***(21)*** described this method as a laboratory procedure which did not define the nature of the material obtained either quantitatively or qualitatively. For these reasons, this product is not very common now. However, this method can be used to prepare aluminum phosphate, aluminum hydroxide, or a mixture of these in a controled manner by taking purified antigens in defined solutions (phosphate solution for preparing aluminum phosphate; hydroxide solution for preparing aluminum hydroxide; phosphate solution and then adjusting pH with sodium hydroxide for getting a mixture of aluminum phosphate and aluminum hydroxide). Using controled conditions, consistent preparations of aluminum adjuvants from lot to lot can be made by this method. Though this method is not routinely used, a procedure to prepare alum-precipitated vaccines from a published method ***(20)*** is described below.

1. Alum has been used at a final concentration of 0.2 to 2.0%, depending upon the antigen and purity required. However, to use this procedure for purified antigens in defined solutions, 1% final concentration would give aluminum compounds in the range that has adjuvant properties. Therefore, add the required volume of 10% sodium alum solution to the antigen solution to achieve the desired final concentration of alum.
2. Adsorption of proteins to aluminum adjuvants depends upon pH ***(3,4,6,12)***, *see* **Note 1**. Therefore, optimal pH of adsorption has to be worked out for the antigen under study. Adjust the pH to the optimal pH.
3. Incubate the mixture at 37°C for 1 h and then at 2–8°C overnight.
4. Centrifuge the precipitate and wash the precipitates twice with physiological saline. If the conditions of adsorption (alum concentration and pH) are not optimal, most of the antigens would be washed away.
5. Resuspend the precipitates in physiological saline to the original volume of antigen. Add 1% thimerosal to a final concentration of 0.01% as a preservative.

3.2. Aluminum Hydroxide

Currently, the most commonly used method for preparation of aluminum adsorbed vaccines is adsorption of antigens onto preformed aluminum hydroxide or aluminum phosphate gels under controled conditions ***(3,15)***. Antigens can also be adsorbed onto these aluminum gels during their preparation (*in situ* adsorption). These preparations made by adsorption onto preformed gels or by *in situ* adsorption are usually referred to as aluminum hydroxide or aluminum phosphate adsorbed or adjuvanted vaccines. Tetanus toxoid adsorbed onto preformed aluminum hydroxide and aluminum phosphate gels had 60% of the potency of vaccine to that adsorbed by *in situ* method **(22)**. Gels of aluminum phosphate and aluminum hydroxide, of clinical grade, are commercially available. Adsorption onto preformed gels, bought from commercial sources or prepared in-house, is carried out by incubating the gel and the antigen, at optimal pH, with slow stirring for a few hours to overnight **(4)** at 4°C to room temperature.

As mentioned earlier, antigens on aluminum hydroxide can either be adsorbed *in situ* during preparation of the gel or adsorbed onto preformed gel. In our experience, it may be preferable to buy aluminum hydroxide from a commercial source and develop an optimal process to adsorb antigens onto aluminum hydroxide, particularly for research laboratories, as this adjuvant sometimes shows variability with regard to size and adjuvant properties when prepared under slightly different conditions, such as order of adding reagents, speed at which the reagents are added and mixed, mixing speed, and scaling-up the production. In this chapter, a procedure for preparing aluminum hydroxide is described. It is recommended that various lots of adjuvant should be characterized to ensure consistency in manufacture of the adjuvant.

3.2.1. In Situ *Adsorption onto Aluminum Hydroxide*

Though it is possible to adsorb antigens *in situ* on to aluminum hydroxide, it is not a common procedure because of suspension of antigens in solutions at extremes of pH. Most of the antigens may not be stable at pH 12–14 (NaOH solution) or pH 3–4 (aluminum chloride/sodium acetate solution). If the antigens are stable, it is recommended that the antigens may be added to sodium hydroxide solution. The method described is for a preparation of *in situ* adsorbed vaccine containing 4 mg/mL of $Al(OH)_3$, having 1.38 mg Al/mL (*see* **Note 3** for doses of aluminum adjuvants).

1. Stir the contents continuously during the procedure at 40 to 60 rpm.
2. First add 0.257*M* NaOH solution (20% of final volume) to a mixing vessel.
3. Add sterile distilled water (50–55% of final volume).
4. Add antigens followed by addition of 0.257*M* aluminum chloride/sodium acetate ($AlCl_3/CH_3COONa$) solution (20% of final volume) to the mixture at a rate of 1–2 L/min. During the addition of this solution, monitor pH and maintain it between 5.5 and 6.5 (optimal pH for tetanus and diphtheria toxoids) or any other range suitable for a particular antigen.
5. Add 1% thimerosal solution to get 0.01% final concentration.
6. Adjust to the final volume with sterile distilled water. Mix the suspension for 2 h.
7. Adjust the final pH to 5.9–6.1 (for tetanus and diphtheria toxoids) or to the optimal pH with 5*N* NaOH or 5*N* acetic acid.

3.2.2. Adsorption onto Preformed Aluminum Hydroxide Gel

Method for preparing aluminum hydroxide gel is the same as described above except without the addition of antigens and thimerosal. The method makes a gel with 4 mg/mL of $Al(OH)_3$ having 1.38 mg Al/mL (*see* **Note 3** for doses of aluminum adjuvants). After final pH adjustment, the aluminum hydroxide gel is sterilized by autoclaving. During sterilization of large volumes of gel by autoclaving, it should be ensured that the gel in the middle of the container gets heated to the appropriate temperature. For obtaining gels of higher concentration, these may be prepared from more concentrated solutions of sodium hydroxide and aluminum chloride/sodium acetate or by centrifuging the gel at 4 mg/mL and suspending it in distilled water or physiological saline in a volume to obtain the required concentration of gel. Alternatively, aluminum hydroxide gel from a commercial source may be purchased. To adsorb antigens onto preformed gels, optimal pH of adsorption for antigens to be adsorbed should be determined in preliminary experiments before adsorption (*see* **Note 1**).

1. Stir the contents continuously during the procedure at 40 to 60 rpm.
2. Add the gel to a mixing vessel and add calculated volume of physiological saline.
3. Adjust pH to 5.9–6.1 (for tetanus and diphtheria toxoids) or to the optimal pH with 5*N* NaOH or 5*N* acetic acid.
4. Add the antigens to the gel solution.
5. Add 1% thimerosal solution to get 0.01% final concentration.
6. Mix solution for 2 h.
7. Check pH again and adjust to optimal pH, if necessary with 5*N* NaOH or 5*N* acetic acid.

3.3. Aluminum Phosphate

Like aluminum hydroxide, aluminum phosphate is the most widely used adjuvant with routine human vaccines. Most of the vaccine manufacturers throughout the world prepare this adjuvant in-house. Usually, antigens are adsorbed onto a preformed gel, which can be made by several methods (two methods are described in this chapter). Adsorption of antigens is also carried out on freshly prepared aluminum phosphate gel ***(23)***. *In situ* adsorption of antigens onto aluminum phosphate is preferable to aluminum hydroxide, because pH of the solution (disodium phosphate) in which the antigens are suspended for making aluminum phosphate is not as high as of sodium hydroxide used for making aluminum hydroxide.

Antigens onto aluminum phosphate gel can either be adsorbed *in situ* during preparation of the gel or adsorbed onto preformed gel. There are several methods of preparing preformed gel of aluminum phosphate *(22,24)*. Some of the preparations may have aluminum hydroxide also as the final pH adjustment is done with sodium hydroxide, which results into formation of aluminum hydroxide if aluminum chloride has not been completely reacted with disodium phosphate. Unlike aluminum hydroxide, aluminum phosphate can be prepared in a consistent way from lot to lot and the quality of gel is not as sensitive to the process of making gel as the manufacture of aluminum hydroxide. However, it is recommended that various lots of adjuvant should be characterized to ensure consistency in manufacture of the adjuvant.

3.3.1. In Situ *Adsorption*

In situ adsorption of antigens on aluminum phosphate has been carried out by suspending purified vaccine antigens in dibasic or tribasic sodium phosphate or phosphate buffer and precipitating with aluminum chloride *(3,7,22)*. This type of reaction can be carried out under controled conditions and results in a consistent product. This procedure does not expose antigens to extreme pH conditions as compared to *in situ* adsorption onto aluminum hydroxide. If the antigens cannot tolerate pH of 8.5–9.5 (pH of disodium phosphate solution), the pH can be adjusted prior to the addition of the antigens. The method described here is for the preparation of *in situ* adsorbed vaccine containing 4 mg/mL of $AlPO_4$, having 0.88 mg Al/mL (*see* **Note 3** for doses of aluminum adjuvants).

1. Stir the contents continuously during the procedure at 40 to 60 rpm.
2. Add 0.144*M* disodium phosphate ($Na_2HPO_4.7H_2O$) solution (20% of final volume) to a mixing vessel.
3. Add sterile distilled water (50–55% of final volume).
4. Add antigens followed by addition of 0.164*M* aluminum chloride/sodium acetate ($AlCl_3/CH_3COONa$) solution (20% of final volume) to the mixture at a rate of 1–2 L/min. During the addition of this solution, monitor pH and maintain it between 5.5 and 6.5 (optimal pH for tetanus and diphtheria toxoids) or any other range suitable for a particular antigen.
5. Add 1% thimerosal solution to get 0.01% final concentration.
6. Adjust to the final volume with sterile distilled water. Mix the suspension for 2 h.
7. Adjust the final pH to 5.9–6.1 (for tetanus and diphtheria toxoids) or to the optimal pH with 5*N* NaOH or 5*N* acetic acid.

3.3.2. Adsorption onto Preformed Gel

There are several methods to prepare aluminum phosphate gels *(22,24)*. One of the methods is the same as described above (**Subheading 3.3.1.**) except without the addition of antigens and thimerosal. The method makes a gel with 4 mg/mL of $AlPO_4$ having 0.88 mg Al/mL. After final pH adjustment, the aluminum phosphate gel is sterilized by autoclaving. During sterilization of large volumes of gel by autoclaving, it should be ensured that the gel in the middle of the container gets heated to the appropriate temperature. For obtaining gels of higher concentration, these may be prepared from more concentrated solutions of disodium phosphate and aluminum chloride/sodium acetate or by centrifuging the gel at 4 mg/mL and suspending it in distilled water or physiological saline in a volume to obtain the required concentration of gel. Alternatively, aluminum phosphate gel from a commercial source, may be purchased. Another method of preparing aluminum phosphate gels at commercial scale has been described by the World Health Organization ***(24)***. This method is given below.

3.3.3. Preparation of Aluminum Phosphate from Potassium Alum–WHO Method ***(24)***

1. Dissolve 854 g alum (potassium aluminum sulphate, $KAl(SO_4)_2.12H_2O$) in 6 L of distilled water and filter it. Keep it at 37°C as it is slightly oversaturated at room temperature.
2. Dissolve 685 g of trisodium phosphate ($Na_3PO_4.12H_2O$) in 6 L of distilled water.
3. Pour 21 L of distilled water in a mixing vessel and both solutions are poured into water with mixing.
4. Centrifuge the contents and wash the precipitates twice with physiological saline (0.85% NaCl).
5. Resuspend the precipitates in 8.1 L of physiological saline, homogenize, adjust pH to 6.0 with 5*N* NaOH and autoclave.
6. This material is sufficient for 66 L of a vaccine at 3 mg/mL of $AlPO_4$, having 0.66 mg Al/mL.

Method of adsorption of antigens onto preformed aluminum phosphate gel is the same as described for aluminum hydroxide (**Subheading 3.2.2.**).

3.4. Storage of Aluminum-Containing Adjuvants

Aluminum adjuvant gels without antigens may be stored at room temperature or 2–8°C in closed aseptic containers. Vaccine antigens adsorbed onto mineral adjuvants are stored at 2–8°C. These should not be frozen (*see* **Note 4**).

3.5. Preclinical Evaluation of Vaccines Adsorbed onto Aluminum Compounds

To achieve consistency in manufacture of aluminum adjuvants, it is important to characterize these adjuvants for physicochemical and adjuvant properties. Though aluminum adjuvants have been used widely with human vaccines, there are still a number of unanswered questions about their mechanism of action (*see* **Note 5**), such as optimal size of the gel particles, degree of adsorption of antigens onto adjuvant, amount of gel used as a dose for humans and animals (*see* **Note 3**) and even type of aluminum adjuvant that shows better adjuvanticity (*see* **Note 6**). During the last several years, physicochemical characteristics of aluminum adjuvants have been studied *(7)*. Though there is no clear understanding between these characteristics and adjuvanticity, most of the regulatory agencies have started requiring information on these characteristics with a view to achieving consistency in manufacture of vaccines adsorbed onto aluminum compounds.

3.5.1. Physicochemical Characteristics

The physicochemical characteristics are very useful in optimizing the adsorption of antigens onto aluminum adjuvants and for formulation of combination vaccines. By controling the physicochemical characteristics of aluminum adjuvants and vaccines adsorbed onto these adjuvants, it would be easy to control the manufacturing process of these vaccines and achieve consistency in production as per current good manufacturing practices (cGMP) requirements.

Stanley Hem and coworkers have extensively studied the physicochemical characteristics of aluminum adjuvants and their effects on the adsorption of proteins onto these adjuvants *(7,19,25–29)*. Aluminum hydroxide has been identified as poorly crystalline aluminum oxyhydroxide with a structure of the mineral boehmite. It has high surface area with an isoelectric point (p*I*) of 11, which favors adsorption of negatively charged proteins at neutral pH. In contrast, aluminum phosphate and alum-precipitated vaccines have been classified as amorphous aluminum hydroxyphosphate with little sulfate. Depending upon the conditions under which these gels are prepared, the molar ratio between aluminum and phosphate of amorphous aluminum hydroxyphosphate varies which results in p*I* values from 5 to 7. So these gels are negatively charged or without any charge at neutral pH. The amorphous nature of these compounds contributes to high surface area and high protein adsorption capacity, mainly for positively charged proteins. That is the reason for poor adsorption of negatively charged diphtheria toxoid onto aluminum phosphate at a neutral pH. But, aluminum phosphate gel with a p*I* close to 7 would be positively charged at pH of 6.0, leading to adsorption of diphtheria toxoid. Therefore, formulation of diphtheria, tetanus, and pertussis (DTP) vaccine with aluminum phosphate is usually done at a pH close to 6.0 to allow maximum adsorption of diphtheria toxoid.

The following are some of the physicochemical tests that would be useful for achieving consistency in manufacture of aluminum adjuvants.

1. Isoelectric Point (p*I*). Information on p*I* or point of zero charge will not only be useful as a test to assess consistency in manufacture, it would be useful to deter-

mine optimal conditions for adsorption of a particular antigen on the gel. The isoelectric point of gels can be determined by Doppler electrophoretic light-scattering analysis (DELSA 440, Coulter, Hialeah, FL) ***(30)***.

2. Size of gel particles. One of the mechanisms of adjuvant action by the aluminum adjuvants is the size of gel particles being in the range that is optimal for adjuvant action (<10 μm) (*see* **Note 5b**). Monitoring size of various lots would give the information on consistency in production and would also help in optimizing the adjuvanticity by optimizing the size, if it is not <10 μm. Size of gel particles can be measured by particle size analyzers.
3. pH. pH of the gel has a direct effect on the charge of the gel, thus affecting the adsorption of antigens.
4. Other physical characteristics evaluated by Stanley Hem and coworkers for aluminum adjuvants include X-ray diffraction, infrared spectroscopy, transmission electron microscopy, and energy dispersive spectrometry ***(7,19,25–29)***, which may be useful for first five lots of adjuvant to prove consistency in manufacture.

3.5.2. Determination of Degree of Adsorption

The immunogenicity of antigens adsorbed onto aluminum adjuvants appears to depend on the degree of antigen adsorption and the dose of adjuvant ***(2,3,6)*** (*see* **Note 3**). There has been a debate on the optimal degree of adsorption and its role in the adjuvanticity of aluminum adjuvants in humans ***(31)*** because there is not much information available on this topic. Vaccines with less adsorption of antigens onto aluminum adjuvants, approx 50% or even lower adsorption, have proved effective in the field and meet all the requirements of the regulatory agencies. Despite these controversies and uncertainty about precise mechanism of action of aluminum adjuvants (*see* **Note 5**), adsorption is still considered to be a very important parameter for the function of these adjuvants ***(3)***. Thus, measuring the degree of adsorption is one of the parameters that can be controled in the formulation process during manufacture of aluminum adsorbed vaccines to achieve consistency in production. Adsorption of 80% or more of tetanus and diphtheria toxoids onto aluminum adjuvants is recommended by the WHO ***(24)***. The United States Minimum Requirements ***(32)*** for adult tetanus and diphtheria toxoid is at least 75% adsorption of diphtheria component on the aluminum adjuvants.

Degree of adsorption can be measured by simply centrifuging the adsorbed vaccine and assaying the supernatant for total protein (by Lowry assay, BCA assay, or other protein assay), antigenicity (flocculation), or polysaccharide (by anthrone or some specific sugar assay) depending upon the nature of the antigen. These assays are not very sensitive, for example, in a 10 μg dose of an antigen with 80% adsorption, quantitating 2 μg may not be very accurate. In these cases, proteins can be precipitated with trichloroacetic acid from supernatants of large sample volumes. Antigens from the supernatant may also be assayed by sensitive methods based on immunochemistry, such as enzyme-linked immunosorbent assay (ELISA) *(23)* and nephelometry assay. These assays can measure antigens at much lower levels (in ng/mL concentrations).

3.5.3. Dissolution of Gels to Release Antigens

Aluminum adjuvant gels are often dissolved to release antigens into solution or antigens are desorbed from the gels for direct measurement of antigens adsorbed onto the gels. This is also done to establish identity of the product, which is one of the tests performed on final products as per the requirements of the regulatory agencies. Antigens can be desorbed by exposing the adsorbed preparations to high salt or phosphate concentrations and/or pH that does not support adsorption. The most commonly used procedure in the vaccine industry is to dissolve the gels with 5–10% sodium citrate solution *(24)*. This procedure (described below) works well with aluminum phosphate gel and dissolves the gel at 37°C within 24 h, but aluminum hydroxide gel is sometimes difficult to dissolve and requires incubation of vaccine preparations at 37°C for 2–3 d.

1. Add 100 mg/mL (10% final concentration) of sodium citrate, granular ($C_6H_5Na_3O_7.2H_2O$) directly to adsorbed preparation in a glass or plastic tube. A 20% solution of sodium citrate in distilled water may also be used to achieve 5–10% final concentration.
2. Mix the solution until all the sodium citrate granules have dissolved.
3. Incubate the tube at 37°C overnight or until clear. With some preparations, the solution remains cloudy, but the toxoid is completely dissolved.

3.5.4. Quantitation of Aluminum Adjuvants

One of the quality-control parameters on vaccines adsorbed onto aluminum adjuvants is to quantitate the aluminum compounds at final bulk or final product stage. There are several wet chemistry and physical methods used for quantitation purposes *(24,33)*. These methods include atomic absorption spectrometry, inductively coupled argon plasma (ICP) emission spectrometry, direct current plasma (DCP) technique, and wet chemistry methods by digestion of the sample and titration of aluminum with copper sulphate. Physical methods, such as atomic absorption spectrometry, ICP, and DCP are more common these days, but in a research laboratory, these instruments may not be available and wet chemistry method gives reliable results. A wet chemistry method from the WHO manual *(24)* for quantitation of aluminum is below.

1. Boil 3 mL of sample in glass tube, in duplicate and add 1 mL of concentrated sulphuric acid and 6 drops of concentrated nitric acid to each tube.
2. Heat tubes and start adding nitric acid dropwise when dense white fumes evolve. Continue to add nitric acid while heating until tubes are colorless.

Table 2
Antibody Response of Mice[a] to Varying Doses of Aluminum Phosphate Adsorbed Tetanus Toxoid Injected Undiluted and Diluted in Saline

Dose Lf (~μg)	Human Dose	Inoculum (μL)	Antibody levels at 4 wk	
			TN[b] (AU/mL)	IgG[c] (EAU/mL)
0.2 (0.6)	1/25th	20[d]	0.50	3.87 (2.60–5.75)
0.2 (0.6)	1/25th	500[e]	0.60	3.81 (1.86–7.79)
0.1 (0.3)	1/50th	10[d]	0.25	2.11 (1.33–3.37)
0.1 (0.3)	1/50th	250[e]	0.38	2.05 (1.34–3.15)
0.05 (0.15)	1/100th	5[d]	0.12	0.46 (0.06–3.67)
0.05 (0.15)	1/100th	125[e]	0.16	1.45 (0.88–2.37)

[a]Four-week-old female outbred (CD-1 strain) mice were injected subcutaneously and bled at 4 wk.

[b]TN=Toxin neutralizing antibodies (tetanus antitoxin) were determined in Antitoxin Units per mL (AU/mL) in the pooled sera ***(23)***.

[c]IgG antibodies to tetanus toxin were determined in the sera of individual mice by ELISA and expressed in ELISA Antitoxin Units/mL (EAU/mL) ***(23)***. Results are shown as geometric mean with 95% confidence intervals in parenthesis.

[d] Undiluted vaccine at 5 Lf/mL.

[e]1 in 12.5 diluted (in saline) vaccine at 0.4 Lf/mL.

Lf, Limes flocculation

3. Cool tubes and add 10 mL of distilled water carefully. If tubes are cloudy, boil until these are clear.
4. Add 2–3 drops of methyl orange indicator and add 50% NaOH until a pink-yellow end point is obtained. Dissolve any precipitates with dilute sulphuric acid.
5. Transfer contents of the tubes separately to two Erlemeyer (250 mL) flasks; wash tubes with 25 mL distilled water and pool washings with the contents in flasks.
6. Add 25 mL 0.01*M* disodium ethylenediamine and 10 mL acetate buffer to each flask.
7. Boil flasks gently for 3 min and add 1 mL of pyridylazonaphthol indicator. Titrate hot solution with 0.01*M* cuprous sulphate until a purple brown end point is reached. Take average titer from two flask readings. Simultaneously treat a flask starting with 3 mL distilled water in place of sample to get the blank titer.
8. Aluminum concentration is determined from the following formula.

$$\text{Mg of aluminum per mL} = (\text{Blank titer} - \text{sample titer}) \times 0.2698/3 \text{ (volume of sample)}$$

3.5.5. Animal Experiments

Most of the biologicals, including vaccines, are evaluated in laboratory animals for potency. Doses of vaccines chosen in animal models are usually several-fold (sometimes 100's-fold) lower than the human doses to get the response on the logarithmic part of the dose-response curve ***(6,34)***. **Tables 2**

Table 3
Antibody Response of Guinea Pigs[a] to Varying Doses of Aluminum Phosphate Adsorbed Tetanus Toxoid Injected Undiluted and Diluted in Saline

			Antibody levels at		
			4 wk	6 wk	
Dose Lf (~µg)	Human Dose	Inoculum (µL)	IgG[b] (EAU/mL)	TN[c] (AU/mL)	IgG[b] (EAU/mL)
0.2 (0.6)	1/25th	20[d]	2.37 (1.63–3.45)	0.50	1.57 (1.17–2.12)
0.2 (0.6)	1/25th	500[e]	1.79 (0.84–3.84)	0.40	1.13 (0.71–1.79)
0.1 (0.3)	1/50th	10[d]	1.44 (0.66–3.16)	0.28	1.17 (0.59–2.31)
0.1 (0.3)	1/50th	250[e]	1.25 (0.95–1.64)	0.25	0.69 (0.53–0.90)
0.05 (0.15)	1/100th	5[d]	0.58 (0.27–1.26)	0.09	0.48 (0.22–1.06)
0.05 (0.15)	1/100th	125[e]	0.24 (0.10–0.55)	<0.09	0.16 (0.05–0.48)

[a]Female outbred (Hartley strain) guinea pigs, 450–550 g were injected subcutaneously and bled at 4 wk and 6 wk.

[b]IgG antibodies to tetanus toxin were determined in the sera of individual guinea pigs by ELISA and expressed in ELISA Antitoxin Units/mL (EAU/mL) ***(23)***. Results are shown as geometric mean with 95% confidence intervals in parenthesis.

[c]TN=Toxin neutralizing antibodies (tetanus antitoxin) were determined in Antitoxin Units per ml (AU/mL) in the pooled sera ***(23).***

[d]Undiluted vaccine at 5 Lf/mL.

[e]1 in 12.5 diluted (in saline) vaccine at 0.4 Lf/mL.

and **3** summarize antibody responses of mice and guinea pigs, respectively, to tetanus toxoid when injected as 1/25th to 1/100th of the human dose. Similar data on antibody responses of mice to diphtheria toxoid are shown in **Table 4**. The most common practice to perform this type of assays is to dilute the vaccine formulations in saline or phosphate-buffered saline (PBS). Dilution of vaccines adsorbed onto aluminum adjuvants, particularly in PBS, desorbs certain antigens that can affect the immunogenicity of the vaccine in animals. Dilution of vaccines decreased the antibody responses of guinea pigs to tetanus toxoid (**Table 3**) and of mice to diphtheria toxoid (**Table 4**) as compared to the injection of undiluted formulations. Therefore, preparations adsorbed onto aluminum adjuvants should not be diluted, particularly in PBS, for immunogenicity studies. Several studies demonstrated lower levels of immunogenicity/potency in mice and guinea pigs using aluminum-adsorbed vaccines diluted in saline compared to those diluted in the aluminum adjuvant ***(35–37)***. It is believed that dilution of adjuvanted vaccines for testing in animals may disturb the composition of the vaccine ***(3,6,34–45)***. Potency tests in animals based on dilution of vaccines ***(46,47)*** do not provide the "true picture" of the immunogenicity of the final formulation ***(5,6,35–37)***. Hence, it is recommended that for animal immunogenicity studies of adjuvanted vaccines, the formulation

Table 4
Antibody Response of Mice[a] to Varying Doses of Aluminum Phosphate Adsorbed Diphtheria Toxoid Injected Undiluted and Diluted in Saline

Dose Lf (~μg)	Human Dose	Inoculum (μL)	Antibody levels at 4 wk IgG[b] (μg/mL)
0.2 (0.5)	1/50th	10[c]	3.30 (0.83–13.2)
0.2 (0.5)	1/50th	500[d]	0.29 (0.02–4.75)
0.1 (0.25)	1/100th	5[c]	1.29 (0.05–33.7)
0.1 (0.25)	1/100th	250[d]	0.11 (0.01–1.04)

[a]Four-week-old female outbred (CD-1 strain) mice were injected subcutaneously and bled at 4 wk.

[b]IgG antibodies to diphtheria toxoid were determined in the sera of individual mice by ELISA and expressed in μg/mL *(85)*. Results are shown as geometric mean with 95% confidence intervals in parenthesis.

[c]Undiluted vaccine at 20 Lf/mL.

[d]1 in 50 diluted (in saline) vaccine at 0.4 Lf/mL.

intended for human use should be injected undiluted or with a minimum dilution, if necessary.

Aluminum compounds are very potent adjuvants for tetanus and diphtheria toxoids in guinea pigs and mice, particularly in outbred CD-1 mice ***(34)***. The antibody responses in mice and guinea pigs after a single dose of aluminum phosphate adsorbed tetanus toxoid are routinely very high and persisted at high levels for up to 1 yr ***(3,48,49)***. Single injection of small doses (0.05 Lf or approx 0.15 μg) of aluminum phosphate adsorbed tetanus toxoid elicited protective levels of antibodies in mice and guinea pigs (**Tables 2** and **3**). In contrast, single injections of tetanus and diphtheria toxoids adsorbed onto aluminum adjuvants do not elicit such high antibodies in humans. Thus, animal models seem not to provide true adjuvanticity of aluminum adjuvants ***(50)***. However, animal immunogenicity studies are essential to develop new vaccines or improve existing vaccines. All these factors should be considered when choosing animal models and model proteins for evaluation of new adjuvants and in interpreting the results. To assess the adjuvanticity of new formulations for humoral response, it is recommended that the formulations should be injected undiluted by intramuscular route (if possible). Otherwise, subcutaneous route should be employed, particularly for in-bred mice, who do not have much muscle. In such cases, it is difficult to ensure that all injections are intramuscular without any leakage of injected material from muscles. In humans, it is recommended that vaccines adsorbed onto aluminum adjuvants should be injected by intramuscular route because of less-adverse local reactions as compared to sc injections ***(13,51)***, but the antibody responses in children to a booster injection given by intramuscular or subcutaneous routes were very similar *(51)*. Therefore, for immunogenicity purposes, aluminum adsorbed vaccines can be injected to animals by im or sc routes.

Antibody responses should be evaluated after a single injection, as the adjuvant effect is not very clear or even absent after the booster injection *(23)*. Good scientific practices on performing antibody assays and problems with animal models have been discussed in detail elsewhere *(2)*.

4. Notes

1. **Table 1** summarizes factors affecting adsorption of antigens onto aluminum adjuvants. Adsorption of antigens onto aluminum adjuvants depends heavily on electrostatic forces between adjuvant and antigen *(3,6,7,19)*. Other interactions including hydrophobic, van der Waals, and hydrogen bonding contribute to the adsorption of antigens on aluminum adjuvants. However, these forces may not suffice to cause adsorption of antigen if the same charge or electrostatic repulsive force is present on antigen and adjuvant. The two most commonly used aluminum adjuvants, aluminum hydroxide, and aluminum phosphate, have different points of zero charge *(7,25)*. At neutral pH, these gels have opposite charges, wherein aluminum phosphate is negatively charged and aluminum hydroxide is positively charged. It is important to select the aluminum adjuvant carefully on the basis of the charge of the antigen at neutral pH or any other desirable pH. Other physical conditions affecting adsorption of antigens on mineral adjuvants include pH, temperature, size of the gel particles, and ionic strength of the reaction mixture *(3,4,6,7,12,15,16,52)*. The pH and ionic strength affect adsorption by altering charge on the gel and the antigens, whereas the temperature may affect the rate of interaction between the gel and the antigen. Size of gel particles affects the surface area of gel available for adsorption: small particles have more surface area than large particles. For example, amount of diphtheria toxoid adsorbed on to aluminum hydroxide gels was inversely proportional to the gel particle size *(52)*.

   Acidic pH of less than 6 has been found optimal for adsorption of several antigens on aluminum adjuvants *(12)*. For example, the optimal pH for adsorption of tetanus and diphtheria toxoid onto aluminum phosphate is 6.0–6.3 *(3)*. The adsorption of diphtheria toxoid onto aluminum phosphate is heavily influenced by pH and the presence of excess phosphate ions in the reaction mixture *(3,6)*. Aluminum phosphate and diphtheria toxoid are both negatively charged at neutral pH resulting in poor adsorption. At pH 6.0, aluminum phosphate is positively charged, thus improving adsorption of negatively charged diphtheria toxoid. *In situ* adsorption of diphtheria toxoid resulted in higher adsorption than the commercial aluminum phosphate preparation *(3,6)*, probably because of trapping of some antigen in the gel. Adsorption of tetanus and diphtheria toxoids onto aluminum hydroxide gel (Alhydrogel) was not sensitive to the conditions of pH and excess phosphate ions *(2,3,6)* because it is positively charged at pH 6.0 and 7.0.

Adsorption of bovine serum albumin onto aluminum hydroxide and lysozyme onto aluminum phosphate was inversely proportional to the ionic strength *(19)*. Excess anions, particularly phosphate ions, and impurities, such as amino acids, peptides, and polysaccharides, reduce protein adsorption, probably by competing with antigen for adsorption sites *(16)*. Multiple-charged negative ions, especially phosphate ions, interfere with the adsorption capacity of aluminum hydroxide and these may be used for eluting adsorbed antigens from the gel *(4)*. Lindblad and Sparck *(16)* recommended avoiding PBS in the reaction mixture for adsorption of antigen onto aluminum adjuvants. In general, a low ionic strength and absence of excess phosphate ions and impurities are recommended for optimal adsorption of antigens on aluminum phosphate gel *(15)*. The temperature of adsorption has been considered important for complete adsorption of antigen onto aluminum phosphate although most of the adsorption, up to 80–90% of diphtheria toxoid, occurred within a few minutes at temperatures ranging from 4 to 45°C *(12)*.

Aluminum hydroxide (Alhydrogel) was capable of adsorbing higher amounts of tetanus toxoid (273.4 Lf or approx 820 µg per mg of gel) and diphtheria toxoid (126.6 Lf or approx 380 µg per mg of gel) than aluminum phosphate (Adjuphos®) (53.5 Lf [Limes flocculation] or approx 161 µg tetanus toxoid/mg gel) at a pH of 6.0 *(3)*. Lindblad and Sparck *(16)* found 10–20 times more adsorption of human serum albumin on aluminum hydroxide than on aluminum phosphate. Therefore, aluminum hydroxide has higher adsorption capacity than aluminum phosphate, particularly for routine childhood vaccine antigens, tetanus, and diphtheria toxoids. The major reason is the charge on these gel at neutral or slightly acidic pH (6.0). As discussed, aluminum hydroxide has strong positive charge at pH 6–7.0, whereas aluminum phosphate has a weak or neutral charge at this pH range. Tetanus and diphtheria toxoids being negatively charged at pH 6–7.0 show strong and more adsorption to aluminum hydroxide than to aluminum phosphate.

There has been some discussion on the desorption of antigen from adjuvant after injection into the body where a physiologically neutral pH and presence of body fluids containing proteins and anions might desorb the antigen from the gel. Earlier studies showed that freshly made preparations of aluminum phosphate adsorbed diphtheria toxoid had more antigen desorption than aged preparations when exposed to neutral pH or serum *(12)*. Thus, aging of aluminum-adsorbed vaccines appears to improve their immunogenicity *(8)*.

2. For preparing any of the adjuvant formulations described in this chapter, use of sterile water for injection for clinical use materials and sterile distilled water free from endotoxin for laboratory use or preclinical materials is required. For convenience purposes, distilled water is mentioned throughout the text where use of such water is required. All chemicals should be of USP, NF, or FCC grades.
3. The dose of mineral adjuvants also affects the overall immunogenicity of vaccines *(15)*. A small amount of adjuvant may be required for complete adsorption of the antigen, but low doses may not provide an optimal adjuvant effect. There appears to be a need for excess free adjuvant for an optimal adjuvant effect

(53,54). In animal studies, as the amount of aluminum adjuvant was increased, the adjuvant effect increased, but only to a certain concentration after which, the adjuvant effect declined *(15,16,35,55–57)*. The reasons for this optimum concentration of adjuvant are unknown. It is speculated that a certain minimum amount of aluminum compound is necessary to form a depot at the site of injection or to optimally stimulate macrophages *(3)*. Excessive amounts of aluminum compounds may suppress immunity by covering the antigen completely with mineral compounds *(58,59)* or through toxicity to macrophages *(60)*.

The usual dose of aluminum used for human vaccines is around 0.5 mg. The upper allowable limits of aluminum adjuvants for injection in humans is 1.25 mg as per WHO regulations *(47)* and 0.85 to 1.25 mg as per United States Food and Drug Administration guidelines *(33)*.

4. Mineral adjuvants cannot be frozen or easily lyophilized *(17,61)* as both of these processes cause the collapse of the gel resulting in gross aggregation and precipitation. Although tetanus toxoid with collapsed aluminum gel precipitates was found to be immunogenic *(62)*, such a vaccine is not clinically acceptable. Successful lyophilization of aluminum adjuvants was reported *(63)*, but lyophilized vaccines containing aluminum adjuvants are not commercially available. Use of a lyophilized DTP vaccine with acellular pertussis components adsorbed onto aluminum adjuvants and stabilized with Haemocoel® and sucrose has also been described *(64)*. Though Haemocoel has been used for lyophilization of International Standards and Reference Preparations of aluminum adsorbed vaccines, it has not been used in human vaccines. The progress in this field is slow as there does not seem to be a need for a lyophilized aluminum adsorbed vaccine in developed countries. With the improvement of cold chain, such a vaccine is also not a priority in developing countries.
5. The mechanism of action of mineral adjuvants is complex and not yet fully understood. It likely involves various mechanisms including formation of depot, increasing targeting of antigens to antigen presenting cells, and nonspecific activation of immune system. All of these mechanisms are discussed below.
   a. Depot Formation. Depot formation by mineral adjuvants, including aluminum compounds, is considered to be one of the important mechanisms of action. The depot concept has generated numerous discussions. Is it a short-term depot, to which macrophages are attracted *(65)*, or a long-term depot from which antigen is released over an extended protracted time? There are also questions regarding site of the depot. Is it formed at the site of injection or in the draining lymph nodes? These questions remain unanswered with evidence to support or contradict theories.

   Glenny et al. *(66)* proposed that aluminum adjuvants act by depot formation at the site of injection, allowing for a slow release of antigen and thus prolonging the time for the interaction between antigen and antigen-presenting cells and lymphocytes. The local depot mechanism was challenged when Holt *(8)* described that antibody formation continued even after removal of adjuvant-antigen depot from the site of injection. In a recent study, approx 90% of radio-labeled aluminum phosphate adsorbed tetanus toxoid disappeared from the site of injection within 24 h of sc injection, whereas tetanus toxoid encapsulated within biodegradable polymer microspheres stayed at the site of injection for prolonged periods ***(6,67)***. However, the amount of aluminum phosphate adsorbed tetanus toxoid at the site of injection was higher than the soluble tetanus toxoid for 4 wk, thus demonstrating some localized depot formation. White et al. ***(68)*** showed that antibody-producing cells in the regional, popliteal, lymph nodes of rabbits injected with 150 Lf of soluble diphtheria toxoid completely disappeared in 3 wk, whereas rabbits injected with 10 Lf of aluminum phosphate precipitated toxoid had antibody producing cells in the nodes at 3–4 wk, suggesting a depot in the draining lymph nodes.

The most direct evidence for a local depot effect comes from experiments in which local granulomas, formed after injection of aluminum adsorbed vaccines, were able to induce immune responses when excised from the site of injection 7 wk later, macerated and injected into other animals ***(69)***. Remarkably, the antigen in the granuloma was apparently not available to the animals for a secondary response, because minute doses of antigen injected adjacent to the granuloma produced a secondary antibody response ***(70)***. White ***(70)*** postulated that antigen at this time is unable to penetrate the fibrous tissue surrounding the granuloma and antibody may react with antigen to form an antigen-antibody precipitate within the fibers of the peripheral zone of the granuloma, thus preventing the diffusion of antigen from granuloma and sequestering it from antigen presenting cells.

b. Targeting to Antigen Presenting Cells. Adjuvanticity of mineral adjuvants may be because of their ability to convert soluble antigens to particulate forms, which are more readily phagocytosed. The particle size of commercially available aluminum adjuvant gels is less than 10 µm, the average size for aluminum hydroxide, Alhydrogel was 3.07 µm and for aluminum phosphate, Adju-phos was 4.26 µm ***(3)***. It has been shown that polylactide glycolide (PLGA) microspheres less than 10 µm are taken up by antigen-presenting cells and provide strong adjuvant effects ***(71)***. Antigen adsorbed onto aluminum hydroxide is more readily taken up by human monocytes than free antigen, and the human monocytes exposed to aluminum hydroxide secrete IL-1 ***(72)***. Adjuvanticity of aluminum gel particles via targeting to antigen presenting cells, emphasizes the importance of degree of adsorption of antigens onto gels.

c. Activation of Immune System. An increased antibody response to a soluble antigen has been observed when aluminum adjuvant was injected at a different site, suggesting a systemic stimulatory effect on immunocompetent cells, possibly by release of inflammatory cytokines ***(73)***. However, these results have not be confirmed. Comparison of the immune responses of mice to diphtheria toxoid and aluminum hydroxide injected at different sites vs soluble diphtheria toxoid alone ***(3)*** demonstrated that both elicited very low and similar antibody levels, even after 2 doses. However, aluminum compounds can induce eosinophilia *(74)* and activate complement *(75)*, which may lead to a local inflammatory response, thus enhancing the antibody response.

Mineral adjuvants augment mainly humoral immune response, particularly IgG1 and IgE antibody responses, through IL-4 *(76)* by activating Th2 type cells *(65,77)*. These adjuvants are not efficient in raising cell-mediated immune responses *(17,65,78)*. The induction of delayed type hypersensitivity by aluminum adjuvants in mice and guinea pigs has not been clearly demonstrated *(15,79)*. Cooper *(77)* described aluminum adjuvants as good stimulants for Th2 type cell-mediated immune response, especially eosinophils. This type of response is similar to that elicited by some helminth parasites *(4)* and this property makes aluminum adjuvants a good candidate for antiparasite vaccines. In a special mouse hybrid model of schistosomiasis, Horowitz et al. *(80)* demonstrated protection in animals injected with sonicated parasite antigen and aluminum hydroxide. In contrast, antigen injected with Freund's Complete Adjuvant (FCA) elicited lower IgE antibodies and lower levels of protection.

6. Aluminum hydroxide has been found to be a more potent adjuvant than aluminum phosphate *(81,82)*. This may be caused by its overall higher adsorption capacity and better adsorption properties of certain antigens at neutral pH *(6)*, *see* **Note 1**. Aluminum hydroxide adjuvanted antigens induced antibody responses that are comparable to FCA *(83,84)*. Diphtheria toxoid adsorbed onto aluminum phosphate under optimal conditions induced antibody levels in rabbits similar to those elicited by the toxoid given with FCA *(85)*. Aluminum hydroxide is a good adjuvant for weak immunogens in mice, but saponin and FCA are more potent adjuvants for strong immunogens *(15,82)*.

Acknowledgment

The authors thank Professor Edgar Relyveld for his comments and suggestions.

References

1. Gupta, R. K., Relyveld, E. H., Lindblad, E. B., Bizzini, B., Ben-Efraim, S., and Gupta, C. K. (1993) Adjuvants—a balance between toxicity and adjuvanticity. *Vaccine* **11,** 293–306.
2. Gupta, R. K. and Siber, G. R. (1995) Adjuvants for human vaccines—current status, problems and future prospects. *Vaccine* **13,** 1263–1276.
3. Gupta, R. K., Rost, B. E., Relyveld, E., and Siber, G. R. (1995) Adjuvant properties of aluminum and calcium compounds, in *Vaccine Design: The Subunit and Adjuvant Approach* (Powell, M. F. and Newman, M. J.. eds.), Plenum, New York, pp. 229–248.
4. Lindblad, E. B. (1995) Aluminium adjuvants, in *The Theory and Practical Application of Adjuvants* (Stewart-Tull, D. E. S., ed.), Wiley, Chichester, pp. 21–35.
5. Relyveld, E. H. (1996) A history of toxoids, in *Vaccinia, Vaccination and Vaccinology. Jenner, Pasteur and their successors* (Plotkin, S. and Fantini, B., eds.), Elsevier, Amsterdam, pp. 95–105.

6. Gupta, R. K. (1998) Aluminum compounds as vaccine adjuvants. *Adv. Drug Delivery Rev.* **32,** 155–172.
7. Hem, S. L. and White, J. L. (1995) Structure and properties of aluminum-containing adjuvants, in *Vaccine Design: The Subunit and Adjuvant Approach* (Powell, M. F. and Newman, M. J., eds.), Plenum, New York, pp. 249–276.
8. Holt, L. B. (1950) *Developments in Diphtheria Prophylaxis.* William Heinemann Medical Books, London, pp. 1–181.
9. Aprile, M. A. and Wardlaw, A. C. (1966) Aluminum compounds as adjuvants for vaccine and toxoids in man: a review. *Can. J. Pub. Health* **57,** 343–354.
10. Relyveld, E. H. (1986) Preparation and use of calcium phosphate adsorbed vaccines. *Dev. Biol. Stand.* **65,** 131–136.
11. Nicklas, W. (1992) Aluminum salts. *Res. Immunol.* **143,** 489–494.
12. van Ramshorst, J. D. (1949) The adsorption of diphtheria toxoid on aluminum phosphate. *Recueil Travaux Chimiques des Pays-Bas* **68,** 169–180.
13 Relyveld, E. H., Bizzini, B., and Gupta, R. K. (1998) Rational approaches to reduce adverse reactions in man to vaccines containing tetanus and diphtheria toxoids. *Vaccine* **16,** 1016–1023.
14. Edelman, R. (1980) Vaccine adjuvants. *Rev. Infect. Dis.* **2,** 370–383.
15. Bomford, R. (1989) Aluminium salts: perspectives in their use as adjuvants, in *Immunological Adjuvants and Vaccines* (Gregoriadis, G., Allison, A. C., and Poste, G., eds.), Plenum, London, pp. 35–41.
16. Lindblad, E. B. and Sparck, J. V. (1987) Basic concepts in the application of immunological adjuvants. *Scand. J. Lab. Anim. Sci.* **14,** 1–13.
17. Alving, C. R., Detrick, B., Richards, R. L., Lewis, M. G., Shafferman, A., and Eddy, G. A. (1993) Novel adjuvant strategies for experimental malaria and AIDS vaccines, in *Specific Immunotherapy of Cancer with Vaccines* (Bystryn, J., Ferrone, S., and Livingston, P., eds.), *Ann. NY Acad. Sci.* **690,** 265–275.
18. Stewart-Tull, D. E. S. (1989) Recommendations for the assessment of adjuvants (immunopotentiators), in *Immunological Adjuvants and Vaccines* (Greogoriadis, G., Allison, A. C., and Poste, G., eds.), Plenum, New York, pp. 213–226.
19. Al-Shakhshir, R. H., Regnier, F. E., White, J. L., and Hem, S. L. (1995) Contribution of electrostatic and hydrophobic interactions to the adsorption of proteins by aluminium-containing adjuvants. *Vaccine* **13,** 41–44.
20. Seal, S. C. and Johnson, S. J. (1941) Studies on the purification of alum-precipitated diphtheria toxoid. *J. Infect. Dis.* **69,** 102–107.
21. World Health Organization (1976) Immunological adjuvants, in *Tech. Rep. Series* no. 595, WHO, Geneva, pp. 3–40.
22. Levine, L., Stone, J. L., and Wyman, L. (1955) Factors affecting the efficiency of the aluminum adjuvant in diphtheria and tetanus toxoids. *J. Immunol.* **75,** 301–307.
23. Gupta, R. K. and Siber, G. R. (1994) Comparison of adjuvant activities of aluminum phosphate, calcium phosphate and stearyl tyrosine for tetanus toxoid. *Biologicals* **22,** 53–63.
24. World Health Organization (1977) Manual for the Production and Control of Vaccines—*Tetanus Toxoid*, BLG/UNDP/77.2 Rev.1.

25. Al-Shakhshir, R., Regnier, F., White, J. L., and Hem, S. L. (1994) Effect of protein adsorption on the surface charge characteristics of aluminium-containing adjuvants. *Vaccine* **12,** 472–474.
26. Hem, S. L. and White, J. L. (1984) Characterization of aluminum hydroxide for use as an adjuvant in parenteral vaccines. *J. Paremteral Sci. Tech.* **38,** 2–10.
27. Masood, H., White, J. L., and Hem, S. L. (1994) Relationship between protein adsorptive capacity and the X-ray diffraction pattern of aluminum hydroxide adjuvants. *Vaccine* **12,** 187–189.
28. Shirodkar, S., Hutchinson, R. L., Perry, D. L., White, J. L., and Hem, S. L. (1990) Aluminum compounds used as adjuvants in vaccines. *Pharmaceut. Res.* **2,** 1282–1288.
29. Seeber, S. J., White, J. L., and Hem, S. L. (1991) Predicting the adsorption of proteins by aluminum-containing adjuvants. *Vaccine* **9,** 201–203.
30. Rinella, J. V., Jr., White, J. L., and Hem, S. L. (1995) Effect of anions on model aluminum-adjuvant-containing vaccines. *J. Colloid Interface Sci.* **172,** 121–130.
31. Corbel, M. J., Griffiths, E., and Winsnes, R. (1997) Workshop on standardization of aluminum adsorbed vaccines—Meeting Report, 21 June 1996, Bergen, Norway. *Biologicals* **25,** 351–353.
32. United States Minimum Requirements (1956) Tetanus and diphtheria toxoids combined precipitated, adsorbed (for adult use), Amendment No. 1, U.S. Dept. Health, Education and Welfare, National Institutes of Health, Bethesda, MD.
33. May, J. C., Progar, J. J., and Chin, R. (1984) The aluminum content of biological products containing aluminum adjuvants: determination by atomic absorption spectrometry. *J. Biol. Stand.* **12,** 175–183.
34. Gupta, R. K., Griffin, P., Jr., Rivera, R., and Siber, G. R. (1998) Development of an animal model to assess the immunogenicity of single-dose tetanus and diphtheria vaccines based on controlled release from biodegradable polymer microspheres. *Dev. Biol. Stand.* **92,** 277–287.
35. Hennessen, W. (1965) The mode of action of mineral adjuvants. *Progr. Immunobiol. Stand.* **2,** 71–79.
36. Hennessen, W. (1967) Mode of action and consequences for standardization of adjuvanted vaccines. *Symp. Series Immunobiol. Stand.* **6,** 319–326.
37. Relyveld, E. H. (1985) Immunological, prophylactic and standardization aspects in tetanus, in *Proceedings of the Seventh International Conference on Tetanus* (Nistico, G., Maestroni, P., and Pitzurra, M., eds.), Gangemi, Rome, pp. 215–227.
38. Lyng, J. (1986) Potency assay of diphtheria and tetanus toxoids. Some theoretical and practical considerations. *Dev. Biol. Stand.* **64,** 47–50.
39. Discussion (1991) Laboratory testing of the diphtheria toxoid and tetanus toxoid components of tetanus toxoid vaccines, diphtheria and tetanus toxoid vaccines, and diphtheria and tetanus toxoids and pertussis vaccines, in *Proceedings of an Informal Consultation on the World Health Organization Requirements for Diphtheria, Tetanus, Pertussis and Combined Vaccines* (Manclark, C. R., ed.), Dept. Health and Human Services, U.S. Public Health Service, Bethesda, MD, DHHS Publication No. [FDA] 91-1174, pp 75–79.

40. Lyng, J., Heron, I., and Ljungqvist, L. (1990) Quantitative estimation of diphtheria and tetanus toxoids. 3. Comparative assays in mice and in guinea pigs of two tetanus toxoid preparations. *Biologicals* **18,** 3–9.
41. Lyng, J. and Heron, I. (1991) Quantitative estimation of diphtheria and tetanus toxoids. 5. Comparative assays in mice and in guinea pigs of two diphtheria toxoid preparations. *Biologicals* **19,** 327–334.
42. Huet, M., Relyveld, E., and Camps, S. (1990) Methode simple de controle de l'active des anatoxines tetaniques adsorbees. *Biologicals* **18,** 61–67.
43. Huet, M., Relyveld, E., and Camps, S. (1992) Simplified activity evaluation of several tetanus vaccines. *Biologicals* **20,** 35–43.
44. Gupta, R. K., Anderson, R., Cecchini, D., Rost, B., Griffin, P., Benscoter, K., et al. (1996) Development of a guinea-pig model for potency/ immunogenicity evaluation of diphtheria, tetanus, acellular pertussis (DTaP) and *Haemophilus influenzae* type b polysaccharide conjugate vaccines. *Dev. Biol. Stand.* **86,** 283–296.
45. Gupta, R. K. and Siber, G. R. (1995) Reappraisal of existing methods for potency testing of vaccines against tetanus and diphtheria. *Vaccine* **13,** 965–966.
46. Aggerbeck, H. and Heron, I. (1995) Adjuvanticity of aluminium hydroxide and calcium phosphate in diphtheria-tetanus vaccines-I. *Vaccine* **13,** 1360–1365.
47. World Health Organization (1990) Requirements for diphtheria, tetanus, pertussis and combined vaccines, in *Tech. Rep. Series* 800, WHO, Geneva, Switzerland, pp. 87–179.
48. Gupta, R. K., Alroy, J., Alonso, M. J., Langer, R., and Siber, G. R. (1997) Chronic local reactions, long term immunogenicity and immunologic priming of mice and guinea pigs to tetanus toxoid encapsulated in biodegradable polymer microspheres composed of poly lactide-co-glycolide polymers. *Vaccine* **15,** 1716–1723.
49. Gupta, R. K., Chang, A.-C., and Siber, G. R. (1998) Biodegradable polymer microspheres as vaccine adjuvants and delivery systems. *Dev. Biol. Stand.* **92,** 63–78.
50. Gupta, R. K. (1995) New advances in vaccine technologies and applications—Meeting Report, 13–15 February 1995, Bethesda, MD, USA. *Vaccine* **16,** 1623–1625.
51. Mark, A., Carlsson, R.-M., and Granstrom, M. (1999) Subcutaneous versus intramuscular injection for booster DT vaccination of adolescents. *Vaccine* **17,** 2067–2072.
52. Souza Santos, P., Vallejo-Freire, A., Furlanetto, R. S., and Andrade, M. C. (1957) Correlation between the adsorption of diphtheria toxoid and alizarin by aluminum hydroxide hydrate gels. *Mem. Inst. Butantan* **28,** 221–231.
53. Jensen, O. M. and Koch, C. (1988) On the effect of $Al(OH)_3$ as an immunological adjuvant. *Acta Pathol. Microbiol. Immunol. Scandinavica* **96,** 257–264.
54. Cooper, P. D., McComb, C., and Steele, E. J. (1991) The adjuvanticity of algammulin, a new vaccine adjuvant. *Vaccine* **9,** 408–415.
55. Prigge, R. (1942) Wirksamkeit und schutzkraft der diphtherie-impfstoffe. *Behringwerk Mitteilungen Nr.* **21,** 75–99.

56. Prigge, R. (1949) Die beziehung zwischen dem antigengehalt der diphtherie-impfstoffe und ihrer wirksamkeit. *Klin. Wschr.* **27,** 685–690.
57. Holt, L. B. (1955) Quantitative studies in diphtheria prophylaxis: an attempt to derive a mathematical characterization of the antigenicity of diphtheria prophylactic. *Biometric* **11,** 83–94.
58. Haas, R. and Thomssen, R. (1961) Uber den entwicklungsstand der in der immunbiologie gebrauch-lichen adjuvantien. *Ergebn. Mikrobiol.* **34,** 27–119.
59. Haas, R., Keller, W., and Kikuth, W. (1955) Grundsatzliches zur aktiven schutzimpfung gegen poliomyelitis. *Dtsch. Med. Wschr.* **80,** 273.
60. Munder, P. G., Ferber, E., Modolell, M., and Fischer, H. (1969) The influence of various adjuvants on the metabolism of phospholipids in macrophages. *Int. Arch. Allergy* **36,** 117–128.
61. Warren, H. S., Vogel, F. R., and Chedid, L. A. (1986) Current status of immunological adjuvants. *Ann. Rev. Immunol.* **4,** 369–388.
62. Menon, P. S., Sahai, G., Joshi, V. B., Murthy, R. G. S., Boprai, M. S., and Thomas, A. K. (1976) Field trial on frozen and thawed tetanus toxoid. *Indian J. Med. Res.* **64,** 25–32.
63. Rethy, L., Solyom, F., Bacskai, L., Geresi, M., Gerhardt, Z., Koves, B., et al. (1985) Design and control of new type vaccines. Efficacy testing of adsorbed and freeze-dried toxoid-virus-bacterium combined vaccines. *Ann. Immunol. Hungarica* **25,** 49–57.
64. Afari, E. A., Kamiya, Y., Nkrumah, F. K., Dunyo, S. K., Akpedonu, P., Kamiya, H., and Fukai, F. (1996) Randomized controlled trial of acellular diphtheria, pertussis and tetanus vaccines in southern Ghana. *Annals Trop. Paed.* **16,** 39–48.
65. Cox, J. C. and Coulter, A. R. (1997) Adjuvants—a classification and review of their modes of action. *Vaccine* **15,** 248–256.
66. Glenny, A. T., Buttle, G. A. H., and Stevens, M. F. (1931) Rate of disappearance of diphtheria toxoid injected into rabbits and guinea pigs:toxoid precipitated with alum. *J. Path. Bact.* **34,** 267–275.
67. Gupta, R. K., Chang, A.-C., Griffin, P., Rivera, R., and Siber, G. R. (1996) *In vivo* distribution of radioactivity in mice after injection of biodegradable polymer microspheres containing ^{14}C-labeled tetanus toxoid. *Vaccine* **14,** 1412–1416.
68. White, R. G., Coons, A. H., and Connolly, J. M. (1955) Studies on antibody production III. The alum granuloma. *J. Exp. Med.* **102,** 73–82.
69. Harrison, W. T. (1935) Some observations on the use of alum-precipitated diphtheria toxoid. *Am. J. Publ. Health* **25,** 298–300.
70. White, R. G. (1967) Concepts relating to the mode of action of adjuvants. *Symp. Series Immunobiol. Stand.* **6,** 3–12.
71. Eldridge, J. H., Staas, J. K., Meulbroek, J. A., Tice, T. R., and Gilley, R. M. (1991) Biodegradable and biocompatible poly (DL-lactide-co-glycolide) microspheres as an adjuvant for Staphylococcal enterotoxin B toxoid which enhances the level of toxin-neutralizing antibodies. *Infect. Immun.* **59,** 2978–2986.
72. Mannhalter, J. W., Neychev, H. O., Zlabinger, G. J., Ahmad, R., and Eibl, M. M. (1985) Modulation of the human immune response by the non-toxic and non-

pyrogenic adjuvant aluminium hydroxide: effect of antigen uptake and antigen presentation. *Clin. Exp. Immunol.* **61,** 143–151.
73. Flebbe, L. M. and Braley-Mullen, H. (1986) Immunopotentiating effects of the adjuvants SGP and Quil A. I. Antibody responses to T-dependent and T-independent antigens. *Cell. Immunol.* **99,** 119–127.
74. Walls, R. S. (1977) Eosinophil response to alum adjuvants: involvement of T cells in non-antigen-dependent mechanisms. *Proc. Soc. Exp. Biol. Med.* **156,** 431–435.
75. Ramanathan, V. D., Badenoch-Jones, P., and Turk, J. L. (1979) Complement activation by aluminium and zirconium compounds. *Immunology* **37,** 881–888.
76. Grun, J. L. and Maurer, P. H. (1989) Different T helper cell subsets elicited in mice utilizing two different adjuvant vehicles: the role of endogenous interleukin-1 in proliferative responses. *Cell Immunol.* **121,** 134–145.
77. Cooper, P. D. (1994) The selective induction of different immune responses by vaccine adjuvants, in *Strategies in Vaccine Design* (Ada, G. R., ed.), R. G. Lands, Austin, TX, pp. 125–158.
78. Alving, C. R., Glass, M., and Detrick, B. (1992) Summary: adjuvants/clinical trials working group. *AIDS Res. Human Retroviruses* **8,** 1427–1430.
79. Bomford, R. (1980) The comparative selectivity of adjuvants for humoral and cell-mediated immunity. II. Effect on delayed-type hypersensitivity in the mouse and guinea pig, and cell-mediated immunity to tumour antigens in the mouse of Freund's incomplete and complete adjuvants, alhydrogel, *Corynebacterium parvum, Bordetella pertussis*, muramyl dipeptide and saponin. *Clin. Exp. Immunol.* **39,** 435–443.
80. Horowitz, S., Smolarsky, M., and Arnon, R. (1982) Protection against *Schistosoma mansoni* achieved by immunization with sonicated parasite. *Eur. J. Immunol.* **12,** 327–332.
81. Berman, P. W., Gregory, T., Crase, D., and Laski, L. A. (1985) Protection from genital herpes simplex virus type 2 infection by vaccination with cloned type 1 glycoprotein D. *Science* **227,** 1490–1492.
82. Bomford, R. (1984) Relative adjuvant efficacy of $Al(OH)_3$ and saponin is related to the immunogenicity of the antigen. *Int. Arch. Allergy Appl. Immunol.* **75,** 280–281.
83. Bomford, R. (1980) The comparative selectivity of adjuvants for humoral and cell-mediated immunity. I. Effect on the antibody response to bovine serum albumin and sheep red blood cells of Freund's incomplete and complete adjuvants, alhydrogel, *Corynebacterium parvum, Bordetella pertussis*, muramyl dipeptide and saponin. *Clin. Exp. Immunol.* **39,** 426–434.
84. Woodard, L. F. (1989) Adjuvant activity of water-insoluble surfactants. *Lab. Anim. Sci.* **39,** 222–225.
85. Gupta, R. K., Varanelli, C. L., Griffin, P., Wallach, D. F. H., and Siber, G. R. (1996) Adjuvant properties of non-phospholipid liposomes (Novasomes®) in experimental animals for human vaccine antigens. *Vaccine* **14,** 219–225.

5

Poly(Lactide-Coglycolide) Microparticles As Vaccine Adjuvants

Derek T. O'Hagan and Manmohan Singh

1. Introduction

Over the last 20 years, the adjuvant effect achieved through the association of antigens with polymeric microparticles has been repeatedly demonstrated *(1,2)*. Encapsulation of antigens into microparticles, including submicron particles (nanoparticles), promotes their entry into lymph nodes and provides a high local concentration of antigen over an extended time-period. Microparticles also promote the interaction of encapsulated antigens with antigen presenting cells (APCs), e.g., macrophages.

The biodegradable and biocompatible polyesters, the poly(lactide-coglycolides) (PLG) are the primary candidates for the development of microparticles as vaccines, because they have been used in humans for many years as suture material and as controled-release delivery systems for peptide drugs *(3)*. However, the adjuvant effect achieved by the encapsulation of antigens into PLG microparticles has been demonstrated only relatively recently (**Fig. 1**) *(4–6)*. Particle size was shown to be an important parameter affecting immunogenicity, because smaller microparticles (<10 µm) were significantly more immunogenic than larger particles (>10 µm) *(6,7)*. The adjuvant effect of microparticles can also be enhanced by their coadministration with additional adjuvants *(5)*. Recent studies have shown that microparticles also exert an adjuvant effect for cell-mediated immunity, including the induction of cytotoxic T cell (CTL) responses following both systemic and mucosal administration *(8,9)*. The induction of CTL responses are important for the eradication of virally infected cells and for immune responses against alternative intracellular pathogens.

From: *Methods in Molecular Medicine, Vol. 42:*
Vaccine Adjuvants: Preparation Methods and Research Protocols
Edited by: D. T. O'Hagan © Humana Press, Inc., Totowa, NJ

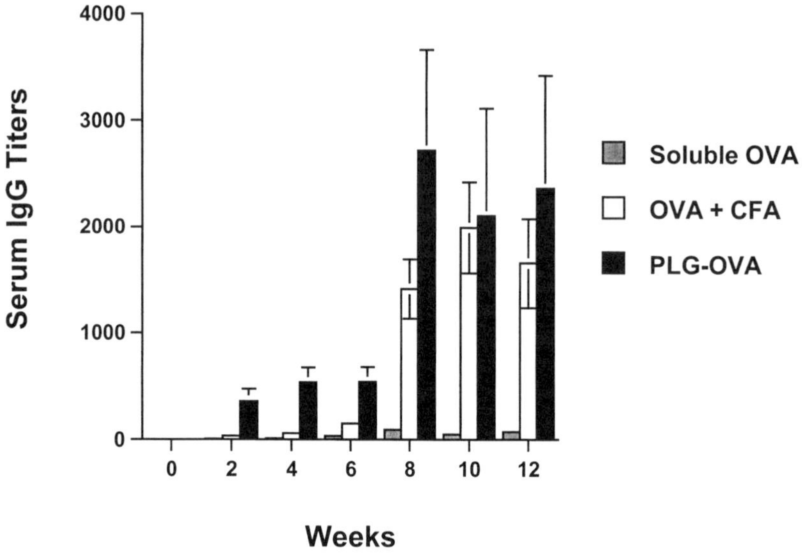

Fig. 1. Serum IgG titers in mice after sc immunization at week 0 and 6 with either soluble ovalbumin (OVA), OVA in CFA, or entrapped in PLG microparticles. Mean ± s.e. is represented at each time-point.

In the long term, one of the most attractive features of microparticles for vaccine development is their ability to control the rate of release of entrapped antigens *(2,**10**)*. Ultimately, this may allow the development of single-dose vaccines, through the preparation of microparticles that release entrapped antigens at the time-points when booster doses of vaccines would normally be administered. The development of a single-dose vaccine would represent a significant step towards the preparation of an ideal vaccine and would result in improved vaccine compliance, particularly in the developing world. In a recent study in rats, a single immunization with tetanus toxoid (TT) entrapped in controled-release microparticles induced comparable immunity to three doses of TT adsorbed to Alum *(**10,11**)*. In addition, a single dose of microparticles with an entrapped peptide *(**12**)* or protein *(**13**)* from HIV-1 induced neutralizing antibodies for at least one year. Nevertheless, further research is needed to promote the stability of antigens during microencapsulation and following in vivo administration.

Mucosal administration of vaccines is an attractive approach, which offers several significant advantages over the traditional approach to vaccine delivery, which normally involves intramuscular injection. The advantages of mucosal delivery include easier administration, reduced side effects, and the potential for frequent boosting without the need for trained personnel. More-

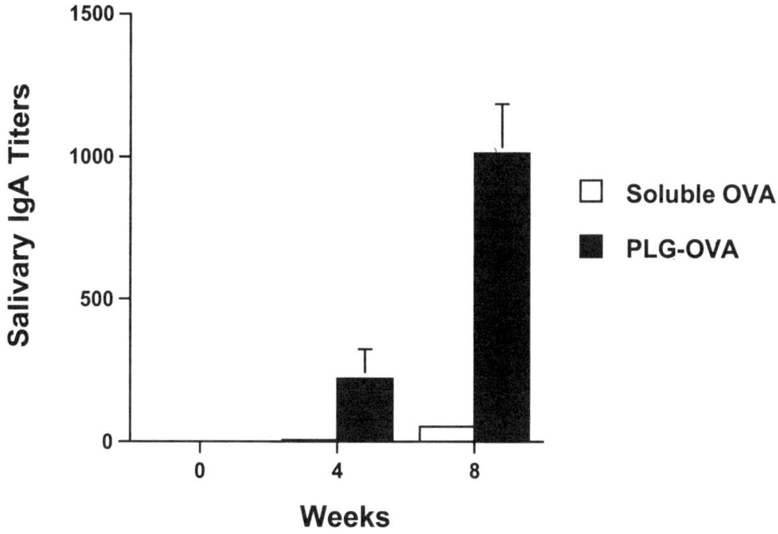

Fig. 2. Salivary IgA titers in mice after oral immunization with either soluble OVA or entrapped in PLG microparticles. Mean ± s.e. is represented at each time-point.

over, mucosal delivery of vaccines is the only effective means to induce immune responses in the mucosal secretions of the body. This is important, because the majority of pathogens initially infect hosts through the mucosal tissues of the gut, the respiratory, or the genital tracts. In addition, because the protective barrier of the skin is not breached during mucosal administration, the potential for the introduction of infection through the use of "dirty" needles is eliminated.

In mice, oral immunization with PLG microparticles induced potent secretory IgA (**Fig. 2**), serum IgG (**Fig. 3**), and systemic CTL (**Fig. 4**) responses *(8,14–16)*. Although, relatively large doses of antigens were used in these studies (at least 100 μg), a single oral dose of 10 μg of fimbriae from *B. pertussis* in microparticles protected mice from intranasal challenge *(17)*. In addition, intranasal immunization with 1–10 μg of *Bordetiella pertussis* antigens in microparticles also induced protective immunity in mice against aerosol challenge *(18,19)*. In primates, intratracheal or oral delivery of microencapsulated inactivated simian immunodeficiency virus (SIV) in parenterally primed animals induced protective immunity against intravaginal challenge with the virus; systemic immunization alone did not protect *(20)*. Also in a primate study, intratracheal immunization induced protection against aerosol challenge with staphylococcal enterotoxin B *(21)*. Recently, microparticles have also been shown to be effective for the oral delivery of plasmid DNA in mice *(22,23)*. However,

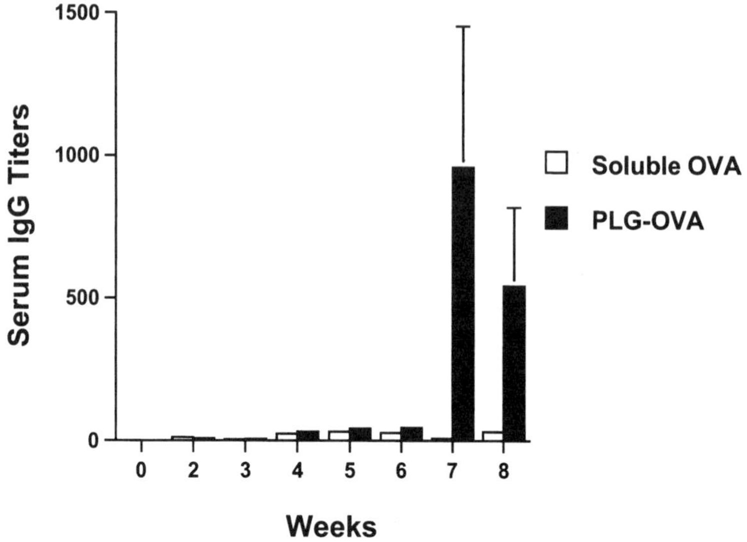

Fig. 3. Serum IgG titers in mice after oral immunization with either soluble OVA or entrapped in PLG microparticles. Mean ± s.e. is represented at each time-point.

a potential limitation to the oral delivery of vaccines in microparticles is the low level of uptake of particles following oral administration *(24)*.

2. Materials

1. Silverson Laboratory Homogenizer equipped with a 1/2- or 3/4-in probe (Silverson Machines Ltd., East Longmeadow, MA) or IKA homogenizer (IKA Works Inc., Wilmington, DE).
2. PLG polymers of various molecular weights with varying monomer ratios of lactic to glycolic acid from Boehringer Ingelheim (Ingelheim, Germany; United States distributors B.I. Chemicals Henley Division, Montvale, NJ). The method described hereunder was carried out with RG 505 (a 50:50-monomer ratio of lactic to glycolic acid) (*see* **Note 1**).
3. Polyvinyl alcohol (PVA), 85–90% hydrolyzed, 12,000–25,000 molecular weight.
4. Methylene chloride high-pressure liquid chromatography (HPLC) grade.
5. Protein estimation kit (Pierce BCA kit).
6. NaOH/SDS solution for hydrolysis: 0.2*N* NaOH with 1% SDS.

3. Methods

3.1. Microencapsulation of Antigens

The process is based on the formation of a primary emulsion (w/o) with the antigen in an aqueous medium and the polymer in a organic solvent and then dispersing this emulsion in an aqueous solution containing an emulsion stabi-

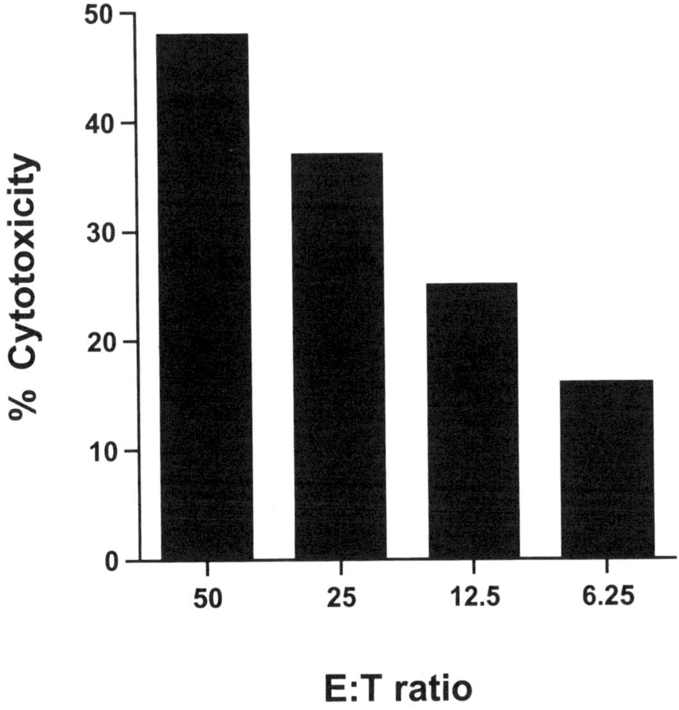

Fig. 4. % Cytotoxicity as a measure of CTL response in mice after oral immunization with PLG-OVA microparticles at various E:T ratios.

lizer (PVA) to form a multiple emulsion (w/o/w). The organic solvent from this multiple emulsion is evaporated at room temperature to form discrete polymer microparticles with entrapped antigen (*see* schematic diagram—**Fig. 5**) ***(10)***. For example, microparticles with an entrapped model protein Ovalbumin (OVA) with a 1% w/w loading level (*see* **Note 12**) are prepared as follows:

1. Weigh 500 mg of the PLG polymer (*see* **Note 1**) and dissolve it in 10 mL of methylene chloride (*see* **Note 2**) to form a 5% polymer solution (*see* **Note 3**) (Solution A).
2. 5 mg of OVA is dissolved in 2.5 mL of PBS buffer (Solution B).
3. 4 g of PVA (*see* **Note 4**) is dissolved in 40 mL distilled water (Solution C).
4. Solution A is added to solution B and homogenized at 10,000 rpm on a silverson or IKA homogenizer for 3 min (*see* **Note 5**). To this primary emulsion, Solution C is added and the resulting emulsion again homogenized at 10,000 rpm for 5 min (*see* **Note 6**).
5. The multiple emulsion is then stirred at 1500 rpm on a magnetic stirrer overnight to allow the methylene chloride to evaporate.

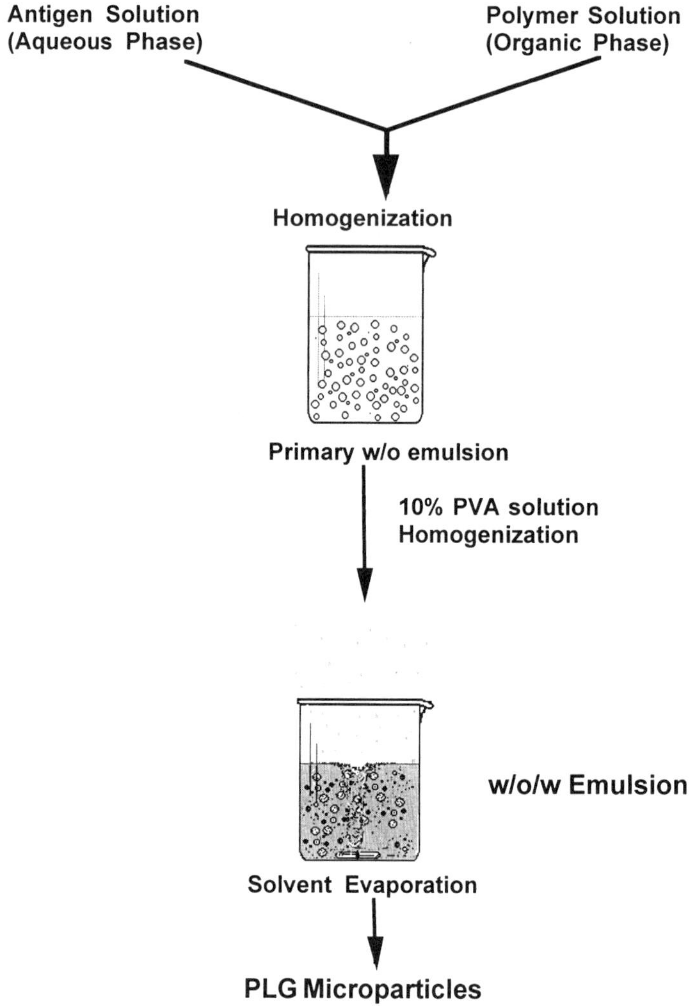

Fig. 5. Preparation of PLG microparticles using the solvent evaporation method of microencapsulation.

6. After overnight solvent evaporation (*see* **Note 7**), the emulsion is centrifuged at 15,000*g* for 45 min.
7. The supernatant is discarded and the pellet is resuspended in distilled water to wash the microparticles. The suspension is centrifuged at 15,000*g* for 45 min again (*see* **Note 8**).
8. After washing, the pellet is suspended in a small volume of distilled water (5 mL) and a small aliquot of this suspension is retained for size determination.

9. The microparticle suspension is frozen in acetone/dry-ice mixture and freeze dried in a lyophilizer overnight (*see* **Note 9**).
10. The dried microparticles are stored in a sealed glass vial in a dessicator for use.

3.2. Determination of Microparticle Size

Microparticles that are less than 10 µm in size are taken up by the APCs and are most suitable for maximum adjuvant effect. Therefore, it is very crucial to monitor the size distribution of all microparticle preparations to achieve a uniform size distribution.

1. The microparticle suspension sample previously retained is used to determine the microparticle size using a particle sizing instrument (Malvern Mastersizer, Malvern, or a Coulter Counter from Coulter Electronics, Hialeah, FL).
2. 50 µL of the microparticle suspension is added to 250 mL of distilled water in the sampling apparatus of a Malvern Mastersizer.
3. The concentration of the microparticles in the sampling port should be enough to give at least a 10% obscuration to laser source.
4. The instrument is calibrated with standards of defined dimensions before measurements.
5. A no-sample blank measurement calibrates the baseline.
6. The sample is added and the measurement made at least three times.
7. The mean diameter of all three measurements is recorded.

3.3. Determination of Antigen Loading Level in the Microparticles

The dose of antigen entrapped in microparticles is calculated based on actual entrapment of the antigen in the microparticles. The determination is most commonly carried out by BCA or Lowry method for protein estimation, but can be validated with amino acid analysis (AAA) or radiolabeling.

1. Weigh 3 10-mg samples of dry microparticles in 3 separate 5-mL glass vials.
2. Add 1 mL of 0.2*N* NaOH/1% sodium dodecyl sulfate (SDS) solution to each vial and place the vials on a constant shaker at room temperature.
3. Similar samples of blank microparticles (no antigen entrapped) are also hydrolyzed to serve as negative controls.
4. The microparticles are allowed to hydrolyze overnight.
5. Using a Pierce BCA kit, a series of dilutions are made with a bovine serum albumin (BSA) standard or the purified native antigen control.
6. 100 µL of the hydrolyzed samples are taken in glass tubes for protein estimation.
7. The BCA reagents are added to all tubes and incubated at 60°C for 20 min.
8. The protein concentration from the microparticle samples are calculated using the BSA standard curve.

3.4. Determination of Surface Properties of Microparticles Using Scanning Electron Microscopy (SEM)

A highly porous or irregular surface of the microparticles can lead to a high burst release or dumping of the antigen. Therefore, it is important to evaluate the surface properties of the microparticles under a scanning electron microscope (*see* **Note 10**).

1. 10 mg of dried microparticles are suspended in 500 μL of distilled water to yield a viscous suspension.
2. 100 μL of this suspension is added on surface of metal stubs used for SEM.
3. The stubs are air-dried and then sputter coated with gold-palladium to a 100 A thickness.
4. The stubs are now mounted on the microscope for scanning.
5. Four or five microparticle fields are identified and scanned on each stub.
6. The SEM photographs are collected at different magnification levels with a size bar imprinted on the micrographs.

3.5. In Vitro Release of Antigens from the Microparticles

To evaluate batch to batch reproducibility among various microparticle formulations, the in vitro release kinetics of the antigen is a good test to use.

1. Several vials containing 10 mg of microparticles and 2 mL of PBS (pH 7.4) are incubated at 37°C on a constant shaking mixer. One vial is withdrawn at each time-point of the in vitro estimation, for instance, day 1, 3, 7, 14, 21, and 28.
2. The microparticle suspension is centrifuged at 5000*g* for 10 min and the supernatant collected.
3. The supernatant is used for protein estimation at various time-points in the release kinetics.
4. Percent cumulative release of the antigen vs time is plotted for each batch of microparticles.

3.6. Estimation of Antigen Integrity

Antigen integrity can be estimated by several methods that evaluate the denaturation, aggregation, and loss of functional activity of the native antigen. Some of the commonly used methods are described below.

3.6.1. Sodium Dodecyl Sulfate-Polyacrylamide Gel Electrophoresis (SDS-PAGE) Analysis of Entrapped Antigens

For gross measurement of aggregation and denaturation estimation of molecular weight of the entrapped antigen by SDS-PAGE analysis is a commonly used method.

1. 10 mg of microparticles are weighed out in a 3-mL glass vial and to this 1 mL of 0.2*N* NaOH/1% SDS solution is added.
2. The microparticles are allowed to hydrolyze overnight at 37°C until a clear solution is obtained.
3. The protein concentration of the antigen solution is carried out using a BCA assay.
4. This antigen solution is then run on a SDS-PAGE gel with known molecular-weight markers using standard protocols and stained for band intensity.
5. The gel is analyzed visibly to look for gross denaturation, changes in molecular weight, and aggregation of antigen.

3.6.2. HPLC and GPC Analysis of Entrapped Antigen

Alternative methods that also address antigen integrity are HPLC or GPC analysis of the entrapped antigen ***(25)***.

1. 10 mg of microparticles are weighed out in a 3-mL glass vial and to this 1 mL PBS is added.
2. The microparticles are allowed to release the "burst" percentage of the antigen load entrapped in them overnight at 37°C .
3. The protein concentration of the antigen solution is carried out using a BCA assay.
4. This antigen solution is then run on a HPLC or GPC system using a set protocol for the given antigen with standard samples.
5. Changes in released antigen, with respect to the starting material, can be quantified using peak height and elution times.
6. Conformational changes, aggregation, and loss of activity can be estimated by this analysis for selected antigens.
7. If the antigen is not sensitive to changes at alkaline pH, the microparticles can be hydrloyzed with 0.2*M* NaOH/5% SDS solution and then the entrapped antigen can be analyzed by GPC or HPLC.

3.6.3. Estimation of Antigen Activity in the Microparticles

Most antigens have a specific enzyme-linked immunosorbent assay (ELISA) or a radioimmunoassay (RIA), which confirms the inherent functional activity of the antigen. These immunoassays can be utilized to check the activity of the released antigen both initially and at later time-point in the in vitro release ***(25)***.

1. Several vials containing 10 mg of microparticles and 2 mL of PBS (pH 7.4) are incubated at 37°C on a constant shaking mixer. One vial is withdrawn at each time-point, for instance, day 1, 3, 7, 14, 21, and 28.
2. The supernatant that contains the antigen is tested on the functional ELISA or RIA to estimate percent activity remaining at each time-point.

3.7. Additional Tests

Additional tests that can be carried out to ensure reproducibility, quality control, and lot-to-lot variation are listed below. These tests need not be performed on routine formulations for in vivo evaluation, but must be considered when preparing for important preclinical experiment, toxicology, and human evaluation *(12)*.

1. Sterility.
2. Endotoxin levels.
3. Bioburden.
4. Moisture content.
5. Residual solvent content (*see* **Note 11**).
6. Microparticle porosity.
7. Residual stabilizer.

4. Notes

1. The choice of the polymer type is dependent on the actual needs of the antigen delivery system. The erosion of the polymer is dependent on two main parameters—molecular weight and monomer ratios; the higher the molecular weight of the polymer, the longer the time it will need to erode in vivo. Also, the monomer ratios of lactic acid and glycolic acid in the polymer backbone effect the erosion. Higher lactic acid content slows erosion rates in comparison to higher glycolic acid content. If the antigen needs to be released quickly, then low molecular-weight polymers such as RG 502H, 502, 503 are used. If the antigen delivery system is meant for long-term delivery than high molecular-weight polymers such as RG 506, 508 are preferred. Also the size of the microparticle required (small – <10 μms or large >10 μms) dictates the polymer type. Higher molecular weights lead to more uniform large microparticles.
2. PLG polymers are soluble in only a limited range of organic solvents and are insoluble in water. The most commonly used solvent for PLG is dichloromethane (DCM), although ethyl acetate and others have also been used. The choice of the solvent is also affected by the respective antigen stability in different solvents (ethyl acetate or acetone can replace methylene chloride), rate of solvent removal (methylene chloride evaporates more rapidly than ethyl acetate), and polymer solubility (polymer solubility is limiting in ethyl acetate and acetone).
3. To prepare antigen entrapped microparticles, certain amount of polymer needs to be present to ensure complete entrapment or particle formation with the antigen. The polymer concentration is selected based on the size of microparticle required. A 4–6% polymer solution is ideal for making small microparticles (<10 μms) whereas a 12–20% polymer solution is required to make >10-μm sized micropartcles.
4. The choice and percentage of the stabilizer is dependent the microparticle size and duration of release required. A 10% PVA concentration provides more

homogeneously dispersed size range than a 1% PVA concentration. Other stabilizers are polyvinylpyrrolidone (PVP) and sodium oleate.

5. Although the antigen in an aqueous solution has been widely used for encapsulation of proteins into PLG microparticles, freeze-dried antigen could also be directly dispersed into the organic phase and emulsified with the aqueous PVA phase to yield a s/o/w system (solid-in-oil-in-water). This modification can be utilized for higher loading levels of antigens. Exposure to solvent can be minimized by the dispersion of antigen into the solvent as a dried solid, although dissolving the antigen in an aqueous phase and the preparation of an emulsion normally limits the direct exposure of the antigen to the organic solvent. This also creates an organic/aqueous interface, which may promote the denaturation of some antigens.
6. In addition to solvent exposure, antigen instability problems may also arise during microparticle preparation as a consequence of the high shear forces used during preparation. The extent of shear applied during microparticle preparation is generally greater as the desired microparticle size decreases. The homogenization speed can be manipulated to suit the individual needs of the formulator. Nevertheless, despite the potential problems, it should be noted that a range of proteins have been successfully entrapped in PLG microparticles prepared by solvent evaporation, without evidence of significant changes in their native structure.
7. The removal of the solvent from the emulsion can either be carried out by evaporation at room temperature, under vacuum, or by extraction in water. Although all methods might lead to uniform microparticles, our laboratory has determined the solvent evaporation method to be more reproducible with several antigens.
8. The number of washings to be carried out will also be determined by the solvent and stabilizer used. For methylene chloride and PVA, 2–3 washes will ensure complete removal of free and unbound PVA and residual solvent.
9. In case the antigen is sensitive to freezing, the collected microparticles may be either air or vacuum dried at room temperature.
10. The scanned surfaces of the microparticles may provide further information about porosity, cracks, and craters in the microparticles present because of insufficient or rapid solvent removal, slow stirring speed, and low polymer concentration.
11. Following microparticle preparation, the presence of residual solvents in the formulation might conceivably affect antigen stability. However, the level of DCM in microparticles prepared by solvent evaporation, was shown to be below the lowest limit of detection using gas chromatography, i.e., <10 ppm ***(12)***. Furthermore, Lupron Depot, a marketed product manufactured by solvent evaporation, contains <50 ppm DCM. Consequently, the level of residual DCM in microparticles is low enough to not represent an issue for protein stability, although it is an important regulatory concern.
12. The loading level of the microparticles are calculated by estimating the amount of protein (antigen) per given weight of the polymer microparticles. Thus, a 1.0% w/w loading level would represent 1 mg of antigen per 100 mg of microparticles.

References

1. O'Hagan, D. T. (1994) Microparticles as oral vaccines, in *Novel Delivery Systems for Oral Vaccines* (O'Hagan, D. T., ed.), CRC, Boca Raton, FL, pp. 175–205.
2. O'Hagan, D. T. (1997) Prospects for the development of new and improved vaccines through the use of microencapsulation technology, in *New Generation Vaccines 2nd Edition* (Levine, et al., eds.), Marcel Dekker, New York, pp. 215–228.
3. Okada, H. and Toguchi, H. (1995) Biodegradable microspheres in drug delivery. *Crit. Rev. Therapeut. Drug Carr. Sys.* **12,** 1–99.
4. O'Hagan, D. T., Rahman, D., McGee, J. P., Jeffery, H., Davies, M. C., Williams, P., et al. (1991a) Biodegradable microparticles as controlled release antigen delivery systems. *Immunology* **73,** 239–242.
5. O'Hagan, D. T., Jeffery, H., Roberts, M. J. J., McGee, J. P., and Davis, S. S. (1991b) Controlled release microparticles for vaccine development. *Vaccine* **9,** 768–771.
6. Eldridge, J. H., Staas, J. K., Meulbroek, J. A., Tice, T. R., and Gilley, R. M. (1991) Biodegradable and biocompatible poly (DL-lactide-co-glycolide) microspheres as an adjuvant for staphylococcal enterotoxin B toxoid which enhances the level of toxin-neutralizing antibodies. *Infec. Immun.* **59,** 2978–2986.
7. O'Hagan, D. T., Jeffery, H., and Davis, S. S. (1993) Long term antibody responses in mice following subcutaneous immunization with ovalbumin entrapped in biodegradable microparticles. *Vaccine* **11,** 965–969.
8. Maloy, K. J., Donachie, A. M., O'Hagan, D. T., and Mowat, A. McI. (1994) Induction of mucosal and systemic immune responses by immunization with ovalbumin entrapped in poly (lactide-co-glycolide) microparticles. *Immunology* **81,** 661–667.
9. Moore, A., McGuirk, P., Adamd, S., Jones, W. C., McGee, J. P., O'Hagan, D. T., and Mills, K. H. G. (1995) Immunization with a soluble recombinant HIV protein entrapped in biodegradable microparticles induces HIV-specific $CD8^+$ cytotoxic T lymphocytes and $CD4^+$ Th1 cells. *Vaccine* **13,** 1741–1749.
10. O'Hagan, D. T., Singh, M., and Gupta, R. K. (1997) Poly(lactide-co-glycolide) microparticles for the development of single-dose controlled-release vaccines. *Adv. Drug Deliv. Rev.* **32,** 225–246.
11. Singh, M., Li, X-M., Wang, H., McGee, J. P., Zamb, T., Koff, W., et al. (1997) Immunogenicity and protection in small animal models with controlled release tetanus toxoid microparticles as a single dose vaccine. *Infec. Immun.* **65,** 1716–1721.
12. O'Hagan, D. T., McGee, J. P., Boyle, R., Gumaer, D., Li, J., Potts, B., et al. (1995) The preparation, characterization and pre-clinical evaluation of an orally administered HIV-1 vaccine, consisting of a branched synthetic peptide immunogen entrapped in controlled release microparticles. *J. Cont. Rel.* **36,** 75–84.
13. Cleland, J. L., Powell, M. F., Lim, A., Barron, L., Berman, P. W., Eastman, D. J., et al. (1994) Development of a single-shot subunit vaccine for HIV-1. *AIDS Res. Hum. Retro.* **10,** S21–S26.

14. Eldridge, J. H., Hammond, C. J., Meulbroek, J. A., Staas, J. K., Gilley, R. M., and Tice, T. R. (1990) Controlled vaccine release in the gut associated lymphoid tissues. I. Orally administered biodegradable microspheres target the Peyer's patches. *J. Cont. Rel.* **11,** 205–214.
15. Challacombe, S. J., Rahman, D., Jeffery, H., Davis, S. S., and O'Hagan, D. T. (1992) Enhanced secretory IgA and systemic IgG after oral immunization with biodegradable microparticles. *Immunology* **76,** 164–168.
16. Challacombe, S. J., Rahman, D., and O'Hagan, D. T. (1997) Salivary, gut, vaginal and nasal antibody responses after oral immunization with biodegradable microparticles. *Vaccine* **15,** 169–175.
17. Jones, D. H., McBride, B. W., Thornton, C., O'Hagan, D. T., Robinson, A., and Farrar, G. H. (1996) Oral immunization with microencapsulated pertussis fimbriae induces protective immunity in mice. *Infect. Immun.* **64,** 489–494.
18. Cahill, E. S., O'Hagan, D. T., Ilum, L., Barnard, A., Mills, K. H. G., and Redhead, K. (1995) Immune responses and protection against bordetella pertussis infection after intranasal immunization of mice with filamentous haemagglutinin. *Vaccine* **13,** 455–462.
19. Shahin, R., Leef, M., Eldridge, J. H., Hudson, M., and Gilley, R. (1995) Adjuvanticity and protective immunity elicited by Bordetella pertussis antigens encapsulated in poly(D,L-lactide-co-glycolide) microspheres. *Infect. Immun.* **63,** 1195–1200.
20. Marx, P. A., Compans, R. W., Gettie, A., Staas, J. K., Gilley, R. M., Mulligan, M. J., et al. (1993) Protection against vaginal SIV transmission with microencapsulated vaccine. *Science* **260,** 1323–1327.
21. Tseng, J., Komisar, J. L., Trout, R. N., Hunt, R. E., Chen, J., Johnson, A. J., et al. (1995) Humoral immunity to aerosolized staphylococcal enterotoxin B (SEB), a super-antigen, in monkeys vaccinated with SEB toxoid-containing microspheres. *Infect. Immun.* **63,** 2880–2885.
22. Mathiowitz, E., Jacob, J. S., Jong, Y. S., Carino, G. P., Chickering, D. E., Chaturvedi, P., et al. (1997) Biologically erodible microspheres as potential oral drug delivery systems. *Nature* **386,** 410–414.
23. Jones, D. H., Corris, S., McDonald, J. C. S., and Farrar, G. H. (1997) Poly (DL-lactide-co-glycolide)-encapsulated plasmid DNA elicits systemic and mucosal antibody responses to encoded protein after oral administration. *Vaccine* **15,** 814–817.
24. O'Hagan, D. T. (1996) The intestinal uptake of particles and the implications for drug and antigen delivery. *J. Anat.* **189,** 477–482.
25. Barackman, J., Singh, M., Ugozolli, M., Ott, G., and O'Hagan, D. (1998) Oral immunization with poly(lactide-co-glycolide) microparticles containing an entrapped recombinant glycoprotein (gD2) from herpes simplex type 2 virus. *S.T.P. Pharma.* **8,** 41–46.

6

Poly(Methyl Methacrylate) Nanoparticles As Vaccine Adjuvants

Jörg Kreuter

1. Introduction

Nanoparticles are solid particles ranging in size from 1 to 1000 nm (1 μm). They consist of macromolecular materials and can be used therapeutically or prophylactically, for example, as adjuvants in vaccines or drug carriers, in which the active principle (drug or biologically active material) is dissolved, entrapped, or encapsulated, or to which the active principle is adsorbed or chemically attached *(1–3)*. One of the first areas of application of nanoparticles was their employment as adjuvants for vaccines. The most frequent method for the preparation of nanoparticles for this purpose was, and still is, emulsion polymerization. The polymers that can be employed for this process include poly(methyl methacrylate) *(4–6)*, polyacrylamide *(7)*, and poly(alkyl cyanoacrylates) *(8,9)*. Among these polymers, poly(methyl methacrylate) proved to be by far the most optimal and suitable material *(10,11)*. Nanoparticles made from polyacrylamide or poly(alkyl cyanoacrylate) possess the disadvantage that they either require large amounts of organic solvents and surfactants for their production, followed by laborious cleaning procedures as in the case of polyacrylamide *(7)*, or their adjuvant effects are very poor *(8,9)*, as with the poly(alkyl cyanoacrylates).

In contrast, poly(methyl methacrylate) (PMMA) nanoparticles exhibit very good adjuvant effects with a considerable number of antigens *(4,6,8,9,12–17)*, their production procedure is simple and easy *(18,19)*, the scale-up of this procedure is unproblematic *(20)*, and the material, PMMA, possesses a very good toxicological safety record, and is slowly biodegradable *(6,9–11,21)*. This good bioacceptability is demonstrated by the fact that this material is in use as an

From: *Methods in Molecular Medicine, Vol. 42:*
Vaccine Adjuvants: Preparation Methods and Research Protocols
Edited by: D. T. O'Hagan © Humana Press, Inc., Totowa, NJ

artificial bone and device material for implantation in humans for more than 50 years *(22,23)*.

It is today's workhorse in bone cements. As a consequence, particles of this material similar in size to nanoparticles are frequently present in patients' bodies as the result of such bone-replacement implants. The latter particles originate from mechanic abrasions of the implants and from interaction with the body's cells. The body burden of particulates from these implants is greater by far than after injection of nanoparticles in amounts required for vaccination (maximally 2.5 mg/vaccination).

Histological examination of the tissue at the injection site 1 yr after im injection of a PMMA nanoparticle-containing influenza vaccine in seven guinea pigs showed no abnormalities *(6)*. Histological reactions such as the appearance of giant cells and eosinophils were the same as with the fluid vaccine control. In a comparative experiment with 24 different adjuvants for an inactivated HIV-2 split whole-virus vaccine, PMMA nanoparticles were among the best-tolerated adjuvants *(9)*.

Experiments with ^{14}C-labeled nanoparticles demonstrated that after im or sc injection, more than 99% of the PMMA nanoparticle adjuvant stays at the injection site *(21,24)*. These experiments also showed that, with time, the PMMA particles were biodegraded and radioactive degradation products were excreted via the feces after a lag period of about 200 d; whereas the urine levels of radioactivity were not increased. After 287 d, 55–71% of the injected dose still remained at the injection site *(21)*. These findings are similar to findings with other biodegradable polymers: the biodegradation of these polymers is also characterized by a lag phase *(25)* during which the molecular weights of the polymers are constantly reduced by the degradation process. However, no significant transport of degradation products and excretion takes place during this time. After the lag period, when a certain considerable lower molecular weight is reached, transport of degradation products combined with their elimination from the body occurs *(25)*. Accordingly, elimination of ^{14}C-label was observable because of bilary excretion *(24,26)* after im and sc injection of ^{14}C-PMMA nanoparticles after the time period mentioned above, i.e., 200 d.

As already mentioned in **Subheading 1.**, emulsion polymerization represents the most important method for the production of nanoparticles for vaccine adjuvants. In the case of PMMA, a special form of emulsion polymerization, i.e., emulsifier free emulsion polymerization (heterogeneous polymerization), is employed. This expression seems to be a contradiction in itself. The reason for the choice of this expression is owing to the earlier assumption that the location of the polymerization was within the micelles formed by the emulsifier that was added to the polymer/water mixture used for emulsion polymerization *(27,28)*. Later it was found that the kinetics of the polymerization process, the particle number, and the particle growth were not different if no emulsifier was present ***(29–35)***. This led to the conclusion that the place of the particle formation and the initial polymerization is located in the aqueous phase.

During the initial phase of polymerization, the generated oligomers grow as more monomer molecules are absorbed and polymerized. At a certain molecular weight or particle size, the oligomers become insoluble, thus forming the small separate particles of the polymer latex.

The particle formation is independent of the rate of polymerization ***(34)***, but dependent on the polymer concentration in the aqueous phase ***(31)***. This indicates that the particle formation is thermodynamically controled. In the case of methyl methacrylate, for instance, particle formation observed by Tyndall light scattering occurs at a polymer concentration of 0.03 g/100 mL water ***(34)***.

The particles are stabilized either by hydrophilic groups present in the polymer or by emulsifier present in the medium. They continue to grow by absorbing more monomer, which is present in the surrounding aqueous phase, in the emulsifier micelles, and/or in the monomer droplets, and which diffuses to the growing nanoparticles. Termination of the polymerization occurs by reaction of the macroradicals with a small radical or with another macroradical either in the aqueous phase or in the precipitated phase, i.e., the polymer particles ***(35)***. Subsequently, if more and more radicals in the aqueous phase become absorbed or terminated, no more new particles are formed and the polymer particles become the main location of polymerization. By absorbing more monomer, the particles grow gradually until the monomer is completely converted to polymer.

In the case of the production of PMMA nanoparticles for the use as adjuvants for vaccines, no surfactants are employed because they would reduce the adjuvant effect ***(9)***.

2. Materials

1. Methyl methacrylate.
2. Sodium hydroxide, analytical grade.
3. Sodium chloride, analytical grade.
4. Potassium peroxodisulfate.
5. Double-neck round-bottom flask, 1 L.
6. Glass stirrer fitting to the above flask.
7. Spiral reflux condenser, 50 cm.
8. Water bath with thermostat.
9. Bath-type ultrasonicator.
10. Photon correlation spectrometer (BI-200 SM with detector BI-DS and digital correlator BI-2030 AT, Brookhaven Instruments Corp., Holtsville, NY).

3. Methods

3.1. Purification of the Monomer

1. The monomer, methyl methacrylate, is generally stabilized by polymerization inhibitors. Remove stabilizers by extraction of 100 mL of methyl methacrylate with 20 mL of a solution of 5 g NaOH and 20 g NaCl in 100 mL distilled water.
2. Repeat this procedure twice to remove all stabilizer.
3. Wash the methyl methacrylate three times with 20 mL distilled water.
4. Store the water-saturated methyl methacrylate at 2–8°C.

3.2. Polymerization

The polymerization can be performed by γ-irradiation or chemical initiation. Gamma-irradiation has the advantage that it can be performed at room or refrigerator (2–8°C) temperature. Initiation by high-energy radiation rests upon the same theories of emulsion polymerization respectively emulsifier-free polymerization *(36,37)*. Chemical initiation has the advantage that it does not require radioactive irradiation facilities. The disadvantage is that temperatures above 65°C have to be employed. For this reason, the polymerization cannot be carried out in the presence of heat-sensitive drugs or biological materials. The polymerization is initiated by the formation of radicals caused by the decay of the initiator at elevated temperatures. Because oxygen interacts with these radicals and inhibits or retards polymerization, it has to be reduced by gassing with nitrogen for 1 h.

3.2.1. Polymerization with Gamma Rays

1. Dissolve a certain amount (between 0.1 and 1.5%) of purified methyl methacrylate in water, saline 0.9%, buffer solution, or in an antigen solution or suspension.
2. This mixture is then irradiated with gamma rays. Oxygen present in the aqueous phase does not have to be removed. A dose rate of about 5–25 gy/min leads to optimal nanoparticle yields (> 98%) with slightly higher yields at lower dose rates *(38)*. Polymerization starts at about 0.3–0.4 kgy and reaches about 85% conversion at 1 kgy, 95% conversion at 2 kGy, and above 98% conversion at 5 kgy. A dose of 25 kgy leads to almost total conversion *(38)* (*see* **Note 1**).

3.2.2. Chemically Initiated Polymerization

1. Degas 1 L of twice-distilled water, saline 0.9%, or a buffer solution by bubbling of nitrogen for 1 h though this solution.
2. Add into a jacketed round- or flat-bottom flask equipped with a stirrer (magnetic stirring bar or tightly fitting glass stirrer) that is closed with the reflux condenser.
3. Nitrogen is then bubbled through the water for 15 min.
4. A certain amount of monomer (*see* **Table 1**) is added and dissolved in the water by stirring at about 80 to 500 rpm.

Table 1
Influence of Monomer Concentration, Initiator Concentration, and Temperature on Particle Size and Molecular Weights of Poly(Methyl Methacrylate) Nanoparticles

Potassium peroxodisulfate concentration (mmol)	Methyl methacrylate concentration (mmol) at two temperatures										
	10		33.75		80		156.25		80		156
	65°C	85°C	65°C	85°C	65°C	85°C	65°C	85°C	65°C	85°C	85°C
	Particle size (nm)								Molecular Weight (M_w)		
0.3	85	72	129	128	181	170	256	262	—	434,000	—
1.65	98	88	151	169	212	193	248	248	—	—	—
3.0	92	72	135	149	223	177	250	258	289,500	220,500	400,000

Source: Adapted from Berg, U., Immunstimulation durch hochdisperse Polymersuspensionen, Diss. ETH Zürich No. 6481, Zürich, Switzerland.

5. Raise the temperature gradually (about 2°C/min) to about 45°C.
6. Dissolve the polymerization initiator potassium peroxodisulfate (**Table 1**) in a small amount of water (this amount should not exceed 4% of the volume of the aqueous monomer solution) and add to the monomer solution (*see* **Notes 2** and **3**).
7. Increase temperature until the desired polymerization temperature (65°C–85°C, *see* **Table 1**) is reached.
8. Keep at this temperature for 2 h.
9. Heat the medium to 90°C in order to enpolymerize trace monomeric residuals *(18)*.

3.3. Particle Size Determination

1. Add 50 mg of lyophilized nanoparticles to 5 mL of dust-free water or to 5 mL of dustfree aqueous 1% surfactant solution and sonicate in an ice-containing bath-type sonicator for at least 1 h.
2. Dilute the above suspension or alternatively a nonlyophilized nanoparticle suspension with dust-free water or the above 1% surfactant solution by a factor of 1:100, and sonicate for another hour.
3. Measure immediately in the photon correlation spectrometer (PCS) (*see* **Note 5**).

3.4. Vaccine Preparation

PMMA nanoparticles can be used in two forms: the vaccine antigen can either be incorporated into the nanoparticles or it can be adsorbed to previously formed particles. In the first case, the polymerization is carried out in presence of the antigen. In this case, polymerization has to be performed by gamma-ray irradiation because this type of polymerization can be carried out at room or refrigerator temperatures. The conditions with antigens are the same as with empty nanoparticles (*see* **Subheading 3.2.1.**). The presence of the antigens did not change the polymerization kinetics ***(37)***, the physicochemical properties of the nanoparticles ***(4–6,12–15)***, or their biodegradation behavior ***(24)***. Doses of about 5 kgy are optimal for incorporation of antigens, doses of 1.5 kgy are sufficient for gamma-irradiation-sensitive antigens. Experiments with a number of inactivated antigens did not reveal any changes of antigenicity or in the level of the antibody response ***(38)***.

3.4.1. Adsorption of the Antigen

Adsorption of vaccine antigens can be performed with nanoparticles produced by gamma-irradiation (**Subheading 3.2.1.**) or by chemical polymerization (**Subheading 3.2.2.**). Suspensions are mixed with the antigen in the desired concentration and are kept for at least 14 h ***(18)***, preferentially under gentle agitation (stirring or shaking).

1. Rewet lyophilized nanoparticles by ultrasonication (45 min or better 3 × 15 min on 3 consecutive days, and store at 2–8°C).
2. If the antigen is not stable against ultrasonication (most antigens are not stable), the nanoparticles have to be rewetted separately using water, saline 0.9%, or a buffer solution and then mixed with the antigen.
3. Nonlyophilized empty nanoparticles or nanoparticles rewetted separately from antigen are mixed with the antigen in concentration that give the final vaccine and nanoparticle adjuvant concentrations.
4. Store this mixture at least for 14 h ***(18)*** before it is used as a vaccine. If possible, the mixture should be shaken or stirred gently during this minimal storage time (*see* **Notes 6–11**).

3.4.2. Incorporation of the Antigen

1. Use antigen instead of water, saline, or buffer and polymerize as descibed in **Subheading 3.2.1.**
2. This preparation can be used directly after preparation (*see* **Notes 6–11**).

3.5. Storage

1. The nanoparticle vaccines can be stored in the refrigerator or, if the antigen withstands lyophilization, in lyophilized form (*see* **Note 4**).

3.6. Conclusions

PMMA nanoparticles are polymeric particulate adjuvants for vaccines. These nanoparticles can easily be manufactured in a reproducible manner in the described particle sizes and with specific surface properties. Scale-up of the production process is also facile *(20)*. PMMA is a material with a good safety record that has been used in humans for more than 50 yr. PMMA nanoparticle adjuvants achieved good antibody responses and good protection against challenge with a number of antigens. Additionally, they also seem to lead to a higher stability of the vaccines containing this type of adjuvant.

4. Notes

1. The particle size of PMMA nanoparticles produced by gamma ray-initiated polymerization is about 120 to 150 nm *(18,39)*. The molecular weights of these particles are between 20,000 and 80,000, depending on the initial monomer concentration and the electrolyte concentration in the surrounding medium *(34,40)*.
2. High initiator concentrations (> 5 mmol) lead to precipitation and flocculation. Lower initiator concentrations lead to the formation of a stable latex *(18)*. In the latter system, the particles are stabilized by electric repulsion generated by the persulfate groups, which are covalently linked to the polymer molecules and are not removable by dialysis.
3. The monomer concentration strongly influences both the molecular weight and the particle size. The temperature effect is less important for the molecular weight and much less significant for the partice size (**Table 1**). The initiator concentration has an opposite effect: increasing initiator concentrations decreases the molecular weight very significantly, but increases the particle size slightly. For this reason, it has to be concluded that the mechanism of the growth of the polymer molecule itself and the mechanism of particle growth and stabilization are different. It can be further concluded that one particle consists of more than one polymer molecule: at a density of 1.06 g/mL and an approximate diameter of 150 nm *(39)*, the molecular weight should be about 10^{11} if one particle would consist of one molecule. However, the observed molecular weights (**Table 1**) demonstrate that one particle consists of about 2×10^5 to 10^7 polymer molecules. The particle formation is, as discussed above in **Subheading 1.**, thermodynamically controlled *(34)*: whereas an increase in initiator molecules leads to a decrease in molecular weight at a given monomer concentration, the particle size will increase because more stabilizing sulfate groups originating from the stabilizer can be formed on the polymer surface.
4. PMMA nanoparticles, as well as nanoparticles-containing vaccines, may be stored in lyophilized form at room temperature or in an aqueous suspension at 2–8°C. Their stability depends on the antigen present. Empty PMMA nanoparticles kept under sterile conditions are stable for at least 5 yr after storage in suspension in the refrigerator or for 25 yr in freeze-dried form at room temperature.
5. Physicochemical Properties: The average particle size of PMMA nanoparticles produced by γ-irradiation is about 130 ± 30 nm *(39)*, their molecular weights, M_{GPC}, M_w, and M_n are listed in **Table 2** *(40)*. The density of these particles is

Table 2
Molecular Weights of Poly(Methyl Methacrylate) Nanoparticles after γ-Ray-Initiated Polymerization

Polymerization medium	M_{GPC}	M_w	M_n
100 mmol/L MMA[a] in PBS; 4°C	20,280	42,400	5655
100 mmol/L MMA[a] in water; 4°C	18,370	37,500	5680
100 mmol/L MMA[a] in water; freeze-dried; 4°C	18,350	36,400	3920

[a]Monomeric methyl methacrylate
Adapted from **ref. *40***.

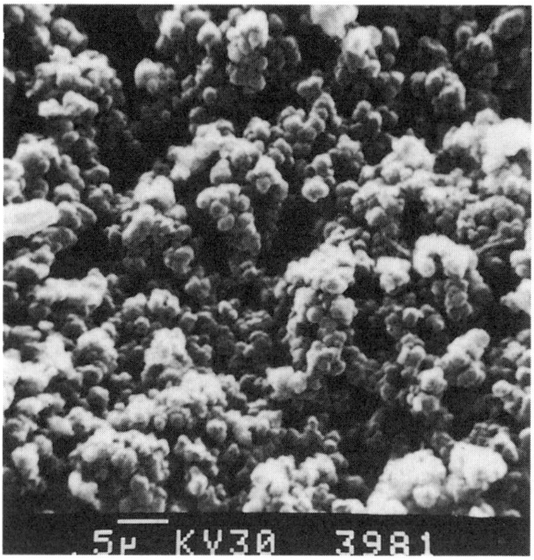

Fig. 1. Scanning electron micrograph of PMMA nanoparticles polymerized by γ-irradiation in water. Marker = 500 nm.

1.06 g/cm^3. Their specific surface depends on their size, in the case of the 130-nm nanoparticles produced by γ-irradiation it was 50 m^2/g, and the electrophoretic mobility in water was –2.75 ± 0.6 μm cm s^{-1} V^{-1} *(39)*. **Figures 1** and **2** show scanning electron microscopy pictures of PMMA nanoparticles produced by gamma-irradiation (5 kgy) in water (**Fig. 1**) or in phosphate-buffered saline pH 7.2 (PBS; **Fig 2**).

The particle sizes and molecular weights of PMMA nanoparticles produced by chemical initiation are listed in **Table 1**. Their density, specific surface area, and electrophoretic mobility depends on the exact polymerization conditions and on the initiator used *(18)*.

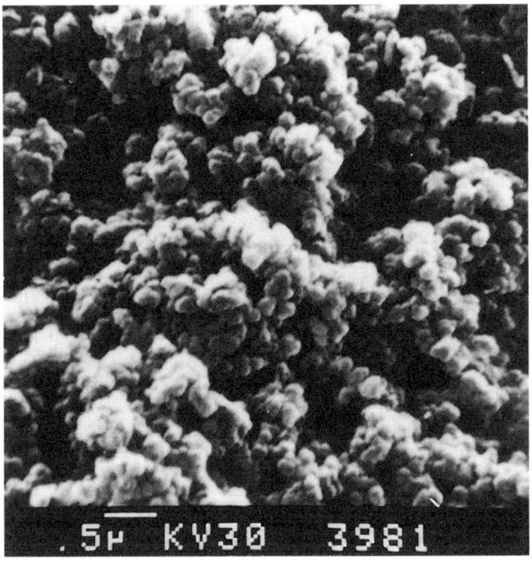

Fig. 2. Scanning electron micrograph of PMMA nanoparticles polymerized by γ-irradiation in PBS, pH 7.2 . Marker = 500 nm.

All PMMA nanoparticles are X-ray amorphous independent from their polymerization method.

6. Vaccination: PMMA nanoparticles can be used in vaccines for im, sc injection, and also perorally. They may be also used in combination vaccines or in combination with other adjuvants *(9)*. The optimal adjuvant concentration with most antigens was 0.5% *(4,8,17)*. Boosting is possible and unproblematic. No allergic or other advers reactions were observed.
7. The adjuvant effect increases with decreasing particle size *(12,15)* and increasing hydrophobicity *(8,9)* (*see* also **Fig. 3**). Consequently, addition of surfactants reduces the adjuvant effect of PMMA nanoparticles *(9)*.
8. The ability to achieve a reproducible small particle size with PMMA nanoparticles is a significant advantage over a number of other adjuvants. With emulsions, the size of the droplets may change from preparation to preparation *(3,12)*. Moreover, the particle size that is relevant for the immune response may be further altered during and after injection: the consistency of the tissue into which the vaccine is injected may yield a smaller droplet size because of friction between the vaccine liquid and the tissue. On the other hand, for instance fatty tissue may induce a coalescence of the droplets resulting in a larger particle size *(3)*.
9. The antibody response, as well as protection in most cases, is especially pronounced after longer time periods with incorporated, as well as with adsorbed

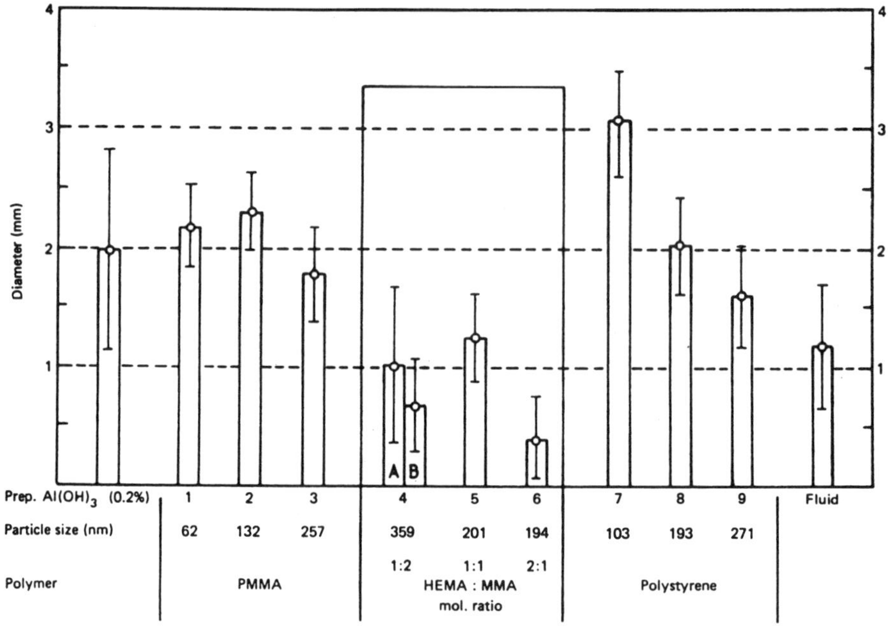

Fig. 3. The antibody titers of the mouse sera were determined by a radial immunodiffusion test (Mancini method) and quantitated by the diameter of the precipitation ring. The figure shows the precipitation ring diameters (antibody response; mean ± ~95% confidence intervals) after immunization of mice with different bovine serum albumin vaccines. The variables shown are size of the adjuvant particles, and copolymer composition: PMMA, poly(methyl methacrylate); HEMA/MMA, 2-hydroxyethyl methacrylate/methyl methacrylate copolymer. The standard deviations of the polymer particle sizes are: preparation 1, 9 nm; preparation 2, 12 nm; preparation 3, 12 nm; preparation 4, 4,83 nm; preparation 5, 12 nm; peparation 6, 17 nm; preparation 7, 35 nm; preparation 8, 2 nm; and preparation 9, 6 nm. Reproduced from Kreuter et al. (1988) *Vaccine* **6,** 255, by permission of the publishers, Butterworth Heinemann Ltd.

virus ***(14)*** (**Fig. 4**). In addition, these PMMA nanoparticle vaccines can increase vaccine stability against temperature inactivation ***(14)***.

10. With some antigens, such as HIV-1, a delayed antibody response may be observed ***(16,17)***. Significantly high antibody titers with HIV-1 were reached after 10 wk, whereas HIV-2 yielded high titers already after 4 wk. Although the HIV-1 antibody titers were about 5 to 10 times lower than with HIV-2, they still were about 10 times higher than those with aluminum hydroxide or with the fluid vaccine, even in comparison to HIV-2.
11. A combination of two or more different carriers or adjuvants may be necessary to induce the optimal immune response ***(9,10)***: In an experiment using a single

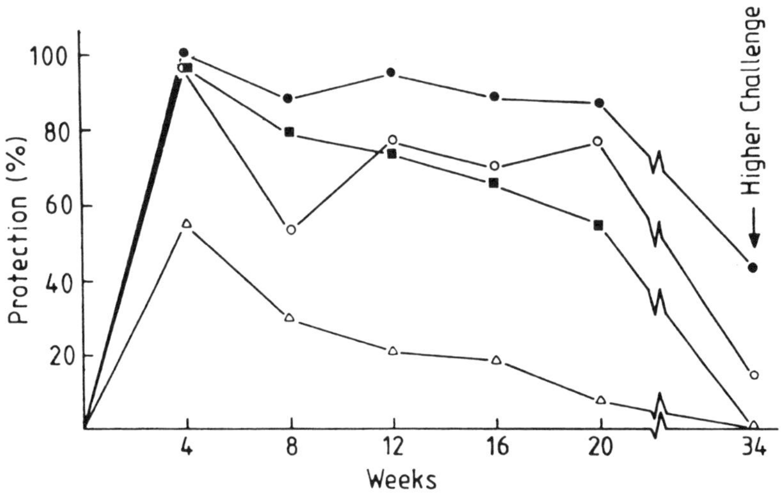

Fig. 4. Protection of mice against infection with a dose of 50 LD_{50} of infectious mice-adapted influenza virus after sc immunization with 20 IU of A_0PR 8 whole virus using the following adjuvants: ● incorporation into 0.5% PMMA; ○ adsorption onto 0.5% PMMA; ■ adsorption onto 0.2% aluminium hydroxide; Δ fluid vaccine without adjuvant. Higher challenge = 250 LD_{50}. Reproduced from Kreuter (1988) *J. Microencapsul.* **5,** 116, by permission of the publishers, Taylor and Francis.

injection of 5 μg antigen and a single time-point determination after 10 wk, PMMA nanoparticles were compared to 24 different adjuvants including different aluminum compounds, Freund's Complete (FCA) and Incomplete (FIA) Adjuvants, liposomes, surfactants, Iscoms, and muramyl peptides (**Fig. 5**). In this experiment, the nanoparticles yielded by far the highest ELISA antibody titers ***(9)***. This experiment also showed that using Western blots, a whole virus vaccine that contained a variety of single antigenic components, some adjuvants were more effective against one antigenic component, whereas other adjuvants were more effective against others. In this experiment, PMMA nanoparticles failed to induce significant antibodies against *gp120* as detected by the Western blot. Only aluminum hydroxide, aluminum phosphate, Aerosil® 200, Aerosil® R972, FCA and FIA adjuvants were able to induce significant antibody responses to *gp120*. This antigen is very hydrophilic and it appears that in an immunogen mixture, as was used in the split virus vaccine, the *gp120* was not able to interact with the very hydrophobic PMMA nanoparticles and, therefore, was unable to induce antibodies in significant amounts. This observation, therefore, demonstrates that the choice of an optimal adjuvant or carrier depends on the physicochemical and biochemical properties of the immunogen. A combination of two or more different carriers or adjuvants may be necessary to induce the optimal immune response ***(9,10)***.

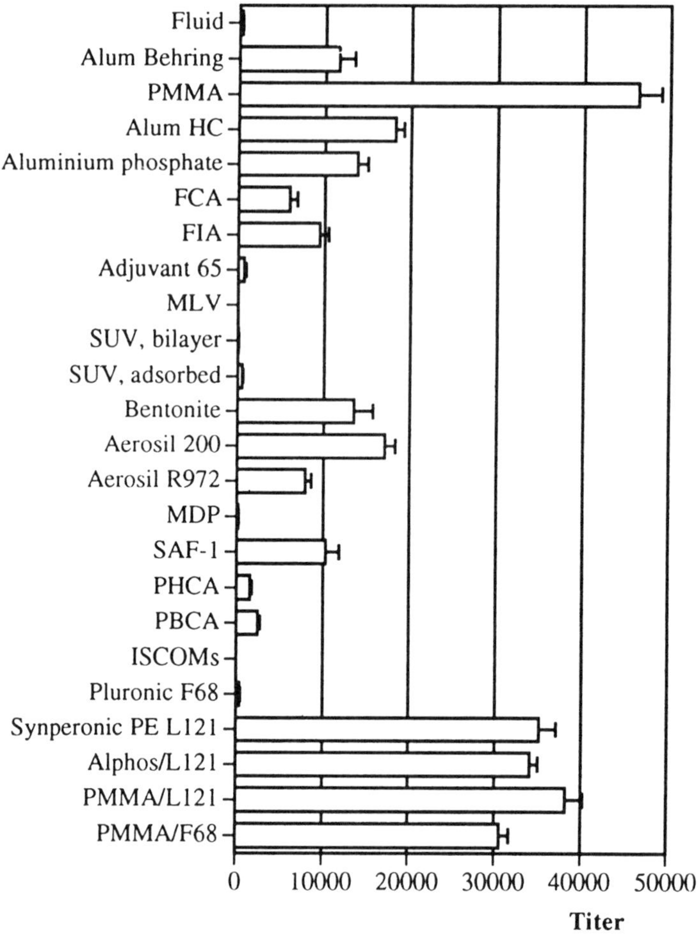

Fig. 5. Serum antibody titers against HIV-2 inactivated split whole virus in mice immunized with 5 μg viral proteins in combination with different adjuvants. Mice immunized with ISCOMs received 0.5 μg protein. PMMA, poly(methyl methacrylate) nanoparticles; Alum HC, aluminum hydroxycarbonate (produced by S.L. Hem, Purdue University); FCA, Freund's complete adjuvant; FIA, Freund's incomplete adjuvant; MLV, multilamellar large vesicles, incorporated antigen; SUV, bilayer, small unilamellar vesicles, protein integrated into the bilayer; SUV, adsorbed, small unilamellar vesicles, protein adsorbed onto the surface; MDP, N-acetyl-L-muramyl-L-alanyl-D-isoglutamine; SAF-l, Syntex Adjuvant Formulation-l; PHCA, poly(hexylcyanoacrylate) nanoparticles; PBCA, poly(butylcyanoacrylate) nanoparticles; ISCOMs, immunostimulating complexes; Alphos/L121, combination of aluminum phosphate and Synperonic® PE L121; PMMA/L121, combination of PMMA and Synperonic® PE L121; PMMA/F68, combination of PMMA and Pluronic® F68. Reproduced from Stieneker et al. (1995) *Vaccine* **13,** 49, by permission of the publishers, Butterworth Heinemann Ltd.

References

1. Kreuter, J. (1994) Nanoparticles, in *Encyclopedia of Pharmaceutical Technology, Vol. 10* (Swarbrick, J. and Boylan, J. C., eds.), Dekker, New York, pp. 165–190.
2. Kreuter, J. (1983) Evaluation of nanoparticles as drug delivery systems I: preparation methods. *Pharm. Acta Helv.* **58,** 196–209.
3. Kreuter, J. (1994) Nanoparticles, in *Colloidal Drug Delivery Systems* (Kreuter, J., ed.), Dekker, New York, pp. 219–342.
4. Kreuter, J. and Speiser, P. P. (1976) New adjuvants on a polymethylmethacrylate base. *Infect. Immunity* **13,** 204–210.
5. Kreuter, J. and Speiser, P. P. (1976) In vitro studies of poly(methyl methacrylate) adjuvants. *J. Pharm. Sci.* **65,** 1624–1627.
6. Kreuter, J., Mauler, R., Gruschkau, H., and Speiser, P. P. (1976) The use of new polymethylmethacrylate adjuvants for split influenza vaccines. *Exp. Cell Biol.* **44,** 12–19.
7. Birrenbach, G. and Speiser, P. P. (1976) Polymerized micelles and their use as adjuvants in immunology. *J. Pharm. Sci.* **65,** 1763–1766.
8. Kreuter, J., Liehl, E., Berg, U., Soliva, M., and Speiser, P. P. (1988) Influence of hydrophobicity on the adjuvant effect of particulate polymeric adjuvants. *Vaccine* **6,** 253–256.
9. Stieneker, F., Kersten, G., van Blois, L., Crommelin, D., Hem, S. L., Löwer, J., and Kreuter, J. (1995) Comparison of 24 different adjuvants for inactivated HIV-2 split whole virus as antigen in mice. Induction of titres of binding antibodies and toxicity of the formulations. *Vaccine* **13,** 45–53.
10. Kreuter, J. (1995) Nanoparticles as adjuvants for vaccines, in *Vaccine Design* (Powell, M. F. and Newman, M. J., eds.), Plenum, New York, pp. 463–472.
11. Vogel, F. R. and Powell, M. F. (1995) A compendium of vaccine adjuvants and excipients: PMMA, in *Vaccine Design* (Powell, M. F. and Newman, M. J., eds.), Plenum, New York, p. 201.
12. Kreuter, J. and Haenzel, I. (1978) Mode of action of immunological adjuvants: some physicochemical factors influencing the effectivity of polyacrylic adjuvants. *Infect. Immun.* **19,** 667–675.
13. Kreuter, J. and Liehl, E. (1978) Protection induced by inactivated influenza vaccines with polymethylmethacrylate adjuvants. *Med. Microbiol. Immunol.* **165,** 111–117.
14. Kreuter, J. and Liehl, E. (1981) Long-term studies of microencapsulated and adsorbed influenza vaccine nanoparticles. *J. Pharm. Sci.* **70,** 367–371.
15. Kreuter, J., Berg, U., Liehl, E., Soliva, M., and Speiser, P. P. (1986) Influence of the particle size on the adjuvant effect of particulate polymeric adjuvants. *Vaccine* **4,** 125–129.
16. Stieneker, F., Kreuter, J., and Löwer, J. (1991) High antibody titres in mice with polymethylmethacrylate nanoparticles as adjuvant for HIV vaccines. *AIDS* **5,** 431–435.

17. Stieneker, F., Löwer, J., and Kreuter, J. (1993) Different kinetics of the humoral immune response to inactivated HIV-1 and HIV-2 in mice: modulation by PMMA nanoparticle adjuvant. *Vaccine Res.* **2,** 111–118.
18. Berg, U. E., Kreuter, J., Speiser, P. P., and Soliva, M. (1986) Herstellung und in vitro-Prüfung von polymeren Adjuvantien für Impfstoffe. *Pharm. Ind.* **48,** 75–79.
19. Kreuter, J. (1985) Poly(alkyl acrylate) nanoparticles, in *Methods in Enzymology, Vol. 112, Drug and Enzyme Targeting* (Widder, K. J. and Green, R., eds.), Academic, Orlando, FL, pp. 129–138.
20. Kreuter, J. (1990) Large-scale production problems and manufacturing of nanoparticles, in *Specialized Drug Delivery Systems* (Tyle, P., ed.), Dekker, New York, pp. 257–266.
21. Kreuter, J., Nefzger, M., Liehl, E., Czok, R., and Voges, R. (1983) Distribution and elimination of poly(methyl methacrylate) nanoparticles after subcutaneous administration to rats. *J. Pharm. Sci.* **72,** 1146–1149.
22. Charnley, J., ed. (1970) *Acrylic Cement in Orthopaedic Surgery.* Livingstone, Edinburgh.
23. Cabanela, M. E., Coventry, M. B., MacCarty, C. S., and Miller, W. E. (1972) The fate of patients with methyl methacrylate cranioplasty. *J. Bone Joint Surg.* **54,** 278–281.
24. Kreuter, J., Täuber, U., and Illi, V. (1979) Distribution and elimination of poly(methyl-2-^{14}C-methacrylate) nanoparticle radioactivity after injection in rats and mice. *J. Pharm. Sci.* **68,** 1443–1447.
25. Schindler, A., Jeffcoat, R., Kimmel, G. L., Pitt, C. G., Wall, M. E., and Zweidinger, R. (1977) Biodegradable polymers for sustained drug delivery, in *Contemporary Topics in Polymer Science, Vol. 2* (Pearce, E. M. and Schaefgen, J. R., eds.), Plenum, New York, pp. 251–289.
26. Nefzger, M., Kreuter, J., Voges, R., Liehl, E., and Czok, R. (1984) Distribution and elimination of polymethyl methacrylate nanoparticles after peroral administration to rats. *J. Pharm. Sci.* **73,** 1309–1311.
27. Fikentscher, H., Gerrens, H., and Schuller, H. (1960) Emulsionspolymerisation und Kunststoff-Latices. *Angew. Chem.* **72,** 856–864.
28. Van der Hoff, B. M. E. (1960) On the mechanism of emulsion polymerization of styrene. II. polymerization in soap solutions below and above the critical micelle concentration and some remarks on the kinetics of emulsion polymerization. *J. Polymer Sci.* **44,** 241–259.
29. Roe, C. P. (1968) Surface chemistry aspects of emulsion polymerization. *Ind. Eng. Chem.* **60,** 20–33.
30. Robb, I. D. (1969) Determination of the number of particles/unit volume of latex during the emulsion polymerization of styrene. *J. Polymer. Sci., Part A-I* **7,** 417–427.
31. Fitch, R. M., Prenosil, M. B., and Sprick (1969) The mechanism of particle formation in polymer hydrosols. I. kinetics of aqueous polymerization of methyl methacrylate. *J. Polymer Sci., Part C* **27,** 95–118.

32. Fitch, R. M. and Tsoi, C. (1970) Polymer colloids: particle formation in nonmicellar systems. *J. Polymer Sci., Polymer Lett.* **8,** 703–710.
33. Fitch, R. M. (1973) The homogeneous nucleation of polymer colloids. *Brit. Polym. J.* **5,** 467–483.
34. Fitch, R. M., Prenosil, M. B., and Sprick, K. J. (1966) The mechanism of particle formation in polymer hydrosols. I. kinetics of aqueous polymerization of methyl methacrylate. *Amer. Chem. Soc., Polymer Preprints* **7,** 707–724.
35. Kreuter, J. (1982) On the mechanism of termination in heterogeneous polymerization. *J. Polymer Sci., Polymer Lett.* **20,** 543–545.
36. Fiquet-Fayard, F. (1959) Polymérization radiochimique du méthacrylate de méthyle (M.A.M.) en solution aqueuse. *J. Chim. Phys.* **56,** 692–698.
37. Acres, G. J. K. and Dalton, F. L. (1963) On Co^{60} gamma ray-initiated emulsion polymerization. *J. Polymer Sci. A* **1,** 3009–3020.
38. Kreuter, J. and Zehnder, H. J. (1978) The use of ^{60}Co-γ-irradiation for the production of vaccines. *Rad. Eff.* **35,** 161–166.
39. Kreuter, J. (1983) Physicochemical characterization of polyacrylic nanoparticles. *Int. J. Pharm.* **14,** 43–58.
40. Bentele, V., Berg, U. E., and Kreuter, J. (1983) Molecular weights of poly(methyl methacrylate) nanoparticles. *Int. J. Pharm.* **13,** 109–113.

7

Aqueous Formulation of Adjuvant-Active Nonionic Block Copolymers

Charles W. Todd and Mark J. Newman

1. Introduction

Despite the recent advances in vaccine technology, there is still a need for safe and effective adjuvants to potentiate the immune responses to subunit immunogens *(1)*. Depending on the disease in question, the vaccine-induced protection may require either a predominantly antibody-mediated response, under the control of (T-helper lymphocyte) Th2-associated cytokines, typically interleukin-4, -5, and -10 (IL-4, -5, -10), or a predominantly cellular response, the Th1 type, characterized by cells producing IL-2, IL-12, and gamma-interferon (γ-IFN), or some combination thereof *(2,3)*. Ideally, a vaccine delivery technology will be compatible with a wide variety of antigens and have the flexibility to achieve this goal of shifting the Th1/Th2 balance of the immune response with minimal formulation changes.

Our approach has been to develop a group of copolymer adjuvants, the Optivax® System, to fill this need. We have produced adjuvant-active nonionic block copolymers that are flexible, linear structures with a core of hydrophobic polyoxypropylene (POP) flanked on both ends by hydrophilic polyoxyethylene (POE) (**Fig. 1**). These molecules can be synthesized with variable ratios of POP and POE with molecular weights ranging from 1 to 20 kilodaltons (kDa). Their adjuvant activity was originally demonstrated in emulsions supplemented with low molecular-weight (2–5 kDa) copolymers *(4–6)*. More recently, we have produced high molecular-weight copolymers (> 9 kDa), which are active in oil-free aqueous formulations *(7–9)*. Preclinical studies showed the adjuvant activity of these compounds and illustrated how the best copolymer could be

From: *Methods in Molecular Medicine, Vol. 42:*
Vaccine Adjuvants: Preparation Methods and Research Protocols
Edited by: D. T. O'Hagan © Humana Press, Inc., Totowa, NJ

$$H\text{-}(O\text{-}CH_2\text{-}CH_2)_a\text{-}(O\text{-}\underset{\displaystyle CH_3}{\underset{|}{C}}H\text{-}CH_2)_b\text{-}(O\text{-}CH_2\text{-}CH_2)_a\text{-}OH$$

Fig. 1. The structure of non-ionic block copolymers. The central core of poly oxypropylene (POP) is sandwiched between two blocks of poly oxyethylene (POE). In copolymer CRL-1005 (5% POE), a ≈ 8 and b ≈ 210; in CRL-2690 (10% POE), a ≈ 16 and b ≈ 210.

selected for a given antigen ***(9)***. Additional studies in rabbits support the safety and lack of toxicity of the copolymers both at the injection site and systemically.

Other preclinical studies provided evidence that copolymers with slightly different structures and physicochemical properties have the ability to shift the balance of the Th1/Th2 cellular immune response (*see* **Subheading 3.4.**). When one of these copolymers, termed CRL-1005, was evaluated in a human clinical trial in combination with a peptide-conjugate antigen, the formulation stimulated strong antibody responses with only minimal local and systemic reactogenicity ***(10)***. In addition to augmenting antibody production, the adjuvant increased the production of cytokines associated with both Th1 and Th2 cellular immune responses. The activity of this copolymer in the clinical setting and the preclinical findings concerning the effects of these polymers on the balance of the Th1/Th2 immune response, thus open the possibility of specifically tailoring the copolymer to the antigen to produce the optimal immune response desired for protection or immunotherapy.

Our high molecular-weight nonionic block copolymers are synthesized from propylene oxide and ethylene oxide by a proprietary method. In a typical reaction, propylene oxide is reacted with propylene glycol, a bifunctional initiator, in the presence of an alkali metal salt catalyst ***(11)***. Close control of the reaction temperature and pressure favors the production of a linear copolymer that grows by addition of monomers to both ends of the molecule. Synthesis with propylene oxide proceeds until the hydrophobic POP core reaches the required size, which for copolymer CRL-1005 is approximately 12 kDa, then polymerization is continued with ethylene oxide to produce hydrophilic blocks of POE on both ends of the central, hydrophobic POP core. In copolymer CRL-1005, POE constitutes about 5% of the molecule by weight. After completing polymerization, the reactive ends of the polymers are quenched with water, the catalyst is adsorbed onto a mixture of magnesium silicate and silicon dioxide, then removed by filtration.

The resulting Optivax copolymers are clear, viscous liquids with apparent viscosities of approximately 4000 centipoise at 25°C. They are amphipathic compounds with inverse solubility characteristics in aqueous media. Below their cloud points (7–12°C), these copolymers are water soluble and form clear solutions that can be filter sterilized. The solution process involves the formation of hydrogen bonds between oxygen atoms and hydroxyl groups in the copolymer and water molecules. When a solution of copolymer is warmed and passes through its cloud point, the increased thermal motion is sufficient to break the hydrogen bonds and as the copolymer molecules come out of solution, they "self-assemble" into microparticles 0.5–2 μm in diameter ***(8,9)***. The process is reversible. Upon storage of a formulation below its cloud point, the copolymer resolubilizes to give a clear solution. If microparticle formation occurs in the presence of antigen, the size and appearance of the particles are different, indicating an association of the copolymer adjuvant with the antigen ***(9)***.

The interaction and incorporation of antigens with adjuvants cover the spectrum from the high efficiency adsorption of antigen onto aluminum compounds ***(12)*** to the very limited physical interaction antigens with saponins such as Qs-21 ***(13)***. As noted above, the interaction of the antigens with the nonionic block copolymers is an association rather than an adsorption or entrapment. At room temperature, the copolymer in the particles is in equilibrium with that in free solution. Therefore, it has been difficult both to separate free antigen from that which is copolymer-bound and thereby to measure the degree of association of copolymer with different antigens.

The change in size and morphology of the copolymer particles formed in the presence of antigen is dependent on the antigen. Formulation of CRL-1005 with human influenza virus vaccine, which is primarily viral hemagglutinin with some neuraminidase, results in the formation of smaller (0.1–0.6 μm diameter) and smoother particles than copolymer alone. In contrast, the association of chicken ovalbumin (OVA) with this copolymer yields slightly larger particles (0.5–3 μm diameter) than CRL-1005 alone ***(8,9)***. The viral antigens are trans-membrane proteins with hydrophobic regions whereas OVA is a hydrophilic molecule. These differences may be affecting the interactions of the respective proteins with the copolymer both in the solution phase and during particle formation and thereby underlie the differences in size and morphology noted in the final antigen/adjuvant formulations.

Particle size is minimally affected by the changes in pH, osmolarity, and buffer salts encountered in physiologically compatible formulations. Aforementioned, particle formation occurs as the copolymer warms through its cloud point. Adding energy at this step, either by immersion of the formulation in a 37°C water bath or vortexing the mixture results in smaller particles. However, these changes have little effect on the adjuvanticity of the final preparation. When such a microparticulate formulation of copolymer and antigen is injected, it is likely that the antigen is presented to the immune system in the particulate

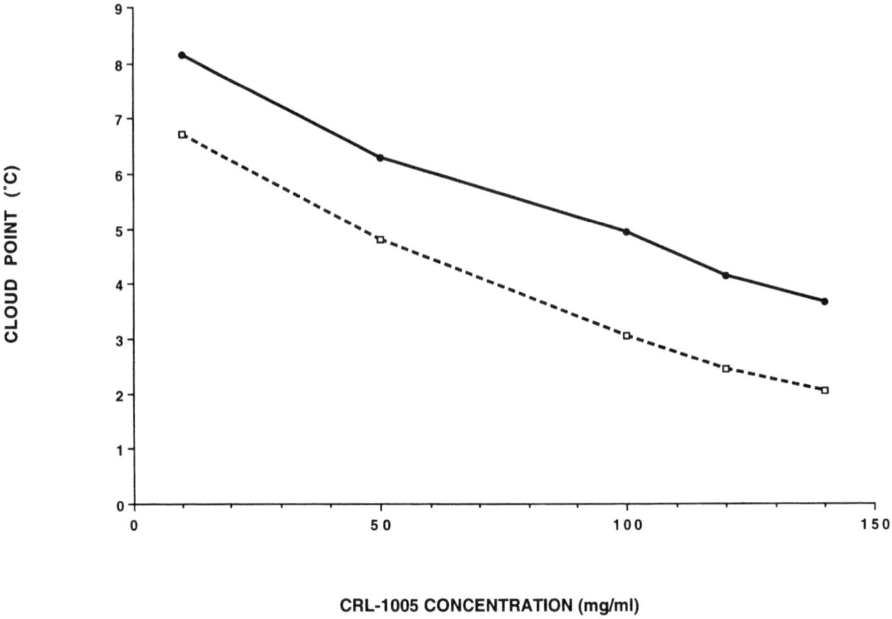

Fig. 2. The effects of CRL-1005 concentration and ionic strength on cloud point. The cloud points of increasing concentrations of CRL-1005 were determined following solubilization in either water (solid line) or 0.15*M* sodium chloride (broken line).

form favored for optimal processing and induction of immune responses *(14)*. These microparticulate suspensions are not emulsions. They are totally oil-free and can be formulated with a wide variety of antigens and subunit vaccine preparations under physiologic conditions.

The two major factors that influence the cloud point of CRL-1005, and that are pertinent to the formulation process, are the concentrations of the copolymer and the cations in the aqueous medium, respectively. A solution of 10 mg/mL CRL-1005 in water has a cloud point of 8.2°C (**Fig. 2**). Increasing the copolymer concentration lowers the cloud point, decreasing it to 3.6°C at 140 mg/mL. The cloud point in physiologic media is also affected by the ionic environment. At identical copolymer concentrations, increasing the concentration of sodium chloride from 0 to 0.15*M* lowers the cloud point by about 1.5°C (**Fig. 2**). This depression is owing to the cation concentration, in this case Na^+, and not the anions *(15)*. The sodium ions are believed to exert their influence by decreasing the interaction between water molecules and the copolymer, thereby weakening the hydrogen bonds *(15)*. For practical purposes, the decreasing cloud point limits solubility in isotonic media to about 100 mg/mL.

2. Materials

2.1. Formulation

1. Copolymer raw material, e.g., CRL-1005, CRL-2690, CytRx Corporation (Norcross, GA).
2. Physiological buffer, e.g., PBS, citrate saline (refer to **Note 1**).
3. Antigen solution, e.g., ovalbumin, tetanus toxoid, influenza hemagglutinin, and so on.

2.2. Copolymer Assay

1. HPLC system (Waters, Milford, MA, or equivalent) equipped with 2 columns (Styragel HR3 + Ultrastyragel 500 Å), in series plus a refractive index detector.
2. Tetrahydrofuran with BHT antioxidant (VWR Scientific, Atlanta, GA).
3. Copolymer Reference Standard (CytRx Corporation).

2.3. Antigen Assay

1. Materials Required: Bio-Rad Detergent Compatible Assay (Bio-Rad, Hercules, CA, Number 500-0112).

2.4. Determination of Particle Size

1. Accusizer 770 and Nicomp 370 Particle Sizers (Particle Sizing Systems, Santa Barbara, CA) or equivalent.
2. Latex Calibration Microspheres (Duke Scientific, Palo Alto, CA).

3. Methods

3.1. Outline of Formulation

The two physicochemical properties of the copolymers that affect the solubilization process are the cloud point of the final solution and the viscosity of the raw material. For the copolymer to go into aqueous solution, its temperature must be below its cloud point, for example, 5.5°C for a 40 mg/mL solution of CRL-1005 in isotonic saline (*see* **Fig. 2**). However, at this low temperature, the increased viscosity of the bulk copolymer and its decreased rate of solubilization combine to slow the dissolution process significantly. To speed up solubilization, we weigh out the copolymer at room temperature, then disperse it by vortexing or stirring into the required amount of buffer to give a heterogeneous suspension of particles and globules ≤ 200 µm in diameter. Upon chilling this suspension on ice with either stirring or agitation, the dispersed copolymer readily dissolves. The final copolymer solution has a viscosity similar to saline and can be sterilized with a 0.2-µm filter provided that the bulk solution and the filter are both kept cold.

3.2. Preparation of Copolymer Solution

1. Weigh out 1 g copolymer into a 50-mL polypropylene centrifuge tube using a polypropylene transfer pipet.
2. Add 19 g buffer to give a 5% (w/w) solution (= 50 mg/mL).
3. Purge the tube head space with nitrogen.
4. Securely cap tube and vortex the formulation to disperse the copolymer into the buffer. Ensure no copolymer is remaining on the side of the tube.
5. Place the tube sideway in crushed ice and agitate on a gyrotory or reciprocal shaker at approx 110 rpm for approximately 1 h to cold solubilize the copolymer. Turn the tube occasionally to ensure thorough dissolution. Check that the copolymer is completely dissolved, then keep the resulting solution on ice.
6. Totally surround a 0.2-µm 115-mL filter to the top of the unit with crushed ice and allow it to chill for at least 15 min.
7. Keeping the filter in the ice, pour the ice-cold clear, copolymer solution into the ice-cold filter and apply negative pressure to filter the solution. Do not try to filter a solution with any cloudiness (*see* **Note 2**).
8. Allow the copolymer to warm slowly to room temperature and go cloudy, then transfer it to a sterile tube. Purge the tube head space with sterile filtered nitrogen, cap, and seal (*see* **Note 3**).

3.3. Preparation of Formulations

1. Using sterile technique and working at room temperature, add appropriate volumes of 50 mg/mL copolymer, antigen, and buffer to give the final formulation for injection (*see* **Note 4**).
2. Chill the formulation on ice until the copolymer dissolves and the preparation goes clear. Leave on ice for 30 min to allow the antigen and copolymer to interact.
3. Allow formulation to warm slowly to room temperature for about 15 min and go cloudy. Mix once more by inversion before injecting animals.
4. Formulations of copolymer and antigen can be kept at 4°C for several days provided they are stored under nitrogen.
5. Although formulation is performed at room temperature when the copolymer is particulate, optimal adjuvant activity is achieved by cold solubilization of the adjuvant with the antigen then allowing particle formation to occur in the presence of antigen.
6. Because the natural state of the copolymer is a viscous liquid, formulations cannot be lyophilized and reconstituted later.

3.4. Dosing and Applications

The copolymers can function as adjuvants over a range of concentrations depending on the antigen and the animal immunized. Whenever possible, we perform a dose-response curve for each new antigen and species to determine the optimal copolymer dose. It is possible to overdose with the copolymer and lose adjuvant activity. The antigen may be diluted out at a high copolymer dose, and

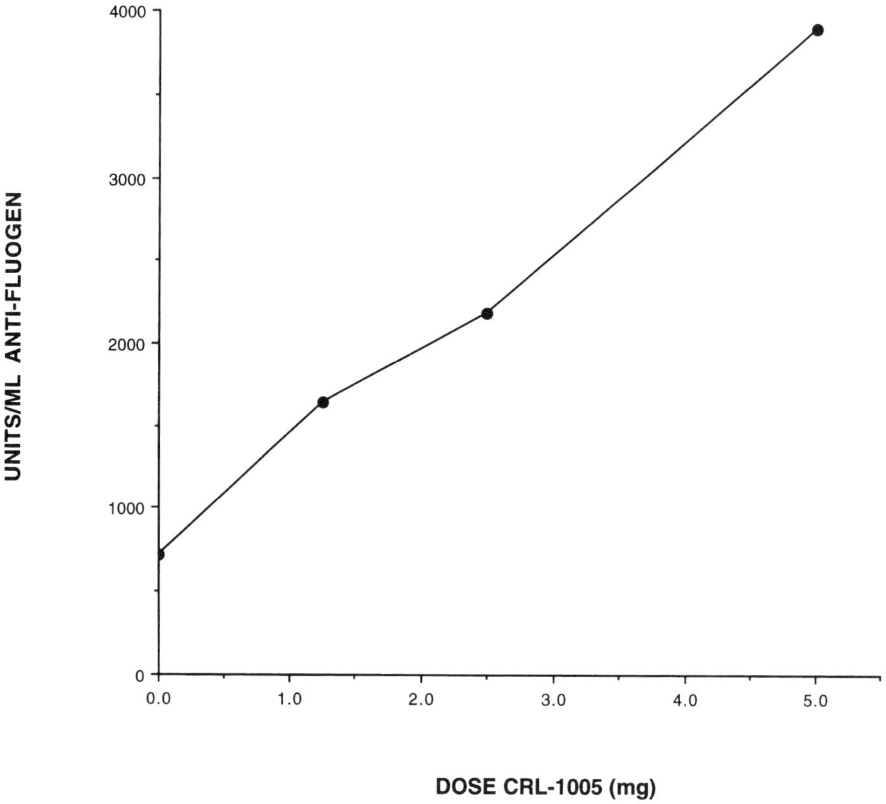

Fig. 3. The serological responses of mice to Fluogen® supplemented with increasing amounts of CRL-1005. Groups of Balb/C mice were immunized on day 0 with 4.5 µg Fluogen HA. The antigen was administered either alone or supplemented with 1.25, 2.5, or 5 mg, respectively, of CRL-1005. Antibody concentrations at day 28 were measured by ELISA against total Fluogen viral proteins and were quantified by interpolation on to a dilution curve of an in-house standard serum which had been assigned 10,000 ELISA U/mL.

consequent high copolymer to antigen ratio, such that antigen presenting cells are saturated with the copolymer and have minimal antigen to process and present.

Working in mice, we have successfully used from 1.25–5 mg CRL-1005 with 4.5 µg of human influenza virus vaccine (**Fig. 3**) and 2.5–5.0 mg copolymer with 15 µg ovalbumin *(8,9)*. For most antigens, we routinely use a 2.5 mg dose in mice, for example, 100 µL of 25 mg/mL copolymer formulated with the appropriate concentration of antigen and a minimum of 28 d between primary and secondary injections. However, for antigens administered in the 0.5–2 µg range, a lower copolymer dose of about 1 mg is preferable.

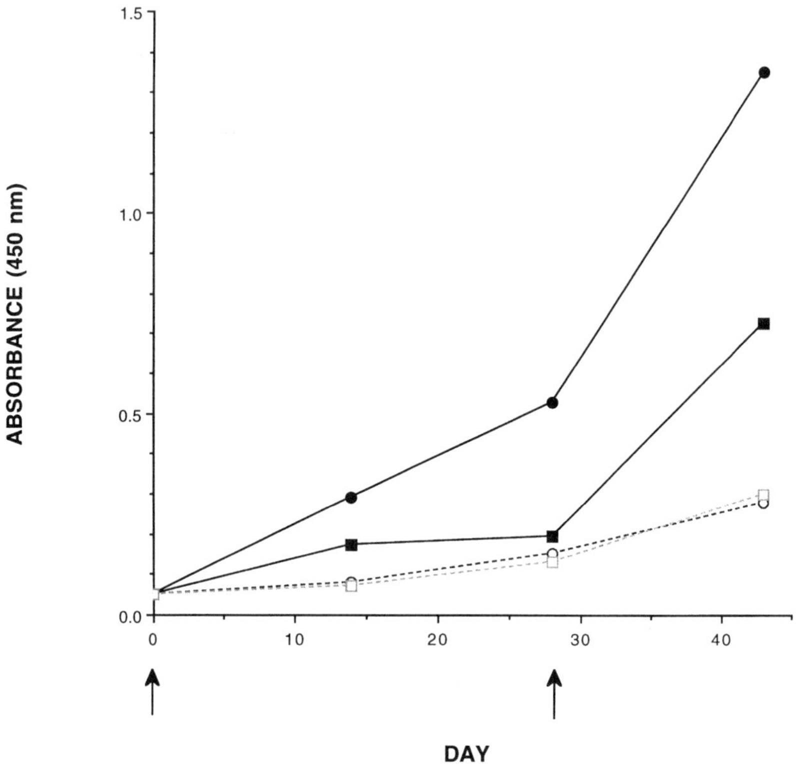

Fig. 4. The kinetics of serum antibody responses induced in rhesus monkeys following two immunizations on days 0 and 28 (↑) with 45 μg Fluogen® HA. Two monkeys were administered the antigen alone (open symbols, dashed lines), and two received antigen supplemented with 25 mg CRL-1005 (filled symbols, solid lines). Antibody concentrations were measured by ELISA against total Fluogen viral proteins and are expressed as absorbance units (450 nm) obtained at a 1/100 serum dilution.

The copolymers also work well in nonhuman primates and people. A 25 mg dose of CRL-1005 with 45 μg human influenza virus hemagglutinin augmented both ELISA-reactive antibody (**Fig. 4**) and functional hemagglutination-inhibition antibody in rhesus macaques compared to unadjuvanted controls *(7)*.

We performed a clinical trial evaluating CRL-1005 as an adjuvant with the peptide conjugate antigen βhCG-CTP37-DT for an immunotherapeutic indication. Certain tumor types display βhCG on their surface and because its expression is normally restricted to the developing fetus, this molecule has been evaluated as a possible target antigen for imunotherapy *(16)*. The synthetic peptide antigen consisted of the 37 carboxy terminal amino acids of βhCG (CTP37) covalently coupled to diphtheria toxoid (DT) at a ratio of approximately 30 CTP37 peptides to each DT molecule. We performed a dose-response escalation, evaluating 4 doses of CRL-1005 at 3, 10, 25, and 75 mg, each with 1 mg of βhCG-CTP37-DT ***(10)***. The copolymer was most effective in the 3–25 mg range giving antibody titers equivalent or superior to those previously seen with the same antigen administered in a water-in-oil emulsion adjuvanted with nor-muramyl dipeptide ***(16)***. A decrease in adjuvant activity at 75 mg in people was consistent with the high dose effect previously noted in mice. At this dose, there was no increase in the rate of local or systemic side effects, supporting the safety of the copolymer.

In addition to the studies cited above, either in collaborations with others or in house, we have formulated the Optivax copolymers with a wide range of viral, bacterial, and protozoal antigens with successful results. The copolymers are effective with whole organisms as well as purified subunits, proteins, and conjugate immunogens containing peptide and carbohydrate determinants.

The copolymer is not believed to cause significant denaturation of antigens. We immunized mice and rhesus macaques with commercial human influenza vaccine adjuvanted with CRL-1005. The sera were positive by ELISA and contained functional antibody with hemagglutination-inhibition activity ***(7)***. In separate experiments, mice were immunized with inactivated mouse-adapted influenza virus adjuvanted with CRL-1005. Upon challenge with live virus, these animals demonstrated protection superior to mice that received the unadjuvanted virus alone. Both these experiments are consistent with a lack of denaturation of the critical neutralizing epitopes on the viral hemagglutinin by the copolymer.

The immune responses in mice have been differentiated into either Th1- or Th2-type based on the cytokine profile induced. The Th1 profile is characterized by the initial production of γ-IFN and IL-12 with an effector phase of T lymphocytes producing IL-2 and γ-IFN, and mediating cytotoxic activity (CTL) ***(17,18)***. In contrast, Th2 responses are influenced by IL-4 with predominantly IL-5 and IL-10-producing T cells in the effector phase that drive antibody production ***(19)***. In general, viral infections elicit a predominantly CTL-mediated Th1 response whereas bacterial and parasitic infections induce antibody-dependent Th2 responses ***(3,19)***. As a consequence, it is critical that immunization achieves the appropriate type of immune response to protect against the indicated pathogen and in this context, the effects of the adjuvant can be critical.

The Optivax copolymers have been evaluated for their abilities to stimulate the immune response differentially. The series used had a POP core of 11 kDa with different amounts of POE. Cytokine profiles were examined in response to the antigen ovalbumin formulated with these copolymers. The adjuvants alum, which induces Th2 responses, and Quil-A saponin, which augments both Th1 and Th2 responses, were included as positive controls. The copolymers

Table 1
The Effects of Different Copolymers on the Augmentation or Induction of Th1 and Th2 Lymphocyte Responses

Adjuvant Used	Th1 cytokine concentrations (pg/mL)		Th2 cytokine concentrations (pg/mL)	
	γ-IFN	IL-2	IL-5	IL-10
Alum	98	0	5550	5120
Quil-A	318	38	5010	6230
5% POE	327	48	6460	6500
10% POE	156	0	5130	4510

Augmentation of OVA-specific cellular immune responses by the use of adjuvants was determined using antigen-driven cytokine production in vitro. Groups of C57Bl/6 mice were immunized on d 0 and d 28 with 25 µg/dose OVA formulated with different adjuvants. The adjuvants alum, which induces Th2 responses, and Quil-A saponin, which augments both Th1 and Th2 responses, were included as positive controls. The experimental adjuvants were copolymers with 11 kDa POP cores and either 5 or 10% POE. Splenic leukocytes were harvested on d 56 and cultured in vitro for 5 d with and without 25 µg/mL OVA using standard techniques. The concentrations of cytokines in culture supernatants were assayed using a commercially-available capture ELISA with the unknowns quantitated against a standard curve (PharMingen, Los Angeles, CA). Data represent (Cytokine concentration in OVA stimulated cultures) – (Cytokine concentration in control cultures).

displayed differential activity (**Table 1**). The more hydrophobic copolymer with 5% POE induced a mixed Th1 and Th2 response of γ-IFN, IL-2, IL-5 and IL-10. In contrast the more hydrophilic copolymer with 10% POE induced a predominantly Th2 profile characterized by lower levels of γ-IFN, undetectable IL-2, and with high concentrations of IL-5 and IL-10 ***(11)***. In separate experiments, Quil-A and the 5% POE copolymer were able to induce CTL, but the 10% copolymer and alum failed to stimulate comparable responses ***(11)***. These experimental data are supported by the observations in the clinical trial where the hydrophilic copolymer CRL-1005 stimulated the secretion of the Th1-associated cytokines γ-IFN and IL-2 as well as the Th2-associated cytokines IL-5 and IL-10 ***(10)***. Although the nature of the response also depends on the antigen, based on these data we believe that with the Optivax system of adjuvants, it may be possible to match the antigen with the appropriate copolymer to elicit the type of response desired for protection or therapy. However, it is not currently possible to predict which copolymers will be optimal for each antigen and further studies will be needed.

3.5. Safety

We have tested the safety of copolymer CRL-1005 in a variety of preclinical and clinical settings both alone and in combination with antigens. All the data generated to date support the safety of this adjuvant technology and the lack of local and systemic toxicity. A preclinical safety/toxicity study in rabbits examined the safety of three intramuscular injections of aqueous CRL-1005 given without antigen at monthly intervals. Five groups of animals, each of 10 males and 10 females, were given the copolymer at 0 (saline control), 12.5 mg, 25 mg, 50 mg, and 80 mg per dose, respectively. The rabbits were monitored for any sign of injection site reactogenicity or systemic effects such as changes in temperature, weight, hematology, and blood chemistry, then examined at sacrifice by gross necropsy and histopathology. There were no clinical signs of toxicity observed during the study and histology revealed no treatment-related changes at the injection sites or in other tissues examined.

As part of the release testing of materials for use in the first Phase 1 clinical trial of CRL-1005, the formulations were evaluated in the General Safety Test required by the United States Food and Drug Administration for vaccines ***(20)***. Because the copolymer and the antigen (βhCG-CTP37-DT) were to be administered im to patients in a 1-mL volume at 4 dose combinations of constant antigen dose and escalating adjuvant doses, the General Safety Test was performed with 0.5-mL and 5.0-mL volumes of the following human doses in mice and guinea pigs, respectively:

1. 1.0 mg βhCG-CTP37-DT + 3 mg CRL-1005
2. 1.0 mg βhCG-CTP37-DT + 10 mg CRL-1005
3. 1.0 mg βhCG-CTP37-DT + 25 mg CRL-1005
4. 1.0 mg βhCG-CTP37-DT + 75 mg CRL-1005

All four formulations passed the General Safety Test.

In addition to the General Safety Test, the copolymer and antigen were tested alone and in combination for their pyrogenicity when injected intravenously into rabbits ***(21)***. The doses of copolymer adjuvant (1.07 mg/kg) and antigen conjugate (14.3 μg/kg) were proportional, on a body-weight basis, to the maximal single human doses (75 mg copolymer + 1 mg antigen) subsequently used in the clinical trial. All three materials tested (CRL-1005 alone, βhCG-CTP37-DT alone, and CRL-1005 + βhCG-CTP37-DT) were nonpyrogenic. Since that study, we have tested another GMP-manufactured lot of aqueous CRL-1005 by both the rabbit pyrogenicity test and the Limulus amebocyte lysate (LAL) gel clot assay ***(22)***. The material was nonpyrogenic by both methods. By the quantitative LAL assay, the endotoxin concentration in the sample was determined to be less than 0.625 endotoxin U/mL, the detection limit for the assay. The four CRL-1005 + βhCG-CTP37-DT formulations tested above were subsequently used in a Phase 1 human clinical trial. All formulations were administered without evidence of significant local or systemic toxicity ***(10)***.

The data summarized above support the safety and lack of toxicity of copolymer adjuvant CRL-1005. The copolymer is not inherently pyrogenic and aqueous clinical materials have been repeatedly manufactured with undetectable endotoxin concentrations. In addition, the General Safety Tests in mice and guinea pigs indicated that large doses of the vaccine formulations have low toxicity. Finally, the preclinical study in rabbits and the Phase 1 clinical trial in humans demonstrate the lack of both local reactogenicity and systemic effects when CRL-1005 is administered intramuscularly. Considering these results, we are confident that copolymer CRL-1005 has a safety profile superior to most of the other new adjuvants currently being evaluated for use in humans.

3.6. Assay of Copolymer Solution to Determine Dosing

The most practical way to measure the concentration of these copolymers in aqueous preparations is by gel permeation chromatography (GPC) with tetrahydrofuran (THF) as the mobile phase. The copolymer is dissolved in the organic phase by diluting the aqueous sample at least 20-fold in THF. Hydrophilic materials such as buffer salts and proteins precipitate out and are removed by filtration, then the copolymer is assayed by size-based GPC with a refractive index detector. The concentration of copolymer in the sample is determined by comparison of the peak areas of the sample and a known concentration of the Reference Standard, respectively.

1. Copolymer Reference Standard. Dissolve 200 mg of Reference Standard in THF, make up to 100 mL to give 2 mg/mL. Add 10 mL of 2 mg/mL copolymer solution to 40 mL THF to give a 0.4 mg/mL solution.
2. Sample preparation. Weigh out 0.8 g of 25 mg/mL aqueous copolymer solution and make up to 50 mL with THF to give a nominal 0.4 mg/mL solution.
3. GPC equipment preparation. Set up and equilibrate the HPLC system for a GPC run. Set up software for the run and prepare the sample queue.
4. System suitability. Make five injections of the reference material. Calculate the standard deviation of the peak response elution time. The Percent Relative Standard Deviation (RSD) should not exceed 3% for any of the standards run.
5. Sample analysis. For each injection (sample or reference standard) to be run, filter the dilution into a 250-μL insert, and load the insert into a 4-mL vial.
6. Cap each vial and place into the sample carrier in the following order: system suitability (five injections of reference standard), duplicate aliquots of each sample preparation and reference standards. Run a reference standard after every four sample injections and at the end of the run.
7. Perform the Analytical run.
8. From the peak areas of the samples compared with the peak areas of the reference standard and its known concentration, determine the concentration of copolymer in the samples.

3.7. Measurement of Protein in the Presence of Copolymer to Determine Antigen Dose

Many protein assays are based on the formation of a colored product following interactions between the reagents and the polypeptide chain. Because these assays are read at room temperature, any determination of protein in the presence of copolymer, which would be in the microparticulate form, would result in a cloudy sample and interference with the determination of color intensity. The Bio-Rad Detergent Compatible Assay is based on the well documented Lowry method and contains sodium dodecyl sulfate (SDS), which solubilizes the copolymer at room temperature, allowing the analysis to proceed.

The assay is performed according to the manufacturer's instructions except that the formulation must initially be diluted to ≤ 2.5 mg/mL copolymer. At this concentration, the SDS in the assay reagents can solubilize the copolymer.

3.8. Measurement of Particle Size

We have used the measurement of particle size to determine the interaction of the copolymers with different antigens and to explore the effects of varying particle size on the adjuvant effect. The Accusizer 770 directly measures both the numbers and sizes of particles ≥ 1 µm by optical sensing based on light obscuration of single particles passing through a photo zone. It reports data as number of particles within a given channel of specified width. In contrast, the Nicomp 370 uses dynamic light scattering at 90° to measure the distribution of particles. It records the Relative Number of particles within a designated size range with the channel containing the greatest number arbitrarily set at 1.0. The Nicomp 370 is best suited for particles ≤ 1 µm. Because the size distribution of the copolymer microparticles ranges from 0.5–3 µm, we use both instruments to analyze copolymer formulations with and without antigen. Both instruments are set up and calibrated with latex microspheres according to the manufacturers instructions.

1. Accusizer 770. Add 10 µL of copolymer suspension to 20 mL filtered PBS in the instrument reservoir. Run particle sizer in Autodilution mode. Print out particle size distribution and channel counts.
2. Nicomp 370. Dilute copolymer suspension 1:10 and inject 3 mL into particle sizer. Run in Autodilution mode with Nicomp data analysis. Collect data until Fit Error and Residual reach acceptable values. Print particle size distribution.

4. Notes

1. Although we have not tested all combinations, from the stand point of pH, ionic strength and buffer components, we believe that the copolymers are compatible with the majority of aqueous buffer formulations that can safely be given orally or parenter-

ally. If required to maintain an antigen in solution, the formulation buffer can contain low concentrations of detergents, for example 0.05% Tween®-80 or Triton® X-100. The detergents should be peroxide-free to avoid initiation of oxidation.
2. Endotoxins are powerful adjuvants, therefore we formulate with water-for-injection and filter sterilize the copolymer solution as quickly as possible to avoid the potential of bacterial contamination.
3. Our studies have indicated that these large nonionic block copolymers can be susceptible to oxidative breakdown. Consequently, we store the raw material under nitrogen at –20°C. Sterile-filtered aqueous copolymer formulations can be stored under nitrogen at 4°C for up to 3 mo. Exercise care during formulation to keep solutions under nitrogen and minimize exposure to atmospheric oxygen. We are evaluating physiologically compatible antioxidant formulations to determine those which will significantly slow any oxidative breakdown.
4. When pipeting copolymer solutions, use extra care. The copolymers have surfactant properties that lower the surface tension, hence solutions tend to drip from pipettes more easily than normal saline, and so on.
5. Working with a contract manufacturer, we have prepared 4 × 2-L GMP batches of clinical grade aqueous CRL-1005 using a modification of the lab-scale protocol. Buffer salts were charged into the receiving vessel and dissolved in a portion of the water. The copolymer was weighed into the buffer with stirring and the formulation made up to final weight with water. The preparation was then chilled to dissolve the copolymer. The critical stage of manufacture was sterile filtration where the copolymer solution had to be kept below its cloud point. The unfiltered bulk, transfer lines, and filter were all chilled to 2.5°C before filtration commenced and maintained at that temperature throughout the process. The filtered bulk was allowed to warm to room temperature before vials were filled. Filled vials were subsequently stored at 5°C.

References

1. Lawrence, D. N., Goldenthal, K. L., Boslego, J. W., Chandler, D. K. F., and La Montagne, J. R. (1995) Public health implications of emerging vaccine technologies, in *Vaccine Design: The subunit and adjuvant approach* (Powell, M. F. and Newman, M. J., eds.), Plenum, New York, pp. 43–60.
2. Scott, P., Pearce, E., Cheever, A. W., Coffman, R. L., and Sher, A. (1989) Role of cytokines and CD4+ T-cell subsets in the regulation of parasitic immunity and disease. *Immunol. Rev.* **112,** 161–182.
3. Seder, R. A. and Paul, W. E. (1994) Acquisition of lymphokine-producing phenotype by CD4+ T cells. *Ann. Rev. Immunol.* **12,** 635–673.
4. Hunter, R. L., Strickland, F., and Kezdy, F. (1981) The adjuvant activity of nonionic block copolymer surfactants. I. The role of hydrophile-lipophile balance. *J. Immunol.* **127,** 1224–1250.
5. Hunter, R. L. and Bennet, B. (1984) The adjuvant activity of nonionic block copolymer surfactants. II. Antibody formation and inflammation related to the structure of triblock and octablock copolymers. *J. Immunol.* **133,** 3167–3175.

6. Hunter, R. L., Olsen, M. R., and Bennet, B. (1995) Copolymer adjuvants and Titermax®, in *The theory and practical application of adjuvants* (Stewart-Tull, D. E. S., ed.), Wiley, London, UK, pp. 51–94.
7. Newman, M. J., Todd, C. W., Lee, E. M., Balusubramanian, M., Didier, P. J., and Katz, J. M. (1997) Increasing the immunogenicity of a trivalent influenza virus vaccine with adjuvant-active nonionic block copolymers for potential use in the elderly. *Mech. Ageing Develop.* **93,** 189–203.
8. Todd, C. W., Pozzi, L.-A. M., Guarnaccia, J. R., Balusubramanian, M., Henk, W. G., Younger, L. E., and Newman, M. J. (1997) Development of an adjuvant-active nonionic block copolymer for use in oil-free subunit vaccine formulations. *Vaccine* **15,** 564–570.
9. Todd, C. W., Lee, E., Balusubramanian, M., Shah, H., Henk, W. G., Younger, L. E., and Newman, M. J. (1997) Systematic development of a block copolymer adjuvant for trivalent influenza virus vaccine, in *Modulation of the Immune Response to Vaccine Antigens* (Brown, F. and Haaheim, L. R., eds.), *Dev. Biol. Stand.* **92,** Karger, Basel, pp. 343–353.
10. Triozzi, P. L., Stevens, V. C., Aldrich, W., Powell, J., Todd, C. W., and Newman, M. J. (1997) Effects of a β-human chorionic gonadotrophin subunit immunogen administered in aqueous solution with a novel noninoic block copolymer adjuvant in patients with advanced cancer. *Clinical Cancer Res.* **3,** 2355–2362.
11. Newman, M. J., Actor, J. K., Balusubramanian, M., and Jagannath, C. (1998) Use of nonionic block copolymers in vaccines and therapeutics. *Critical Rev. Therap. Drug Carrier Sys.* **15,** 89–142.
12. Hem, S. L. and White, J. L. (1995) Structure and properties of aluminum-containing adjuvants, in *Vaccine Design: The subunit and adjuvant approach* (Powell, M. F. and Newman, M. J., eds.), Plenum, New York, pp. 249–276,
13. Kensil, C. R., Wu, J-Y., and Soltysik, S. (1995) Structural and immunological characterization of the vaccine adjuvant QS-21, in *Vaccine Design: The subunit and adjuvant approach* (Powell, M. F. and Newman, M. J., eds.), Plenum, New York, pp. 525–541.
14. Reis e Sousa, C., Stahl, P. D., and Austyn, J. M. (1993) Phagocytosis of antigens by Langerhans cells in vitro. *J. Exp. Med.* **178,** 509–519.
15. Karlström, G., Carlsson, A., and Lindmann, B. (1990) Phase diagrams of nonionic polymer-water systems. Experimental and theoretical studies of the effects of surfactants and other cosolutes. *J. Phys. Chem.* **94,** 5005–5015.
16. Triozzi, P. L., Gonchour, D., Martin, E. W., Aldrich, W., Powell, J., Kim, J. A., et al. (1994) Clinical and immunological effects of a synthetic β-human chorionic gonadotrophin vaccine. *Int. J. Oncol.* **5,** 1447–1454.
17. Manetti, R., Parronchi, P., Guidizi, M. G., Piccinni, M.-P., Maggi, E., Trinchieri, G., and Romagnani, S. (1993) Natural killer cell stimulatory factor (interleukin 12 [IL-12]) induces T helper type 1 (Th1)-specific immune responses and inhibits the development of IL-4-producing Th cells. *J. Exp. Med.* **177,** 1199–1204.
18. Seder, R. A., Gazzinelli, R. T., Sher, A., and Paul, W. E. (1993) Interleukin-12 acts directly on CD4+ T cells to enhance priming for interferon gamma produc-

tion and diminishes interleukin 4 inhibition of such priming. *Proc. Natl. Acad. Sci. USA* **90,** 10,188–10,192.

19. Swain, S. L., Weinberg, A. D., English, M., and Huston, G. (1990) IL-4 directs the development of Th2-like helper effectors. *J. Immunol.* **145,** 3796–3806.
20. *Code of Federal Regulations* 21 CFR 610.11 (1993) 46–48.
21. *United States Pharmacopeia* **23,** (1995) 1718–1719.
22. *United States Pharmacopeia* **23,** (1995) 1696–1697.

8

Liposomes As Immunological Adjuvants and Vaccine Carriers

Gregory Gregoriadis, Brenda McCormack, Mia Obrenovic, Yvonne Perrie, and Roghieh Saffie

1. Introduction

The need for an effective and safe immunological adjuvant or vaccine carrier that could promote appropriate immune responses to vaccines is well recognized *(1,2)*. This is especially true for most of the subunit vaccine and synthetic peptide antigens, which are not only costly or available in small quantities (e.g., recombinant DNA products), but also weakly or nonimmunogenic. However, presently available immunological adjuvants (e.g., complete and incomplete Freund's adjuvants, bacterial endotoxins, polyanions, mineral adsorbents, and so on) can induce local or systemic toxicity, form unacceptable granulomas, lack efficiency, or have short-term effects. An additional hazard with some of the adjuvants is the production of vaccine-related allergic reactions in a minority of recipients, including those already sensitized to the antigen *(1,2)*.

A role for liposomes as immunological adjuvants was first established in 1974 *(3)* when strong humoral immune responses to liposome-entrapped diphtheria toxoid were observed after injection into mice. It was of interest to note that, unlike other adjuvants, there were no granulomas at the site of injection *(3,4)*. Moreover, there were no hypersensitivity reactions in preimmunized animals when the antigen was given in the entrapped form *(5)*. In the ensuing years, extensive work in this laboratory and elsewhere has shown that liposomal adjuvanticity applies to a wide variety of bacterial, viral, protozoan, tumor, and other antigens *(6,7)*. In much of this work *(7)*, protective immunity

From: *Methods in Molecular Medicine, Vol. 42:*
Vaccine Adjuvants: Preparation Methods and Research Protocols
Edited by: D. T. O'Hagan © Humana Press, Inc., Totowa, NJ

in animal models was achieved on immunization with the relevant liposome-entrapped antigens (for a list of antigens used in conjunction with liposomes composed of a variety of lipids with or without coadjuvants, *see* **ref.** *7*). It is generally accepted ***(7)*** that liposomal adjuvanticity is observed regardless of the type of association (within the vesicles or attached onto their surface) of the antigen with liposomes.

Recent developments suggest that many of the problems encountered in conventional vaccines may be circumvented by the approach of genetic immunization ***(8–10)***. It has now been established that intramuscular injection of naked, antigen-encoding plasmid DNA leads to humoral and cell-mediated immune responses against the antigen. Experimental evidence ***(8–10)*** indicates that immunity results from the uptake of DNA by muscle cells, episomal DNA expression, extracellular release of the generated antigen followed by its uptake by antigen presenting cells (APC). It is also conceivable that some of the injected DNA is taken up directly by APC. Some of the disadvantages ***(8–10)*** of naked DNA immunization include participation of only a minor fraction of muscle cells in the uptake of DNA, exposure of the latter to deoxyribonuclease in the interstitial fluid, which in turn, necessitates the use of relatively large quantities of DNA, and often, the need to inject the plasmid into regenerating muscle so as to enhance immunity. Work ***(9,11)*** from our laboratory has shown that the use of liposome-entrapped plasmid DNA encoding the S region of hepatitis B surface antigen (HBsAg) may circumvent some of the difficulties, as it would eliminate the involvement of muscle cells and facilitate ***(7,12)*** instead the uptake of DNA by APC infiltrating the site of injection or in the lymphatics. At the same time, liposomes would protect DNA from nuclease attack ***(13)***. Moreover, transfection of APC with liposomal DNA could be promoted by the judicial choice of vesicle surface charge, size and lipid composition, or by the coentrapment, together with DNA, of other appropriate plasmids (for instance, those expressing relevant cytokines) or immunostimulatory sequences. Indeed, we have shown ***(9,11,14–16)*** already that (1) a variety of plasmid DNAs can be entrapped in neutral, anionic, or cationic liposomes, with entrapment yield being greatest when a cationic lipid is included as a liposomal component; entrapment yield does not appear to depend on the plasmid used ***(9)***, and (2) immunization of mice by a variety of routes with DNA entrapped in (cationic) liposomal or niosomal (vesicles made of nonionic surfactants) leads to much greater humoral (on the basis of splenic interleukin-4 and plasma IgG subclasses) and cell-mediated (splenic interferon-γ) immune responses than responses obtained with naked DNA or DNA that was complexed with preformed similar liposomes or niosomes. It appears that the intramuscular and subcutaneous routes are more effective in promoting immunogenicity to the encoded antigen. However, additional work with other plasmids and a variety of vesicle formulations is needed in order to optimize the system.

1.1. Liposomes: Background Research

Liposomes are vesicles made up of one or more concentric lipid bilayers alternating with aqueous spaces ***(12)***. The lipid components are usually phospholipids or other amphiphiles such as nonionic surfactants, often supplemented with cholesterol and other charged lipids. Bilayers can be in a "fluid" or "rigid" state at ambient temperature (*Ta*), depending on the nature of the amphiphile. The fluid state is achieved with amphiphiles that have a gel–liquid crystalline transition temperature (*Tc*) [the temperature at which the acyl chains melt] below *Ta*, whereas the rigid state requires amphiphiles with a *Tc* above *Ta*. Owing to their ability to entrap water- and lipid-soluble molecules in their aqueous and lipid phases, respectively, liposomes have been used since 1970 ***(17)*** as a delivery system for a great variety of pharmacologically active agents in therapeutics ***(12)***. Drug delivery with liposomes or other systems can circumvent many of the problems associated with direct drug use, for instance, toxicity as a result of indiscriminate drug action, premature drug inactivation or excretion, and inability of drugs to reach the target intracellularly. So far, medical applications ***(12)*** investigated include antimicrobial and cancer therapy, vaccines, metal detoxification, gene therapy, and enzyme or hormone therapy. In this respect, in vivo use of liposomes has been made by every conceivable route, including the intravenous, intramuscular, subcutaneous, intrathecal, intratracheal, oral, intranasal, and topical (skin and a variety of mucosal tissues) routes ***(7,12)***. Indeed, liposomes, more than any other system, have met with considerable success with several injectable liposome-based products (including a vaccine) already licensed in the United States and/or Europe and elsewhere ***(12)***.

Advances in liposome technology account for much of the progress in biomedical and other uses of liposomes ***(18)***. Such technology has evolved from the "classic" methods of the 1960s to a great variety of sophisticated techniques developed to meet particular needs. Some of these techniques provide formulations with a high entrapment yield (i.e., a high drug-to-lipid mass ratio) and are amenable to scale up. Only a few techniques, however, are applicable to water-soluble drugs, regardless of their size, charge, solubility, and other physical characteristics. Indeed, the variety and complexity of techniques for the production of drug-containing liposomes is now so great that no one laboratory has hands-on experience with all of them. Here, we describe some of the liposome technology as applied to vaccines (as such or supplemented with coadjuvants) and developed in our laboratory ***(13,19–28)*** over the last 15 years. The technology is characterized by high-yield vaccine entrapment in vesicles of an average size that ranges from about 100 nm to several microns, under conditions that preserve the biological activity of such labile agents as antigens, plasmid DNA, or attenuated microbes.

2. Materials

2.1. Entrapment of Peptide, Protein, and DNA Vaccines

2.1.1. Materials

Materials (all more than 98% pure) required for the preparation of liposome-entrapped vaccines include:

1. Egg phosphatidylcholine (PC).
2. Phosphatidic acid (PA).
3. Phosphatidylglycerol (PG).
4. Phosphatidylserine (PS).
5. Dioleylphosphatidylethanolamine (DOPE).
6. Phosphatidylethanolamine (PE).
7. Distearoyl phosphatidylcholine (DSPC).
8. Cholesterol (CHOL).
9. Triolein (TO).
10. Stearylamine (SA).
11. 1,2-*bis* (hexadecylcycloxy)-3-trimethylamino propane (BisHOP).
12. N[1-(2,3-dioleyloxy) propyl]-N,N,N-triethylammonium (DOTMA).
13. 1,2-dioleyloxy-3-(trimethylamonium propane) (DOTAP).
14. 3 (N,N,-dimethylaminoethane)-carbamyl cholesterol (DC-CHOL).
15. Sepharose (CL) 4B.
16. Polyethyleneglycol 6000 (PEG 6000).

2.1.2. Solutions

1. Thirty-two µmol of phospholipid and 32 µmol of CHOL are dissolved in chloroform (2–5 mL) or a chloroform/ethanol mixture (2:1 v/v) if required. For the preparation of negatively charged liposomes, 3.2 µmol of PA, PS, or PG; and for positively charged liposomes 3.2–8 µmol of SA, BisHOP, DOTMA, DOTAP, or DC-CHOL is also added to the chloroform. Greater or smaller amounts of charged lipids can be used depending on the required amount of surface charge on the vesicles.
2. The water-soluble vaccine (up to 10 mg) in the absence or presence of a coadjuvant (e.g., interleukin(IL-)-2, 12, or 15) is dissolved in 2 mL distilled water (H_2O) or 10 m*M* sodium phosphate buffer pH 7.2 (phosphate buffer; PB) as needed. The composition, pH, and molarity of buffer can be varied providing that this does not interfere with vesicle formation or yield of vaccine entrapment. The amount of added vaccine (and coadjuvant) can be increased or decreased proportionally to the total amount of lipid used (*see* **Subheading 2.1.2.**, **Solution 1**).

2.2. Entrapment of Large Particles, Viruses, or Bacteria Into Giant Liposomes

2.2.1. Materials (see **Subheading 2.1.1.***)*

2.2.2. Solutions

1. PC or DSPC, CHOL, PG and TO (4:4:2:1 molar ratio; 9 µmol total lipid) in 1.0 mL $CHCl_3$.
2. Lipids as in solution A dissolved in 0.5 mL diethyl ether.
3. 0.15*M* sucrose in H_2O.
4. 0.2*M* sucrose in H_2O.
5. 5% glucose in H_2O.
6. 0.1*M* sodium phosphate buffer supplemented with 0.9% NaCl, pH 7.0 (PBS).
7. Discontinuous sucrose gradient (e.g., for *Bacillus subtilis*) prepared by the use of two solutions containing 59.7 and 117.0 g of sucrose, respectively, per 100 mL H_2O in swing-out bucket centrifuge tubes.

3. Method

3.1. Entrapment of Peptide, Protein, and DNA Vaccines

1. The solution of lipids (**Subheading 2.1.2.**, **Solution 1**; however, for DNA entrapment, the preferred lipid composition is 16 µmol PC, 8 µmol PE, and 4 µmol cationic lipid; molar ratio of 8:4:2) is placed into a round-bottomed spherical Quick-fit flask (usually 50 mL vol) and the solvent is evaporated using a rotary evaporator. The lipid film formed on the walls of the flask is then flushed for about 60 s with oxygen-free nitrogen (N_2) to ensure complete solvent removal and to replace air.
2. Distilled H_2O (2 mL) (**Subheading 2.1.2.**, **Solution 2** can be used instead if **step 3** below is not detrimental to the vaccine or to the coadjuvant) is added into the flask, together with a few glass beads, and the mixture is shaken vigorously by hand or mechanically (usually for a few minutes) until the lipid film has been transformed into a milky suspension. This process is carried out above the *Tc* of the phospholipid (>*Tc*), preferably by prewarming the H_2O or **Subheading 2.1.2.**, **Solution 2** before their addition into a prewarmed flask within a shaking water bath. The liposome emulsion is allowed to stand at >*Tc* for about 1–2 h, whereupon multilamellar liposomes of diverse sizes are formed.
3. The milky suspension, devoid of glass beads, is sonicated at >*Tc* with frequent intervals of rest using a titanium probe that is slightly immersed into the emulsion. Sonication is carried out under N_2 delivered through plastic tubing. A slightly opaque to clear suspension of small unilamellar vesicles (SUV) (30–80 nm in diameter) is produced. The time required to produce SUV and the size of the vesicles depends on the amount and type of lipid used, the volume of the suspension and the diameter of the probe. For the amounts of lipid in **Subheading 2.1.2.**, **Solution 1**, a clear or slightly opaque suspension is usually obtained within up to

four sonication cycles, each lasting 30 s, with 30 s rest intervals in between, using a sonication probe of 0.75-in diameter.

4. Following sonication, the generated SUV are allowed to rest at >*Tc* for about 1–2 h, mixed with H_2O (when **Subheading 2.1.2.**, **Solution 2** was used in **step 2**) or with **Subheading 2.1.2.**, **Solution 2** (when H_2O was used in step B), rapidly frozen in liquid nitrogen and freeze-dried overnight under vacuum (<0.1 torr) in a Hetosicc freeze-dryer.
5. Water (0.1 mL per 16–32 µmol of phospholipid) previously warmed to >*Tc* is added to the freeze-dried material which is then swirled vigorously at >*Tc*. It is essential that the volume of H_2O is kept at a minimum, i.e., enough H_2O to ensure complete wetting of the powder. The sample is kept at >*Tc* for about 30 min. The process is repeated with 0.1 mL H_2O and, 30 min later at >*Tc*, with 0.8 mL PB (prewarmed at >*Tc*) and the sample is allowed to stand for 30 min at >*Tc*. This leads to the generation of multilamellar liposomes.
6. The suspension containing the multilamellar liposomes (dehydration–rehydration vesicles; DRV) with entrapped (and unentrapped material) is centrifuged at 40,000*g* for 60 min at 4°C. The liposome pellet obtained (vaccine-containing DRV) is suspended in H_2O (or PB) and centrifuged again under the same conditions. The process is repeated once again to remove the remaining unentrapped vaccine. The final pellet is suspended in 2 mL H_2O or PB. When the liposomes are to be used in vivo, NaCl is added to a final concentration of 0.9%.
7. Vaccine (and coadjuvant) entrapment in DRV liposomes is monitored by measuring the vaccine in the suspended pellet and pooled supernatants. The easiest and probably most accurate way to monitor entrapment is by using a radiolabeled vaccine (e.g., ^{125}I for a protein and ^{35}S or ^{32}P for DNA). When a radiolabel is not available or cannot be used, quantitative analysis should be employed. To that end, a sample of the liposome suspension is treated with Triton X-100 (up to 5% final concentration) or isopropanol (1 : 1 volume ratio), both of which solubilize the bilayers and free the entrapped material. In cases where the detergent, the solvent, or the solubilized liposomal lipids interfere with the assay of the material, lipids must be extracted. Long-term experience in this laboratory has shown that entrapment values can range from about 20 to nearly 100%, depending on the amount and the type of lipid and vaccine used (**Table 1**). Highest values are achieved when the net charge of vaccines is opposite to that of the charged lipid component of liposomes (**Table 2**). However, as some of the liposome-associated vaccines may have interacted (e.g., hydrophobically) with the liposomal surface during the entrapment procedure, actual entrapment of the solute (as opposed to surface-bound solute) should be determined. In the case of (radiolabeled) DNA or proteins, this can be achieved by the respective use of deoxyribonuclease ***(13)*** or a proteinase ***(25,26)***. These will degrade most of the external material on incubation at 37°C for periods of time that depend on the nature of the substrate. Upon ultracentrifugation as above, radioactivity recovered in the supernatant from the degraded material should provide a measure of vesicle surface-adsorbed vaccine biodegradation by the enzyme.

Table 1
Entrapment of Peptides and Proteins in DRV Liposomes

Material	Amount used (mg)	Phospholipid used (μmol)	Entrapment (% of used)
Tetanus toxoid	2.00	16	40–82
Bovine serum albumin	2.00	16	40–45
RIVE	0.05	16	29–31
A/Sichuan	0.05	16	38–45
rHBsAg	0.20	16	31–33
LV39	0.20	16	74–82
Interleukin-2	Up to 10^6 units	16	60–70
Poliovirus 1-VP2 peptide	0.22	16	74–82
Poliovirus-VP2 peptide	0.22	16	62–68
HBsAg S peptide	1.00	32	42–45
HBsAg S pre-S_1 peptide	1.00	32	46–48

Note. Materials were entrapped as described in the text. RIVE, reconstituted influenza virus envelopes; A/Sichuan, A/Sichuan influenza virus hemagglutinin and neuraminidase; rHBsAg, recombinant hepatitis B surface antigen; LV39, *Leishmania major* antigen (mixed isolate); HBsAg, full-length hepatitis B surface antigen. Synthetic S peptide had a 110-137 amino acid sequence; synthetic pre-S_1 peptide sequence was 15–48.

8. This step and the one following are required when vaccine-containing DRV liposomes must be converted into smaller vesicles (down to about 100 nm *z* average diameter). To that end, the liposomal suspension obtained in **step 5** (i.e., before the separation of the entrapped from the nonentrapped vaccine) is diluted with H_2O to 10 mL and then passed for a number of cycles through a Microfluidizer 110S (Microfluidics) with the pressure gage set at 60 psi throughout the procedure to give a flow rate of 35 mL per min. The number of cycles used depends on the vesicle size required (**Table 3**) or the sensitivity of the entrapped vaccine. For instance, plasmid DNA will be denatured (as judged by gel electrophoresis) when microfluidized for more than three cycles using the above conditions ***(13)***. It has also been observed ***(20)*** that the greater the number of cycles, the lower the amount of drug or vaccine is retained by the vesicles. Alternatively, samples can also be microfluidized after the removal of unentrapped vaccine as in **step 6**. In this case, however, drug retention by the liposomes is reduced ***(20)***. It is likely that the presence of unentrapped material during microfluidization diminishes solute leakage, possibly by reducing the osmotic rupture of vesicles and/or the initial concentration gradient across the bilayer membranes ***(20)***.
9. Reduction of the volume (about 10 mL) of the microfluidized sample can, if needed, be effected by covering the sample (in dialysis tubing) with PEG 6000 flakes within a flat container. Removal of excess H_2O from the tubing is relatively rapid (within 30–60 min) and it is therefore prudent to monitor the sample

Table 2
Incorporation of Plasmid DNA into Liposomes by the Dehydration-Rehydration Method

	Incorcopated plasmid DNA (% of used)					
Liposomes	pGL2	pRc/CMV HBS	pRSVGH	pCMV4.65	pCMV4. EGFP	VR1020
PC, DOPE[a]	44.2	55.4	45.6	28.6		
PC, DOPE[b]	12.1		11.3			
PC, DOPE, PS[a]	57.3					
PC, DOPE, PS[b]	12.6					
PC, DOPE, PG[a]			53.5			
PC, DOPE, PG[b]			10.2			
PC, DOPE, SA[a]	74.8					
PC, DOPE, SA[b]	48.3					
PC, DOPE, BisHOP[a]	69.3					
PC, DOPE, DOTMA[a]	86.8					
PC, DOPE, DC-Chol[a]		87.1	76.9			
PC, DOPE, DC-Chol[b]			77.2			
PC, DOPE, DOTAP[a]		80.1	79.8	52.7	71.9	89.6
PC, DOPE, DOTAP[b]		88.6	80.6	67.7		81.6
PC, DOPE, DODAP[a]			57.4			
PC, DOPE, DODAP[b]			64.8			

^{35}S-labeled plasmid DNA (10–500 µg) was incorporated ([a]) into or mixed ([b]) with neutral (PC, DOPE), anionic (PC, DOPE, PS, or PG) or cationic (PC, DOPE, SA, BisHOP, DOTMA, DC-Chol, DOTAP, or DODAP) dehydration-rehydration vesicles (DRV). Incorporation values for the different amounts of DNA used for each of the liposomal formulations did not differ significantly and were therefore pooled (values shown are means of values obtained from 3–5 experiments). PC (16 µmol) was used in molar ratios of 1:0.5 (neutral) and 1:0.5:0:25 anionic and cationic liposomes). PC, egg phosphatidylcholine; DOPE, dioleoyl phosphatidylethanolamine; PS, phosphatidylserine; PG, phosphatidylglycerol; SA, stearylamine; BisHOP, 1,2-*bis* (hexadecylcycloxy)-3-trimethylaminopropane; DOTMA, N[1-(2,3-dioleoyloxy)propyl]-N,N,N, triethylammonium; DC-Chol, 3 -(N,N-dimethylaminoethane) carbonyl cholesterol; DOTAP, 1,2-dioleoyl-3(trimethylammonium) propane; DODAP, 1,2-dioleoyl-3-dimethylammonium propane. Plasmid DNAs used encoded luciferase (pGL2), hepatitis B surface antigen (S region) (pRc/CMV HBS), human growth hormone (pRSVGH), mycobacterium leprosy protein (pCMV 4.65), "fluorescent green protein" (pCMV 4.EGFP) and schistosome protein (VR1020).

regularly. On reaching the required volume, the sample is treated for the separation of entrapped from the unentrapped vaccine. This is carried out by molecular sieve chromatography using a Sepharose CL 4B colum, with vaccine-containing liposomes eluting at the end of the void volume. Vaccine content within liposomes is estimated as in **step 7** and expressed as % of vaccine in the original preparation obtained in **step 6**. (As the sample is microfluidized following **step 5**, i.e., before the estimation of entrapment, a small portion of the sample to be

Table 3
z-Average Mean Size (nm) of Microfluidized DRVs[a]

	Number of cycles				
DRVs and medium	1.8	3.5	5.2	7.1	10.6
Washed					
Water	463.5	149.9	115.0	121.9	114.7
PBS	447.4	198.6	168.1	159.5	155.7
Unwashed					
Water	473.9	132.9	116.9	116.6	101.9
PBS	456.3	186.2	186.7	169.8	159.9

[a]maltrose-containing washed or unwashed DRVs (32 μmol PC) were microfluidized in the presence of water or PBS for up to 10.6 cycles, and samples were measured for vesicle size (diameter in nanometers) by dynamic light scattering (photon correlation spectroscopy). Polydispersity indexes ranged from 0.503 to 0.653 (water) and from 0.517 to 0.653 (PBS).

microfluidized is kept aside for the estimation of entrapment according to **step 6**). Vesicle size measurements are carried out by photon correlation spectroscopy as described elsewhere *(13,26)*. Vesicle size obtained after 10 cycles of microfluidation is about 100–160 nm in diameter, depending on whether microfluidization was carried out in H_2O or PB, using unwashed or washed liposomes (**Table 3**).

3.2. Entrapment by Large Particles, Viruses, or Bacteria Into Giant Liposomes

1. One mL of solution 3 is mixed by vortexing for 45 s with solution 1.
2. The resulting water-in-chloroform emulsion is mixed by vortexing for 15 s with solution B and 2.5 mL solution 4
3. The water-in-oil-in water emulsion formed is placed in a 250-mL conical flask and the organic solvents are evaporated by flushing N_2 at 37°C, while the sample is gently agitated in a shaking incubator. This generates (sucrose-containing) giant liposomes.
4. The giant liposomes are washed by centrifugation over solution 5 in a bench centrifuge at 600*g* for 5 min, and the liposomal pellet is resuspended in 1 mL PBS.
5. The resuspended pellet of giant liposomes is mixed with 1 mL of a suspension of particulate matter (e.g., killed or live *B.subtilis* spores or killed Bacille Calmete-Guerin (BCG) bacteria). The suspended mixture is then freeze-dried overnight under vacuum (<0.1 torr) in a Hetosicc freeze-dryer.
6. The freeze-dried material is rehydrated, with 0.1 mL H_2O at 20°C (rehydration of liposomes containing the "high melting" DSPC at >*Tc* does not have a significant effect on the percent entrapment of materials; **ref.** *27*), swirled vigorously and allowed to stand at >*Tc* for 30 min. The process is repeated after the successive addition of 0.1 mL PBS, and of 0.8 mL PBS 30 min later (1 mL total suspension volume).

Table 4
Entrapment of *Bacillus subtilis* and Tetanus Toxoid in Giant Liposomes

	Entrapped material (% of that used)[a]	
	B.subtilis	Tetanus toxoid
Liposomes		
PC, cholesterol, PG, TO	26.7Å12.1 (7)	8.4Å2.6 (4)
DSPC, cholesterol, PG, TO	21.3Å8.9 (6)	11.1Å1.9 (4)

[a] ^{125}I-labeled *B.subtilis* and tetanus toxoid were entrapped in giant liposomes as described. Results, based on radioactivity measurements, are expressed as percentages (ÅSD) of material used for entrapment. In one experiment, entrapment of ^{125}I-labeled BCG in PC giant liposomes was 27.8%. Numbers in parentheses denote numbers of preparations.

7. Separation of the entrapped particulate material from unentrapped material (e.g., *B.subtilis*) is carried out by sucrose gradient centrifugation by placing the suspension (1 mL) on top of the sucrose gradient (solution 7) followed by centrifugation for 1.5 h at 90,000*g* in a Dupont Combi Plus ultracentrifuge using a swing-out bucket. One-mL fractions are then pipeted out from the top of the gradient and assayed for spore or bacteria content. As with proteins and DNA (*see* **Subheading 2.2.2., item 7**), it is convenient to use radiolabelled (e.g., ^{125}I-labeled) spores or bacteria to monitor content. In the case of *B.subtilis* spores or BCG bacteria, these are recovered at the bottom fraction of the gradient when unentrapped. In contrast, entrapped material is recovered mostly in the top seven fractions of the gradient in association with liposomes ***(21)***.
8. Pooled fractions containing the entrapped spores or bacteria are dialysed exhaustively against PBS until all sucrose has been eliminated. The dialyzed material is centrifuged as in step 4 and the liposomal pellet resuspended in 1 mL PBS for further use. Typical values of *B.subtilis* or BCG entrapment are shown in **Table 4**.

4. Notes

1. The dehydration-rehydration procedures for the entrapment of vaccines (e.g., peptides, proteins, plasmid DNA) and other macromolecules or particulates such as spores, bacteria, and viruses as outlined here are straightforward, mild, and thus compatible with labile materials. Normally, the time required to obtain the final formulation of a liposome-entrapped vaccine is short and does not exceed 2 d. Moreover, it has been shown ***(27)*** that vaccine-containing liposomes as prepared here can be freeze-dried (for storage) in the presence of a cryoprotectant without significant loss of material from within the vesicles on reconstitution with 0.9% NaCl. With both procedures, the most important step is that of rehydration (**Subheading 3.1., step 5** and **Subheading 3.2., step 6**): it is important that water added during the initial rehydration is kept to a minimum volume.
2. The immunoadjuvant action of liposomes with water soluble antigens such as tetanus toxoid appears to be greater when low melting phospholipids (i.e., those with a low *Tc*) are used in the liposome formulation or when the weight ratio of

Table 5
Incorporation of Tetanus Toxoid and Interleukins into Liposomes

Antigen	Interleukin	Tetanus toxoid (% entrapped)	Interleukin (% entrapped)
Tetanus toxoid	—	30–55%	
Tetanus toxoid	IL-2	43.0	48.9
Tetanus toxoid	IL-15	31.7	32.3

Tetanus toxoid (20–50 μg) without or with recombinant interleukin 2 (2–5 × 10^5 U) or simian recombinant interleukin 15 (2.5 × 10^4 U) were entrapped or co-entrapped in dehydration-rehydration vesicles (DRV liposomes) composed of 16 mol PC and equimolar cholesterol. For details on entrapment measurements *see* **refs. *31*** and ***32***.

Table 6
The Effect of IL-2 on Immune Responses Against Liposomal Tetanus Toxoid

	IgG ($\log_{10}$ reciprocal end point dilution)		
Liposomal preparation	IgG_1	IgG_{2a}	IgG_{2b}
(A) Entrapped toxoid	2.7Å0.4	1.3Å0.0	2.4Å0.0
(B) Coentrapped toxoid and IL-2	4.1Å0.4	3.3Å0.5	3.7Å0.7[a]
(C) Separately entrapped toxoid and IL-2	2.5Å0.0	13Å0.0	2.0Å0.0

Mice were immunized on days 0 and 29 with 0.1 μg tetanus toxoid entrapped alone (A), together with IL-2 (145 U) (B) or in mixture with separately entrapped IL-2 (145 U) (C) and bled on day 39. Liposomes were composed of 16 mol PC and equimolar cholesterol. The toxoid was used in amounts (e.g., 0.1 μg) that were too low for liposomes to exhibit significant immunoadjuvant action. Secondary responses (shown in the table) to the toxoid entrapped together with IL-2 in the same liposomes (B) were significantly greater (10–15-fold; P<0.01–0.05), than those observed with groups A and C.

[a]Values were not significantly different (for more details, *see* **ref. *31***).

phospholipid to entrapped antigen is high ***(22,29,30)***. It should be noted, however, that a plethora of publications ***(7)*** since 1974 have successfully employed a great variety of lipid compositions for a wide range of antigens. It is generally accepted that there is no liposomal composition that is ideal for all antigens and that the characteristics of a liposomal formulation should be optimized for a given antigen. However, liposomal adjuvanticity can be augmented further by the coentrapment together with the antigen of cytokines such as IL-2 ***(31)***, or IL-15 ***(32)***. Coentrapment of cytokine with the antigen is straightforward and values of entrapment for each of the two proteins are not interfered with by each other's presence (**Table 5**). Interestingly, the coadjuvant action of both cytokines is present when coentrapped with the antigen, but not when separately entrapped ***(31,32)*** (**Table 6**).

3. Entrapment of plasmid DNA into liposomes by the present method is, as expected, most efficient when a cationic lipid is one of the liposomal components, which include PC and DOPE (**Table 2**). Both the fusogenic DOPE and the cationic lipid are known to promote DNA transfection by mechanisms which are hitherto unclear. Recent in vivo work ***(9,11,14–16)*** with two different antigen-encoding plasmid DNAs has clearly shown that humoural and cell-mediated immune responses to the encoded antigen are, as already mentioned, much greater than those seen with the naked or complexed plasmid. It appears that responses are similar regardless of the cationic lipid used ***(11)***, but are best when PE is included in the liposomal formulation ***(15)***.

Acknowledgement

We thank Concha Perring for excellent secretarial assistance.

References

1. Gregoriadis, G., Allison A. C., and Poste, G., eds. (1993) *Vaccines: Recent Trends and Progress*. Plenum, New York.
2. Powel, M. F. and Newman, M. J., eds. (1995) *Vaccine Design:The Subunit and Adjuvant Approach*. Plenum, New York.
3. Allison, A. C. and Gregoriadis, G. (1974) Liposomes as immunological adjuvants. *Nature* **252,** 252.
4. Manesis, E. K., Cameron, C. H., and Gregoriadis, G. (1978) Incorporation of hepatitis-B surface antigen (HB_sAg) into liposomes. *Biochem. Soc. Trans.* **6,** 925–928.
5. Gregoriadis, G. and Allison, A. C. (1974) Entrapment of proteins in liposomes prevents allergic reactions in preimmunised mice. *FEBS Lett.* **45,** 71–74.
6. Alving, C. R. (1991) Liposomes as carriers of antigens and adjuvants. *Immunol. Meth.* **140,** 1–13.
7. Gregoriadis, G. (1990) Immunological adjuvants: a role for liposomes. *Immunol. Today* **11,** 89–97.
8. Chattergoon, M., Boyer, J., and Weiner, D. B. (1997) Genetic immunization: a new era in vaccines and immune therapeutics. *The FASEB J.* **11,** 754–763.
9. Gregoriadis, G. (1998) Genetic vaccines: strategies for optimization. *Pharmaceut. Res.* **15,** 661–670.
10. Davis, H. L., Whalen, R. G., and Demeneix, B. A. (1993) Direct gene transfer in skeletal muscle in vivo: factors influencing efficiency of transfer and stability of expression. *Hum. Gene Ther.* **4,** 151–156.
11. Gregoriadis, G., Saffie, R., and de Souza, B. (1997) Liposome-mediated DNA vaccination. *FEBS Lett.* **402,** 107–110.
12. Gregoriadis, G. (1995) Engineering targeted liposomes: progress and problems. *Trends in Biotechnol.* **13,** 527–537.
13. Gregoriadis, G., Saffie, R., and Hart, S. L. (1996) High yield incorporation of plasmid DNA within liposomes: Effect on DNA integrity and transfection efficiency. *J. Drug Targeting* **3,** 469–475.

14. McCormack, B. and Gregoriadis, G. (1998) Liposome-mediated DNA immunization with a plasmid encoding a Mycobacterium leprae antigen. *J. Liposome Res.* **8,** 48–49.
15. Perrie, Y. and Gregoriadis, G. (1998) Liposome-mediated vaccination: the effect of vesicle composition. *J. Liposome Res.* **8,** 95–96.
16. Obrenovic, M. M., Perrie, Y., and Gregoriadis, G. (1998) Entrapment of plasmid DNA into niosomes: characterization studies. *J. Pharm. Pharmacol.* **50,** S155.
17. Gregoriadis, G. and Ryman, B. E. (1972) Lysosomal localization of fructofuranosidase-containing liposomes injected into rats. Some implications in the treatment of genetic disorders. *Biochem. J.* **129,** 123–133.
18. Gregoriadis, G., ed. (1993) *Liposome Technology*, 2nd edition, vol. I-III. CRC Press, Boca Raton, FL.
19. Kirby, C. and Gregoriadis, G. (1984) Dehydration-rehydration vesicles (DRV): a new method for high yield drug entrapment in liposomes. *Biotechnology* **2,** 979–984
20. Gregoriadis, G., da Silva, H., and Florence, A. T. (1990) A procedure for the efficient entrapment of drugs in dehydration-rehydration liposomes (DRV). *Int. J. Pharmaceut.* **65,** 235–242.
21. Antimisiaris, S., Jayasekera, P., and Gregoriadis, G. (1993) Liposomes as vaccine carriers: incorporation of soluble and particulate antigens in giant vesicles. *J. Immunol. Meth.* **166,** 271–280.
22. Gregoriadis, G., Davis, D., and Davies, A. (1987) Liposomes as immunological adjuvants: antigen incorporation studies. *Vaccine* **5,** 143–149
23. Garcon, N., Gregoriadis, G., Taylor, M., and Summerfield, J. (1988) Targeted immunoadjuvant action of tetanus toxoid-containing liposomes coated with mannosylated albumin. *Immunology* **64,** 743–745.
24. Gregoriadis, G., Wang, Z., Barenholz, Y., and Francis, M. J. (1993) Liposome-entrapped T-cell peptide provides help for a co-entrapped B-cell peptide to overcome genetic restriction in mice and induce immunological memory. *Immunology* **80,** 535–540.
25. Senior, J. and Gregoriadis, G. (1989) Dehydration-rehydration vesicle methodology facilitates a novel approach to antibody binding to liposomes. *Biochim. Biophys. Acta* **1003,** 58–62.
26. Skalko, N., Bouwstra, J., Spies, F., Stuart, M., Frederik, P. M., and Gregoriadis, G. (1998) Morphological observations on liposomes bearing covalently bound protein: studies with freeze-fracture and cryo-electron microscopy and small angle X-ray scattering techniques. *Biochim. Biophys. Acta* **1370,** 151–160.
27. Gursel, I., Antimisiaris, S. G., Jayasekera, P., and Gregoriadis, G. (1995) in *Liposomes in Biomedical Applications* (Shek, P., ed.), Harwood Academic, pp. 35–50.
28. McCormack, B. and Gregoriadis, G. (1996) Comparative studies of the fate of free and liposome-entrapped hydroxypropyl-β-cyclodextrin/drug complexes after intravenous injection into rats: Implications in drug delivery. *Biochim. Biophys. Acta* **1291,** 237–244.
29. Davis, D. and Gregoriadis, G. (1987) Liposomes as adjuvants with immunopurified tetanus toxoid: influence of liposomal characteristics. *Immunology* **61,** 229–234.

30. Davis, D. and Gregoriadis, G. (1989) Primary immune response to liposomal tetanus toxoid in mice: the effect of mediators. *Immunology* **68,** 277–282.
31. Gürsel, M. and Gregoriadis, G. (1997) Interleukin-2 as a co-adjuvant for liposomal tetanus toxoid: the effect of cytokine and antigen mode of localization in the vesicles. *J. Drug Targeting* **5,** 93–98.
32. Gürsel, M. and Gregoriadis, G. (1997) Interleukin-15 acts as an immunological co-adjuvant for liposomal antigen in vivo. *Immunol. Lett.* **55,** 161–165.

9

Immunopotentiating Reconstituted Influenza Virosomes (IRIVs)

Reinhard Glück

1. Introduction

Immunization is the most effective defense mechanism against microbial infections today. Although highly effective vaccines are currently available for a number of infectious diseases, vaccine formulations can still be improved in a number of important areas. Issues of safety, stability, delivery, and combining vaccines to several pathogens need to be addressed. For many diseases, a greater understanding of microbial pathogenesis and the basis for protective immunity is still needed. The ability to induce antigen-specific humoral and cell-mediated immunity is crucial to the development of effective prophylactic and therapeutic vaccines.

In the past, vaccine development was mainly empirical, and based on attempts to mimic natural infection. Vaccinology has entered a new era, which might be linked to rational drug design vs brute force screening. The development of new or improved vaccines will rely on a sophisticated understanding of the molecular biology, mechanisms of pathogenesis, and interactions with the immune system particular to a given pathogen. As information continues to accumulate, it is becoming increasingly obvious that the immune response to natural infection by microbial pathogens does not define the limits of the possible immune responses to those antigens. It may also not represent the optimal protective response. Pathogens can influence the spectrum of the immune response, often subverting the capacity of the immune system to aggressively interfere with the infectious process *(1)*. In addition, certain aspects of the natural immune response contribute to or are largely responsible for pathogenesis associated with natural infection (e.g., inflammation or immune suppression).

From: *Methods in Molecular Medicine, Vol. 42:*
Vaccine Adjuvants: Preparation Methods and Research Protocols
Edited by: D. T. O'Hagan © Humana Press, Inc., Totowa, NJ

These detrimental responses are often separable from, and even antagonistic to, responses necessary for protection. Thus, it is crucial to develop an understanding for the mechanisms through which pathogens can drive various effector arms of the immune response (e.g., through antigen processing and presentation, cytokine induction, and TH1 vs TH2 helper T-cell responses). Subunit immunogens containing subsets of pathogen proteins formulated, adjuvanted, and delivered in a variety of ways, represent powerful tools for dissecting and manipulating the immune response to complex pathogens. In challenge models, they can be utilized to determine the correlates of protective immunity and immune response pathogenesis. Information from such studies are supportive of custom designing subunit vaccines capable of eliciting protective immunity while avoiding undesirable side effects.

One of the major unsolved problems in vaccinology is immune potentiation, that is, making small antigens or molecular vaccines sufficiently immunogenic. This problem is all the more difficult when one considers the possibility of using peptides rather than proteins as the basis for vaccines to induce protection against diseases.

The basic requirement for a vaccine is a structure capable of T-cell responses and of eliciting antibodies that react with a protein on the pathogen surface that is known to be a target for protective immunity. The structure that induces these antibodies can be either a whole protein (purified from the pathogen or prepared by recombinant technology), or a portion of this protein, i.e., peptide (prepared by chemical synthesis). In the case of bacterial pathogens, purified polysaccharides can often serve as the antigen to induce protective antibodies against the microorganism. The induction of a full immune response, i.e., memory response, requires cooperation between T lymphocytes, which recognize epitope on the protein and B lymphocytes that recognize the structure of the protein.

Studies with enveloped viruses have indicated that cognate help for B cells recognizing surface glycoproteins can be provided by Th epitopes that reside within the virus particles *(2)*. Thus, Th lymphocytes can recognize sites on proteins other than those recognized by B cells. In principle, one should therefore be able to design vaccines in which structural B epitopes are associated in a noncovalent fashion with a source of T epitopes. Covalent conjugation is traditionally used when trying to elicit antibodies against peptides or polysaccharides. In these cases, the hapten or B epitope is covalently bound to proteins such as tetanus toxoid. The immunogenicity of the carrier protein may, however, have undesired consequences such as carrier suppression. The coupling procedure may also lead to an alteration of the peptide structure or to the formation of adducts against which the immune response may be preferentially directed.

Because of their membranous structure, virosomes are capable of combining numerous epitopes (both B and T, as well as whole proteins or polysaccharides) within the same structure. In addition to this ability to copresent multiple antigens, the natural targeting of virosomes to macrophages makes them an ideal candidate for copresentation of various epitopes.

In this chapter, we shall review preparation, characterization, and current advances in virosome design and immunological effects of different vaccine antigens in humans. We shall discuss the adjuvant effect of these so-called immunopotentiating reconstituted influenza virosomes in connection with classical viral and bacterial antigens, with synthetic and recombinant peptide antigen vaccines, and finally with DNA nucleotides. We shall present immunological results from preclinical and clinical trials. Finally, we shall give an overview of product licensing and product distribution worldwide of immunopotentiating reconstituted influenza virosome (IRIV) based vaccines.

1.1. The Virosomal Vaccine Approach

The most significant impediment to the use of synthetic peptides as vaccines has been that they are only weak or nonimmunogenic when injected by themselves into animals *(3,4)*. This property has necessitated the use of carriers, usually large, highly "immunogenic" proteins, to which the peptides are covalently coupled. These carriers, although helpful in producing an initial antibody response, have no relationship to the pathogen against which the vaccine is designed and therefore do not elicit pathogen-specific T-cell help. Therefore, when an individual who has been vaccinated with a peptide-carrier complex is challenged with the pathogen, a primary rather than a secondary (faster, stronger, higher affinity) response results. Also, booster immunizations often lead to a stronger antibody response to the carrier and a diminishing one to the peptide. In addition, these peptide-carrier complexes must usually be combined with other adjuvants (for example, Freund's) to enhance the response to the peptide. These adjuvants frequently induce undesirable side effects which make them unacceptable for use in humans *(3–14)*.

It has been hypothesized that anchorage of a peptide in a liposomal bilayer might mimic the normal presentation of antigen on an infectious agent (i.e., multivalent and projecting outward from an anchor on the surface of the cell) and thereby potentiate the immune response to the peptide. To test this hypothesis, peptides were covalently linked to a phospholipid, providing a hydrophobic anchorage into the phospholipid bilayer.

It has been found that when molecules capable of stimulating T-helper cells (either viral envelope proteins or peptides representing defined Th cell epitopes) are integrated into the same phospholipid matrix as a B-cell epitope, a highly efficient immunogen is produced *(15,16)*. Sequences not recognized by T-helper cells do not elicit antibody responses, even when formulated into peptide-phospholipid complexes *(17)*.

Current concepts regarding the mechanisms through which peptide epitopes are presented to CD8+, major histocompatibility complex (MHC) Class I -restricted cytotoxic T lymphocytes (CTL) indicate that a crucial aspect of this process is the capacity to introduce antigen into the cytoplasm (but not endosomes) of antigen-presenting cells *(18)*. This explains, at least in part, the success of live-attenuated and live-vector vaccines for stimulating cell-mediated immune responses.

In order to obtain a similar mechanism, methods have been introduced for integrating lipid-linked peptides (membrane proteins) into the lipid bilayer of large, mainly unilamellar liposomes *(19)*. For example, glycoproteins of influenza and parainfluenza type I (Sendai) viruses maintain their receptor-binding activities and receptor-induced endocytosis when reconstituted into protein lipid vesicles (virosomes) *(20,21)*. In addition, water-soluble materials can be encapsulated within the aqueous interior of such vesicles at high efficiency. It could even be shown that these vesicles act as effective delivery vehicles for drugs, proteins, and DNA. Using a liposome based system they were employed to achieve the first stable gene transfer in animals *(22,20)*.

Virosomes proved to also be highly effective immunogens in mice, rabbits, and monkeys *(23,24)*. This included the ability to stimulate strong CD8+ CTL responses to lipid bilayer-integrated glycoproteins or lipid-linked peptides, as well as to encapsulated peptides, proteins, and formalin-fixed whole viruses *(17,23,24)*.

1.2. Immunopotentiating Reconstituted Influenza Virosomes

Twenty years after the discovery of the immunological adjuvant properties of liposomes *(25)* and the ensuing multitude of related animal immunization studies *(26)*, liposomes as adjuvants have come of age *(27,28)* with the first liposome-based vaccine against hepatitis A being licensed for use in humans. Vaccines based on novasomes (nonphospholipid biodegradable, pausilamellar vesicles formed from single-chain amphiphiles, with or without other lipids) have also been licensed for the immunization of fowl against Newcastle disease virus and avian reovirus *(29)*.

As forementioned, the way in which liposomes induce immune responses to antigen is not clear, but has been attributed to a depot effect (slow release of antigen and the ability of vesicles and the associated antigen to migrate to regional lymph nodes following local injection). In the case of liposomes, further improvement of adjuvanticity has been achieved by the use of coadjuvants such as lipopolysaccharides, positively or negatively charged lipids, interleukin 2 (IL-2), and by ligand-mediated targeting to antigen-presenting cells *(29)*.

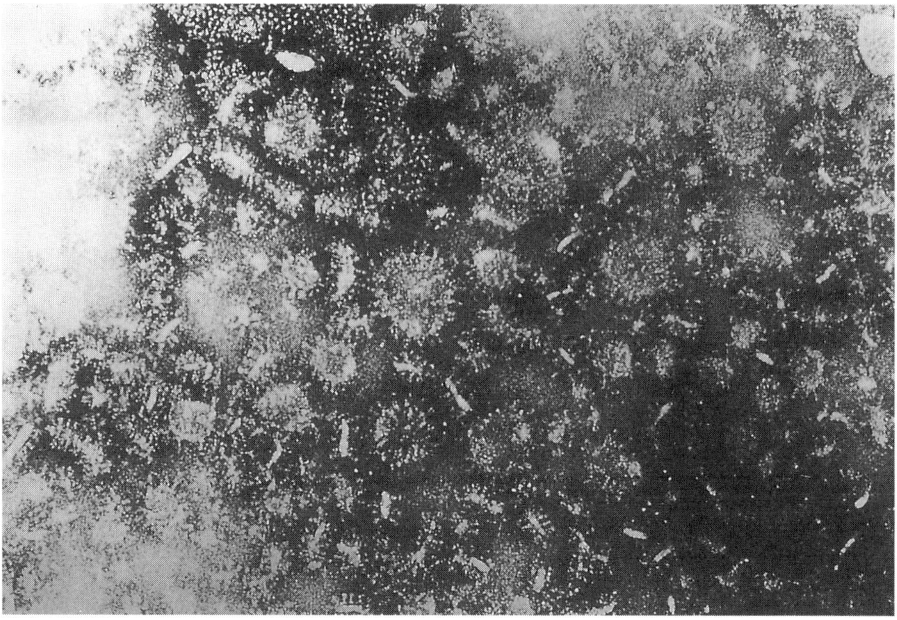

Fig. 1. Transmission electron micrograph of IRIV (× 100,000). The electron micrograph of the IRIVs shows spherical unilamellar vesicles with a mean diameter of ~150 nm. The vesicles show spike projections of ~15 nm, which originate from influenza glycoproteins (E. M. by T. Wyler, Berne).

The approach adapted for the IRIV vaccines is of particular interest, as it combines several components that are known to contribute to immunostimulation and that are at the same time harmless.

IRIVs are spherical, unilamellar vesicles with a mean diameter of ~150 nm. They show short surface projections of 10–15 nm (**Fig. 1**). IRIVs are prepared by detergent removal of influenza surface glycoproteins and a mixture of natural and synthetic phospholipids containing 70% egg yolk phosphatidylcholine (EYPC), 20% synthetic phosphatidylethanolamine (PE), and 10% envelope phospholipids originating from H1N1 influenza virus (A/Singapore/6/86) *(28)* (**Fig. 2**).

EYPC is known to be well tolerated in humans and is an important constituent in commercial solutions for iv applications in undernourished persons. EYPC has been used in nearly all liposomal preparations that were produced for the enhancement of immune responses. PE was chosen for two reasons; first, antigens can be covalently coupled to virosomes via the free aminoacid groups of PE *(30)*, also, it has been shown that liposomes containing PE are able to directly stimulate B cells to produce antibodies without any T-cell

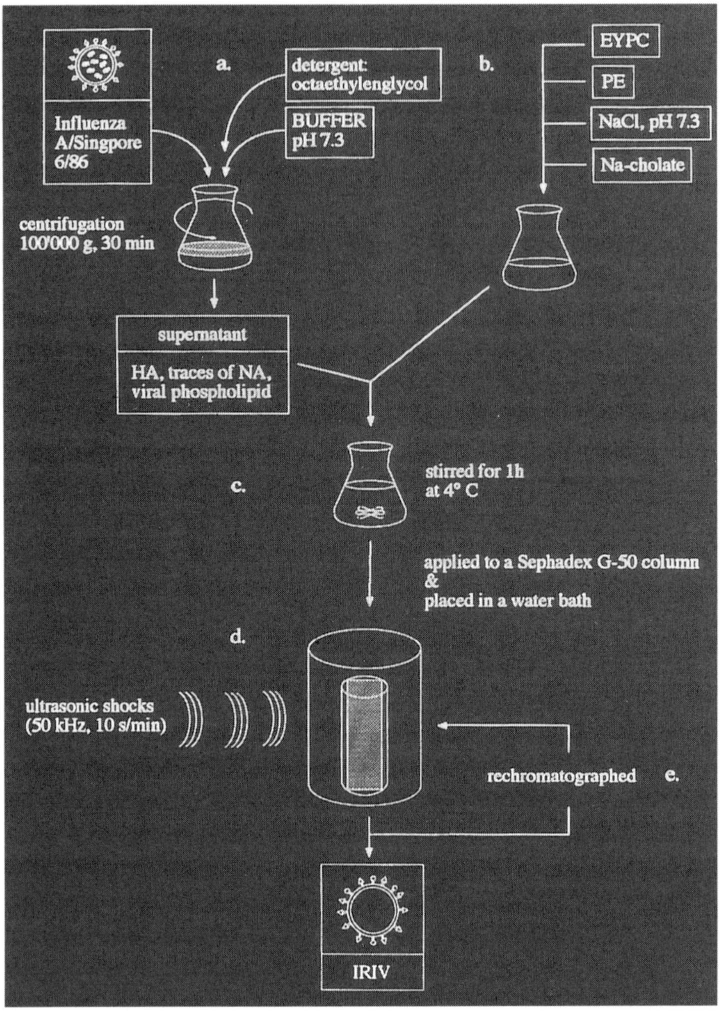

Fig. 2. Production scheme for IRIVs EYPC, egg yolk phosphatidylcholine; PE, phosphatidylethanolamine; HA, hemagglutinin; Na, neuraminidase.

determinant being present *(31)*. There were several reasons for including influenza virus envelope glycoproteins: the hemagglutinin (HA) plays a key role in the mode of action of the IRIVs. HA is the major antigen of influenza virus, containing epitopes on both HA1 and HA2 polypeptides, and is responsible for the fusion of the virus with the endosomal membrane *(32,33)*. The HA1 globular head groups contain the sialic acid site for HA and it is therefore expected that the IRIVs bind to such receptors of antigen-presenting cells (e.g.,

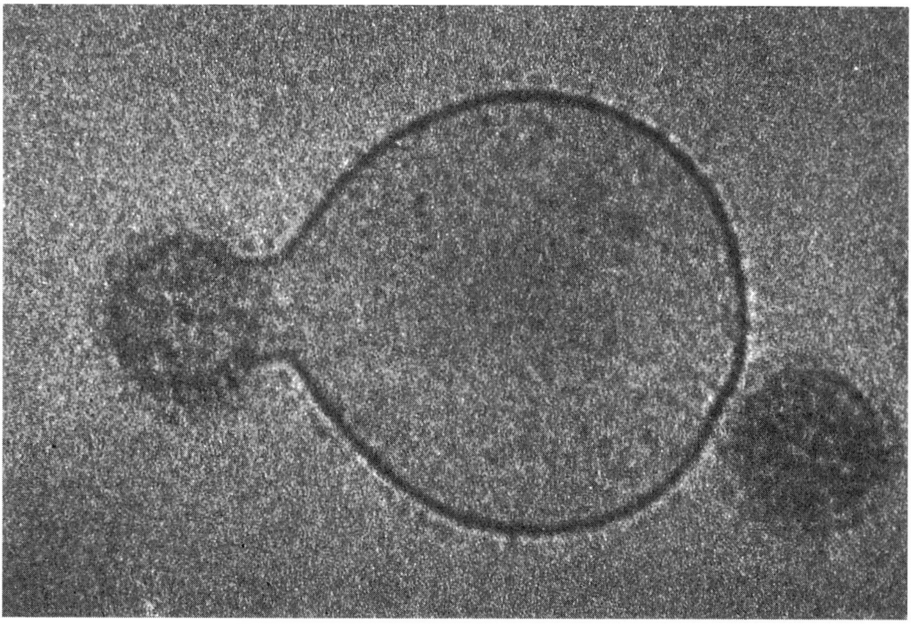

Fig. 3. Electron micrograph of a fusion event between an influenza virosome and an artificial membrane at pH 5.0. (With kind permission of Dr. P. M. Frederik, University of Limburg, Maastricht, The Netherlands.)

macrophages, lymphocytes) initiating a successful immune response. The entry of influenza viruses into cells occurs through HA-receptor-mediated endocytosis *(34)*. It is likely that this mechanism also functions with the IRIV particles. The HA2 subunit of HA mediates the fusion of viral and endosomal membranes, which is required in order to initiate infection of cells. At the low pH of the host-cell endosome (~pH 5.0), a conformational change occurs in the HA that is a prerequisite for fusion to occur. Fusion activity tests have shown that there was no difference of activity between influenza virus and IRIV (**Fig. 3**). It is expected that this mediates the rapid release of the transported antigen into the membranes of the target cells *(35)* (**Fig. 4**).

Further immunopotentiating effects have recently been described for the influenza virus HA: studies provide evidence for an alternative stimulation of peritoneal B lymphocytes by HA, a so-called B-cell "superstimulatory" antigen *(35)*. This finding implies that the B-cell superstimulatory influenza virus glycoprotein has been evolutionarily adapted to activate not only conventional B2 cells, but in addition, a B-cell subset that represents a major weapon in the first line of defense against invading microorganisms. The great potency of B1 cells to build up an immediate immune response against microbial antigen

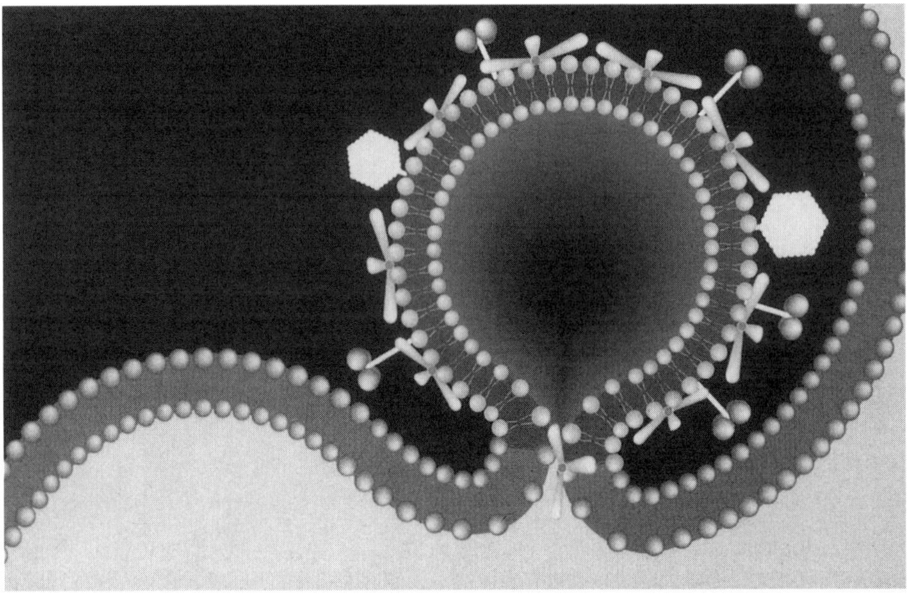

Fig. 4. Computergraph of fusion event between IRIV carrying two hepatitis A particles and the endosomal membrane at pH 5.0. Note the change of conformation of the HA-trimer, which is a prerequisite for exposing the internalized fusion peptide and induction of fusion.

is paralleled by its increased susceptibility to cross react with "third party" antigen. This phenomenon has been further investigated by showing that this new example of B-cell stimulation by multivalent type-2 antigen (e.g., HA) seems to be mediated by a phosphatidyl-inositol- and Ca^{2+} -independent signaling pathway *(36)*. In addition, it has been reported that B-cell superstimulatory influenza virus (H2-subtype) induced B-cell proliferation by a protein kinase C (PKC)-activating, Ca^{2+} -independent mechanism.

Furthermore, influenza A virus has been described as a model system for the study of viral antigen presentation to CTL *(37)*. In the clinical part of this chapter, the potent effect of IRIV designed influenza vaccine on the cellular immune system is mentioned.

The second influenza glycoprotein exposed on the IRIV surface, the enzyme neuraminidase (NA), is a tetramer composed of four equal, spherical subunits that are hydrophobically embedded in the membrane by a central stalk. The entire enzymatic activity takes place in the region of the head. NA catalyzes the cleavage of N-acetylneuraminic acid (sialic acid) from bound sugar residues *(38)*. In the mucus, this process leads to a decrease in viscosity and allows the influenza virus easier access to epithelial cells. In the area of the cell membrane, the same process leads to destruction of the HA receptor. The consequence of this is, first, that newly formed virus particles do not adhere to the host cell membrane after budding, and second, that aggregation of the viruses is prevented. NA therefore allows the influenza virus to retain its mobility. In terms of the IRIV, these characteristics of NA can, in theory, be utilized in that, after coupling with HA, IRIVs not taken up by phagocytosis could be cleaved off again and would therefore not be lost. Also, the reduction in viscosity of the mucus could be useful in connection with the development of a nasal IRIV vaccine.

Recently, a chimeric influenza virus has been constructed that expressed the highly amino acid sequence ELDKWA of *gp41* of human immunodeficiency virus type 1 (HIV-1) ***(39)***. Muster et al. could demonstrate that intranasal immunization of mice with this chimeric virus was also able to induce a humoral immune response at the mucosal level. They concluded that influenza virus can be used to efficiently induce antibodies against antigens from foreign pathogens by mucosal immunization.

The excellent characteristics of IRIVs as adjuvants have been demonstrated in several systems. IRIVs were first utilized in the manufacture of a hepatitis A vaccine. This contains formalin-inactivated and highly purified hepatitis A viruses (HAV) of strain RGSB, cultured on human diploid cells, which are electrostatically coupled to the IRIV vesicle ***(28)***. The surface spikes (HA and NA) of three currently circulating influenza strains were jointly inserted in the vesicle membrane of the IRIVs and successfully tested clinically. A combined hepatitis A/hepatitis B vaccine was also produced, based on IRIVs. The highly purified, inactivated hepatitis A virions and the hepatitis B surface antigens (HBsAg) genetically engineered in yeast were together covalently coupled to the surface of the IRIV ***(40)***. Finally, combination vaccines were developed, for example, a combined diphtheria-tetanus-hepatitis A vaccine. For this, the diphtheria toxoid, the alpha-tetanus toxoid, the beta-tetanus toxoid, and the inactivated hepatitis A virion were covalently bound via crosslinker molecules to the IRIV surface. A "supercombined" vaccine based on IRIV was developed also, containing covalently bound HAV, Hbs Ag, diphtheria, alpha- and beta-tetanus, as well as HA and NA from three different influenza strains ***(41,42)***.

2. Materials

1. Sterile bench: Class 100, according to US Fed.Std. 209e.
2. Ultracentrifuge: Beckman L5.
3. Fixed angle rotor: Type 45 Ti.
4. Fixed angle rotor: Type 19.
5. Refrigerator: Type UKS 5000 (Frigidaire).

6. Rotation mixer: Turbula Type T2c.
7. Ultrasonificator: Zehfeld.
8. Centrifuge tube assembly: For rotor Type 45 Ti (Beckman 355622).
9. Centrifuge tube assembly: For rotor Type 19 (Beckman 334205).
10. Bottles: 500-mL volume, screw cap.
11. Bottles: 250-mL volume, screw cap.
12. Filter: 0.22 µm, 5.0 µm.
13. Syringes: 50 mL.
14. Cylinders: Volume 100 mL, 250 mL.
15. Pipets: Volume 10 mL.
16. Physiological saline: NaCl 0.9%.
17. Octaethyleneglycol: OEG-solution 100 m*M* in saline.
18. Phosphatidylcholine: Lecithin EPC grade (Lipoid GmbH, D-67065 Ludwigshafen).
19. Phosphatidylethanolamine: Kephalin (Berchtold, Biochemisches Labor, CH-Berne).
20. Polystyrol beads: Bio-Beads (SM-2 Adsorbent, washed).
21. Thiomersal: Thiomersal 1%.
22. Water for injection: H_2O for injection, sterile.

3. Methods

3.1. Production of a Commercialized Influenza Virosome Vaccine (see Note 2*)*

1. At the Swiss Serum and Vaccine Institute, Berne, influenza seed virus solution is inoculated into 11-d-old embryonated hens' eggs from flocks under veterinary control. The inoculated eggs are incubated for a further 50–60 h at 33–35°C, depending on the strain. During this period, they are illuminated for a second time (after 40 h) to eliminate dead eggs. After incubation, the eggs are cooled overnight at 1–4°C; they are then opened under laminar flow and the allantoic fluid is aspirated into sterile steel tanks. After centrifugation, the virus suspension is filtered by step filtration, through a filter of 0.65 µm and 0.22 µm, directly into a new 200-L steel tank. The filtered virus suspension is concentrated about fourfold with a molecular filter system (polysulphone membranes), and then purified and concentrated by sucrose density-gradient ultracentrifugation. The virus-containing fraction is diluted and dialyzed against PBS pH 7.4 to reduce the sugar content to less than 1%. Subsequently, inactivation is performed with beta-propiolactone (BPL) at a final concentration of 1 : 2000. Inactivated concentrates are tested for haemagglutinin content by the single radial diffusion test (SRD), sterility, absence of replicating virus (inactivity), total protein, residual BPL, ovalbumin, and endotoxin.
2. Three monovalent influenza bulks, currently H1N1, H3N2, and B are pooled and used as the starting material for the manufacture of the influenza subunit

virosomes. The pool is pelleted in a fixed-angle ultracentrifuge at about 60,000*g* for 1 h. The supernatant contains residual soluble proteins and is discarded. The pellet is dissolved in 100 m*M* octaethylene glycol (OEG) solution and the viruses are thereby disintegrated. Subsequently, the influenza glycoproteins and the viral envelope phospholipids are separated from other virus constituents by a further fixed-angle ultracentrifugation at 100,000*g* for 1 h. This time, the supernatant is processed further and the pellet is discarded. This double ultracentrifugation makes use of the various properties of the unwanted constituents so that a particularly high degree of purity is achieved. After the first ultracentrifugation, dissolved unwanted constituents (e.g., solubilized viral and egg substrate proteins) in the supernatant are discarded. After the second ultracentrifugation, the other unwanted nonsolubilized constituents are pelleted and discarded and the purified supernatant is further processed. After this purification of the glycoproteins and envelope phospholipids, the lecithin is added and solubilized.

The safety of the egg lecithin is particularly important here, because it is of natural origin and the suspension is not subjected to further inactivation. The lecithin from egg yolk (phosphatidyl choline) is obtained from the company Lipoid in Germany, and is used by other producers of pharmaceutical products for parenteral use. Chemical analysis of the composition, particle-size measurement, solubility measurements, and microbiological purity are tested by the manufacturer. The manufacture of the egg lecithin is validated with regard to virus elimination. This validation was performed in cooperation with the "Freie Universität Berlin," Germany, whereby the initial solution was spiked with Newcastle disease virus, adenovirus of birds (serotype I celovirus), and reovirus of birds. None of these viruses could be recovered from the product after manufacture.

3. Liposomes carrying the influenza subunits at the surface are formed spontaneously during the removal of the octaethyleneglycol (OEG) detergent by chromatography. As shown by electron micrographic studies, the distribution of influenza subunits at the liposomal surface is not regular. This means that some of the vesicles are more densely spiked than others (**Fig. 1**). The detergent-free suspension containing virosomal influenza subunits is filtered through a 5-µm filter for separating the chromatographic matrix substance from the suspension. The filtered pool is subsequently tested for HA content, purity, absence of detergent, and phospholipid, and then diluted with PBS-NaCl pH 7.4 to yield the final bulk.

3.2. Production of a Commercialized IRIV-Hepatitis A Vaccine (see Note 1*)*

1. The RG-SB HAV strain is cultured on MRC-5 human diploid cells. The virus is purified from disrupted cells by ultrafiltration, extraction in *n*-heptane to remove lipids, and 30% sucrose cushion ultracentrifugation. HAV is inactivated by treatment with formalin (0.25% wt/vol) at 37°C for 10 d. Inactivation is confirmed by

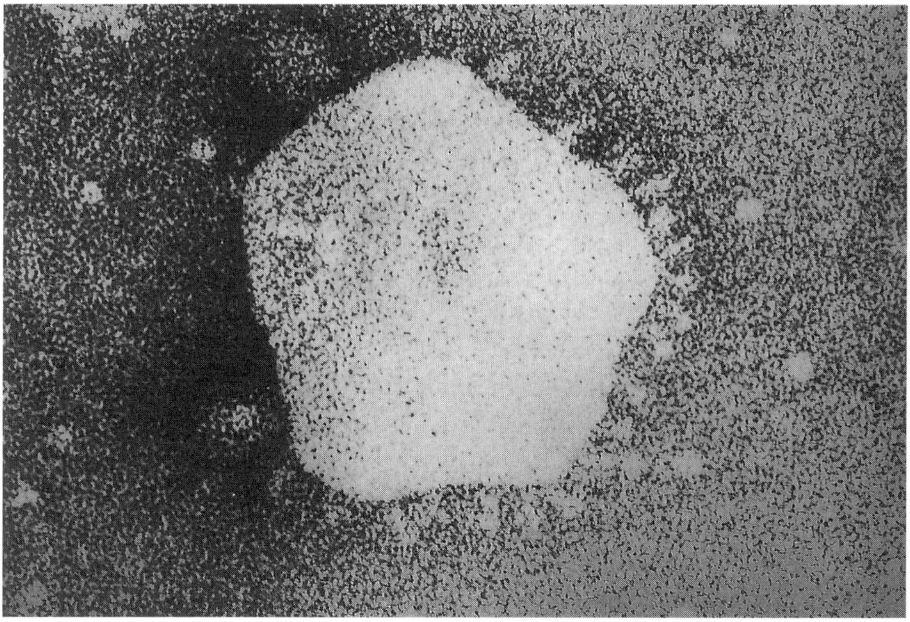

Fig. 5. Electronmicrograph of an IRIV vesicle carrying two hepatitis A virion particles. The influenza glycoproteines (on the right) hemagglutinin and neuraminidase form spikes that protrude 13.5 nm from the IRIV-membrane. The HAs are not activated by the low endosomal pH. The attached two inactivated hepatitis A virions (dark particles on the left) have a diameter of about 25 nm. For comparison, *see* also **Fig. 4**.

lack of viral replication after prolonged incubation of the formalin-treated viral concentrate on MRC-5 cells. The purified HAV concentrate is filtered and the HAV antigen concentration is determined by radioimmunoassay. HAV antigen content is expressed as radioimmunoassay units (RU).

2. The IRIVs are produced as described for the virosomal influenza vaccine with the exception that only one monovalent influenza virus pool (A/ Singapore H1N1) is used for the preparation of IRIVs and in addition to phosphatidylcholine (PC), phosphatidylethanolamine (PE) is added to the phospholipid mixture in a ratio of 4:1. The purified, inactivated HAV suspension with a known amount of antigen is ultrafiltrated (dialyzed) against a physiological saline solution (0.9% NaCl). An appropriate quantity of the IRIV suspension is added to the dialyzed suspension and gently mixed at 25°C for 24 h to allow the HAV to adsorb onto the surface of the IRIV *(30)* (**Fig. 5**). This bulk suspension is diluted with sterile saline solution to a final concentration of 2000 RU HAV antigen/mL (one dose is equivalent to 0.5 mL) and bottled.

3.3. Preparation of Multicombined Virosomal Vaccines by Covalent Coupling of the Antigen (*see* Notes 3, 4, and 5)

1. Antigens (hepatitis A, hepatitis B, diphtheria toxoid, tetanus toxoid, and sPf66 malaria synthetic peptide) are bound to IRIV surface by phosphatidylethanolamine (PE) whose free amino group allows a covalent coupling.
2. PE is dissolved in methanol and 0.1% (v/v) triethylamine is added. The solution is then mixed with γ-maleimidobutyric acid N-hydroxy-succinimide ester (GMBS) (Pierce Chemical Company, Rockford, IL) (ratio PE : GMBS = 2 : 1) which is previously dissolved in dimethylsulfoxide (DMSO). After 15 min incubation at 25°C, the solvents are evaporated for 1 h under vacuum in a speedvac centrifuge.
3. In order to obtain a reduced antigen protein with free cysteine residues, the antigens are treated with 40 mmol/1 DL-dithiothreitol (DTT) for 5 min at 20°C. The DTT is removed using a Sephadex G10 column (Pharmacia LKB Biotechnology, Uppsala, Sweden) and OEG (Fluka Chemicals, Switzerland) is added at a final concentration of 100 mmol/L. The evaporated PE-GMBS is then mixed with the antigen solution at appropriate ratios for 1 h, unbound GMBS is then captured by cysteine. The reactions are monitored by thin-layer chromatography. Additional PC and PE (final ratio 4 : 1) are added to the previously crosslinked PEGMBS and this mixture is dissolved in PBS containing 100 m*M* OEG. This solution is mixed with a A/ Singapore influenza OEG solution as described in the section for virosomal hepatitis A vaccine. Virosomes are then formulated by detergent removal using Bio-Rad SM Bio-Beads (Richmond, CA).

3.4. Preparation of Oligonucleotides Containing Cationic Virosomes (*see* Note 6)

Virosomes are prepared as described for the production of commercial IRIV-hepatitis A vaccine. Instead of PC and PE the cationic N-[1-(2,3-dioleyloxy) propyl]-N,N,N-trimethyl-ammonium methylsulfate (DOTAP) is added to the influenza envelope glycoproteins (HA and NA) and phospholipids. Encapsulation of oligonucleotides into DOTAP-virosomes is performed as follows: cationic virosomes are added to each of the following oligodeoxy-nucleotide phosphorothioates (OPTs): antisense FITC.OPT, sense FITC-OPT, and FITC-OPT. These OPTs are dissolved and the solutions are then treated by sonication for 2 min at 26°C. Nonencapsulated OPT are separated from the virosomes by gel filtration on a High Lead Superdex 200 column (Pharmacia, Uppsala, Sweden). The column is equilibrated with sterile PBS. The void volume fractions containing the DOTAP virosomes with encapsulated OPT is eluted with PBS and collected.

After the virosomes have been fully dissolved in 0.1*N* NaOH containing 0.1% (v/v) Triton X-100, virosome-entrapped FITC-OPT concentrations are determined fluorometrically. For calibration of the fluorescence scale, the fluorescence of empty DOTAP virosomes that had also been dissolved in the above detergent solution is set to zero.

3.5. Entrapment of Mumps Plasmid DNA into Virosomes (*see* Note 7)

cDNA encoding HN antigen of the Urabe *Am*9 strain of the mumps virus is cloned into *Bam*HI site of the plasmid pcDNA3 (InVitrogen, San Diego, CA), which is driven by the CMV promoter. The constructs are grown in DH5a cells and plasmid DNA is purified by QIAGEN EndoFree Plasmid Kit (QIAGEN, Chattsworth, CA) as described by the manufacturer. Influenza virosomes and plasmid encapsulation are prepared as described under OPT containing cationic virosomes. Nonencapsulated plasmid is separated by gel filtration on a High Load Superdex 200 column (Pharmacia).

3.6. Prospects for the Future

Because it is not clear which (if any) animal species or strain correlates with human immunity ***(54)***, products that show promise in an animal system need to be tested in humans for both safety and immunogenicity. Virosomes have been extensively given to humans of all ages in the context of vaccine formulations. Therefore, such efforts should prove exciting for the successful application of the molecular approach to new and improved vaccines.

There are several ways to increase adjuvant activity over that observed with alum, the only adjuvant in approved products licensed by the FDA ***(56)*** and which is far from ideal: (i) by developing an adjuvant vaccine formulation that is more dispersable, therefore improving transfer of antigens to draining lymph nodes; (ii) by using immunostimulants that help to trap and activate appropriate cells within these lymph nodes; (iii) by providing for a physical or chemical association of these immunostimulants with vaccine antigens so that both are delivered simultaneously to lymphoid tissues; and (iv) by using substances and molecules selected on the basis of prior documented safety when parenterally administered to humans. Virosomal preparations and specially IRIV-designed vaccines and similar formulations seem to do all four and, therefore, hold promise as immunopotentiating delivery systems for whichever vaccine is approved next.

3.7. Summary and Conclusion

IRIVs have been shown to act as an efficient and highly effective means of enhancing the immune response to a variety of vaccine antigens, thus illustrating their use as vaccine delivery systems. Their use is not limited to a certain type of antigen. IRIV-based vaccines comprising viral glycoproteins, bacterial

Table 1
Kinetics of the Immune Response Following Immunization with Various Hepatitis A Vaccine Formulations

	Geometric mean titer (% ≥20 IU/ml)				
Vaccine[a] formulation	Day 0	Day 14	Day 28	Day 180	Day 352[b]
Fluid	<20	16 (30)	388 (100)	211 (80)	39 (50)
Al $(OH)_3$	<20	21 (44)	871 (100)	535 (95)	57 (60)
IRIV	<20	140 (100)	831 (100)	1,499 (100)	655 (100)

[a]One dose of each vaccine formulation contained 1000 radioimmunoassay units of HAV antigen and was administered to 40 healthy adults.

[b]Data from 14, 10, and 22 subjects immunized with fluid, Al $(OH)_3$ or IRIV vaccines, respectively.

toxoids, inactivated virus, recombinant proteins, synthetic peptides, and DNA-plasmids or polynucleotids, have been formulated. The safety profile of IRIV vaccines has been excellent. Compared to alum-adsorbed vaccines, they elicit far fewer local reactions. Both local and systemic reactions reported to date have been predominantly mild and transient. Additionally, immunization with IRIVs does not induce a serum antiphospholipid antibody response, even after repeated doses of vaccine have been administered *(57)*, IRIV-based vaccines can readily be made on a commercial scale economically. As noted above, several additional vaccines are undergoing clinical evaluation. Furthermore, a number of novel vaccine antigens are being incorporated into IRIVs in an attempt to develop a variety of new viral, bacterial, and parasitic vaccines.

4. Notes

1. Clinical evaluation of IRIV hepatitis A vaccine: Initial studies *(28)* compared the safety and the kinetics of the immune response induced by three different hepatitis A vaccines: (i) fluid; (ii) alum-adsorbed; and (iii) IRIV, all of which contained the same amount of inactivated hepatitis A antigen. Local reactions occurred at a significantly reduced rate in the IRIV group as compared to recipients of the alum-adsorbed vaccine. Similar results were obtained upon expanded testing in which IRIV vaccine was compared to a commercial alum-adsorbed vaccine *(43–45)*. The IRIV vaccine induced a more rapid immune response evidenced by a statistically higher rate of seroconversion at day 14 accompanied by a higher geometric mean titer (GMT) (**Table 1**). By 4-wk postimmunization, comparable immune responses were attained by all three vaccines. However, there was a significantly greater decline in antibody levels in the groups immunized with the alum-adsorbed or fluid vaccines. One year after immunization, all persons immunized with the IRIV vaccine still possessed anti-HAV antibody levels ≥ 20 mIU/mL. In contrast, only 60 and 50% of subjects who received the alum-

Table 2
Attainment of Protective Anti-HA Antibody Levels Following Immunization in Subjects with Nonprotective Baseline Antibody Titers[a]

Type of vaccine	No. of subjects with protective levels of antibody after vaccination (%)		
1992/1993 season	**H1N1 A/ Singapore 6/86**	**H3N2 A/ Beijing 353/89**	**Yamagata B 16/88**
Subunit	12/49 (41)	12/14 (86)	7/30 (23)
	$p = 0.0049$	$p = > 0.05$	$p = 0.006$
IRIV	42/58 (72)	27/31 (87)	31/57 (54)
1993/1994 season	**H1N1 A/ Singapore 6/86**	**H3N2 A/ Beijing 32/92**	**Panama B 45/90**
Subunit	13/28 (46)	14/26 (54)	10/12 (83)
	$p = 0.03$	$p = 0.0041$	$p = 0.64$
IRIV	25/34 (74)	27/28 (96)	16/17 (94)

[a]Protective anti-HA antibody titer: ≥ 40 ***(58)***.

adsorbed or fluid vaccine, respectively, did so. Expanded testing of the IRIV-formulated hepatitis A vaccine in adult and pediatric populations have found that ≥95% of subjects will achieve protective titers with 1 mo of receiving a single dose of vaccine ***(43–46)***. This single-dose immunization schedule has proved to be effective at controling hepatitis A outbreaks and endemic disease ***(43,47)***. This vaccine was first licensed for use in 1995 under the trade name Epaxal Berna.

2. Clinical evaluation of IRIV influenza vaccine: Several trivalent IRIV-formulated influenza vaccines have been tested in elderly patients ***(48,49)***. In one study the IRIV-formulated vaccine was found to elicit significantly higher fourfold rises in anti-HA antibody levels over baseline to all three vaccine strains compared to both commercial subunit and whole virion vaccines ***(48)***. Peak postimmunization antibody levels were also found to be significantly higher than commercial vaccines. Of greater clinical importance is the percentage of subjects with nonprotective levels of baseline antibodies who attained protective levels following immunization. As shown in **Table 2**, the IRIV vaccine was far more effective than a commercial subunit vaccine in achieving this goal. The IRIV vaccine was found to be superior to standard vaccine formulations, especially when the baseline titers were very low ***(48,49)***. This vaccine was first licensed for use in 1997 under the trade name Inflexal V Berna.

Currently, an IRIV-type influenza vaccine is undergoing phase III clinical testing when administered by the intranasal route with the native heat-labile toxin of *Escherichia coli* being incorporated into the formulation as a mucosal adjuvant.

Table 3
Immunization Scheme

Diphtheria	Di-Anatoxal	Di-Anatoxal Inflexal-Priming	Di-IRIV	Di-IRIV Inflexal-Priming
day 0		Inflexal Berna		Inflexal Berna
day 21	Di-Anatoxal	Di-Anatoxal	Di-IRIV	Di-IRIV
day 42	Bleeding and Di-Anatoxal	Bleeding and Di-Anatoxal	Bleeding and Di-IRIV	Bleeding and Di-IRIV
day 52	Bleeding	Bleeding	Bleeding	Bleeding
Tetanus	**Te-Anatoxal**	**Te-Anatoxal Inflexal-Priming**	**Te-IRIV**	**Te-IRIV Inflexal-Priming**
day 0		Inflexal Berna		Inflexal Berna
day 21	Te-Anatoxal	Te-Anatoxal	Te-IRIV	Te-IRIV
day 42	Bleeding and Te-Anatoxal	Bleeding and Te-Anatoxal	Bleeding and Te-IRIV	Bleeding and Te-IRIV
day 52	Bleeding	Bleeding	Bleeding	Bleeding

Anatoxal: Commercial vaccine, alum adsorbed.
Inflexal: Commercial whole virus influenza vaccine.

Preliminary results indicate that intranasal administration can elicit a significant rise in serum anti-HA antibody titers ***(50)***, as well in mucosal (salivary and nasal wash) IgA titers.

3. Immunogenicity of IRIV- vs alum-adjuvanted diphtheria and tetanus toxoid vaccines in influenza primed mice: The immunogenicity and protective efficacy of two different toxoid vaccines were compared in mice ***(51)***. Because nearly all humans can be considered to be seropositive to influenza the mice were previously primed with a commercial flu vaccine. In one formulation, toxoids (diphtheria or tetanus) were adsorbed to alum, whereas in the other formulation, toxoids were crosslinked to IRIVs. A preimmunization with influenza antigens considerably enhanced the antitoxoid antibody response when the IRIV formulation was administered (**Table 3**). After two immunizations with the IRIV- or alum-based vaccines, the IRIV-based formulation induced a higher humoral immune response than toxoids adsorbed to alum (**Table 4**). Using an in vitro test, diphtheria toxin neuralizing antibodies were tested. IRIV-formulated diphtheria toxoid (Di-IRIV) induced a significantly ($p = 0.002$) higher titer of diphtheria toxin neutralizing antibodies than alum-formulatd diphtheria toxoid (Di-alum). Tetanus challenge experiments showed, that the IRIV based tetanus vaccine induced a threefold higher titer of protective antibodies than the tetanus toxoid adsorbed to alum (**Table 5**). Therefore, the IRIV-based formulations appeared to be superior than the alum-based vaccines in terms of immunogenicity and protective efficacy.

Table 4
Antibody Titers to Different Toxoid Vaccine Formulations

Diphtheria	Di-Anatoxal	Di-Anatoxal Inflexal-Priming	Di-IRIV	Di-IRIV Inflexal-Priming
number of mice	10	5	10	10
day 42 (GMT after 1 immunization)[a]	5043	3566	<8	395
day 52 (GMT after 2 immunizations)[a]	32,768	37,641	4467	57,052
Tetanus	**Te-Anatoxal**	**Te-Anatoxal Inflexal-Priming**	**Te-IRIV**	**Te-IRIV Inflexal-Priming**
number of mice	10	5	10	10
day 42 (GMT after 1 immunization)[a]	5793	5793	512	1663
day 52 (GMT after 2 immunizations)[a]	32,768	23,170	18,820	65,536

[a]Results are expressed as the geometric mean of reciprocal serum dilutions.

Table 5
Titers of Neutralizing Antibodies to Different Toxoid Vaccine Formulations

Neutralizing antibodies to diphtheria toxin (vero cell test)	Di-Alum	Di-IRIV Influenza-Priming
number of mice	10	10
day 52 (GMT)[a]	239	1176
Neutralizing antibodies to tetanus toxin (challenge)	Te-Alum	Te-IRIV Influenza-Priming
day 52 (GMT)[a]	200	600

[a]Results are expressed as the geometric mean of reciprocal serum dilutions.

4. Immunogenicity of an IRIV-SPf66 malaria peptide vaccine in mice: IRIVs were used as a delivery system for the synthetic peptide-based malaria vaccine SPf66. The reduced SPf66 peptide molecules containing terminal cysteine residues were covalently attached to kephalin with the heterobifunctional crosslinker γ-maleimidobutyric acid N-hydroxysuccinimide ester. The SPf66-kephalin was

Table 6
Comparison of Immunogenicity of IRIV-SPf66 (10 μg) with Alum-SPf66 (10 μg) in Mice. Immunization day 0 and day 21. Bleeding on day 43. All Mice were Primed with Influenza-Antigen.

SPf66-IRIV		SPf66-Alum	
mouse no.	units	mouse no.	units
1	2,500	21	71
2	10,000	22	59
3	12,500	23	<15
4	100	24	77
5	14,289	25	<5
6	3,333	26	4,167
7	2,000	27	20,000
8	1,000	28	909
9	2,222	29	56
10	3,448	30	59
13	1,250	31	27
15	200	32	<15
16	2,500	33	<15
17	1,667	34	250
18	3,448	35	434
19	1,961	36	<15
20	12,500	37	<15
		38	50
		39	3,571
		40	<15
		41	<15

incorporated into IRIVs and BALB/c mice were immunized twice by sc injection with peptide-loaded virosomes. Titers of elicited anti-SPf66 IgG were determined by ELISA. These titers were significantly higher and the required doses of antigen were lower, when mice had been preimmunized with unmodified virosomes. SPf66-IRIV elicited far more consistently high anti-SPf66 antibody responses than SPf(66)$_n$ adsorbed to alum (**Table 6**). mAb produced by four B-cell hybridoma clones derived from a SPf66-IRIV immunized mouse crossreacted with *Plasmodium falciparum* blood stage parasites in immunofluorescence assays. All four mAb were specific for the merozoite surface protein 1 (MSP1)-derived 83.1 portion of SPf66. Sequencing of their functionally rearranged kappa light chain variable region genes demonstrated that the four hybridomas were generated from clonally related splenic B cells. BIAcore relative affinity measurements together with these sequencing data provided evidence for the selection of somatically mutated affinity matured B cells after repeated immunization with SPf66-IRIV.

Table 7
Studies 1–4. Demographic Data (yr/mo) of the Study Population

	Study 1		Study 2		Study 3	Study 4
	Combined	Single	Combined	Single	Combined	Combined
n	7	7	23	23	15	15
Female	3	5	7	10	4	4
Male	4	2	16	13	11	11
Age mean	27/01	24/05	23/03	24/01	25/04	22/10
Min	22/10	22/11	21/01	21/08	21/09	21/00
Max	32/11	25/09	25/06	34/03	28/00	28/00

The results indicate that IRIVs are a suitable delivery system for synthetic peptide vaccines and thus have a great potential for the design of molecularly defined combined vaccines targeted against multiple antigens and development stages of one parasite, as well as against multiple pathogens ***(52)***.

5. Phase I clinical testing of a multivalent combined IRIV vaccine in human volunteers: The objective of this study was to produce a fivefold combined vaccine against hepatitis A and B, diphtheria, tetanus, and influenza A/B, and to show that, in principle, IRIVs can serve as carriers for multiple antigens, which have good immunogenicity and are well tolerated. A total of four studies were carried out.

   Either the combined vaccine or the corresponding adequately tested alum-adsorbed single vaccines were tested for reactogenicity and immunogenicity in young adults.

   A hepatitis A and B combination on an IRIV base showed the same immunogenicity and toleration as the single vaccines. However, with the simultaneous coupling of all five vaccines on the same IRIV or the binding of Di-Te and HAV on different IRIVs there was a suppression of the humoral immune response against HAV ($p = 0.03$). The possibility that epitope-specific suppression had occurred could be ruled out. The suppression of the response against HAV could be circumvented by halving the quantity of Di-Te antigen in the combined vaccine so as to avoid antigenic competition. Surprisingly, the immunogenicity of Di-Te vaccination in the combination proved superior to that of a separate vaccination.

   By reducing the diphtheria and tetanus toxoid subunit molecules per IRIV particles, it was possible not only to increase significantly the immune response to these antigens but also to remove completely the antigenic competition phenomenon. Once the optimum composition of the vaccine had been achieved (careful dosing of antigens per IRIV particle), an immunological effect clearly superior to that of comparable, aluminium-adsorbed products was obtained ***(40)*** (**Table 8**).

   The tolerability of this "supercombi vaccine" was significantly better than the commercial alum adsorbed products (**Table 9**).

6. Delivery to cancer cells of antisense L-*myc* oligonucleotides incorporated in cationic virosomes: Antisense OPTs of L-*myc* were encapsulated into reconstituted influenza-virus-A envelopes (virosomes) ***(53)***. The envelopes of the virosomes

Table 8
IRIV-Combination Vaccine vs Single Alum Vaccines

Immunogen	Adjuvant	Day 0 GMT[a]	Day 0 *p*	Day 28 GMT[a]	Day 28 *p*
Alpha DT	Alum	0.4 IU/mL	0.4	0.7 IU/mL	0.00007
	IRIV	0.8 IU/mL		3.2 IU/mL	
Alpha TT	Alum	4.3 IU/mL	0.07	13.1 IU/mL	0.00002
	IRIV	6.6 IU/mL		45.2 IU/mL	
Hbs	Alum	292 IU/mL	0.4	6373 IU/mL	0.002
	IRIV	343 IU/mL		13,204 IU/mL	
HAV	Alum	8.0 mIU/mL	0.6	252 mIU/mL	0.08
	IRIV	7.0 mIU/mL		361 mIU/mL	

[a]Geometric mean titers (alum $n = 26$, IRIV $n = 27$) for diphtheria, tetanus, hepatitis B, and hepatitis A.

Table 9
Comparison of Side Reactions. Combined Commercial Diphtheria, Tetanus, Hepatitis A, and Hepatitis B Vaccines vs an IRIV Supercombined with the Same Antigens

Side Reactions	Commercial Vaccines	IRIV Supercombined
Pain grade 2 or 3	82%	24%
Induration	41%	23%
Redness	37%	9%
Redness average		
Area	left: 3800 mm^2 right: 1034 mm^2	2 mm^2
Swelling	48%	27%
General symptoms		
(Headache, nausea)	78%	28%

consisted of a single positively charged (cationic) lipid bilayer. Binding of cationic virosomes to cellular receptors that are membrane glycoproteins or glycolipids containing terminal sialic acid is mediated by the HA of the influenza virus. After internalization through receptor-mediated endocytosis, cationic virosomes fuse efficiently with the membranes of the endosomal-cell compartment and as a consequence the encapsulated OPT are delivered to the cell cytoplasm. Examination by fluorescence microscopy of the cellular uptake of cationic virosomes containing fluorescein-labeled OPT showed rapid and efficient incorporation of virosomes (**Figs. 6** and **7**). Addition of cationic virosomes (75-150 l) containing antisense L-*myc* OPT in the picomolar range to small-cell-lung-cancer (SCLC) cell cultures that expressed highly the L-*myc* oncogene led to

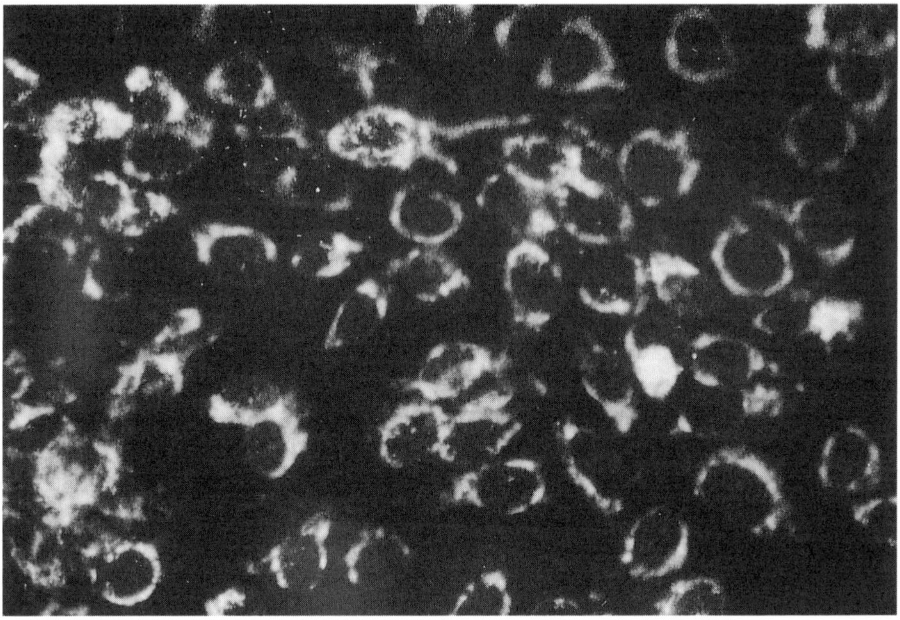

Fig. 6. Cellular uptake of antisense-FITC-L-*myc* virosomes by NCI-H209 cells: 1×10^4 cells were seeded in a chamber slide in 0.3 mL of medium containing 10% FCS. Cells were incubated with 50 µL of virosomes for 5 min, then washed and viewed under fluorescence microscopy.

strong inhibition of thymidine incorporation in a concentration-dependent manner. Virosome-entrapped sense L-*myc* OPT and random-order OPT had only minimal effects on the thymidine uptake. Cells of SCLCc cell line NCl-H82 expressing a very low level of L-*myc* were not affected by antisense-L-*myc* virosomes. In Western blot analysis, expression of L-*myc* protein was suppressed in the antisense-virosome-treated NCl-H209 cells, but not in untreated control NCl-H209 cells. These results suggest that cationic virosomes may have great protential as an efficient delivery system for antisense oligonucleotides in cancer therapy.

7. Intranasal immunization of mice with mumps DNA entrapped into virosomes: We immunized intranasally groups of mice with (a) naked DNA encoding HN antigen of mumps virus (group C) or (b) with DNA entrapped into virosomes after preimmunization with virosomes (group A) or (c) without preimmunization (group B). A control group (H) was immunized intranasally with live Urabe mumps virus. As shown in **Table 10**, the geometric mean titer (GMT) of IgG in the group of mice which had received the preimmunization (A), was higher than that reported in the groups B and C of mice ***(54,55)***. The group of mice immunized intranasally with naked DNA developed a very low level of IgG, whereas

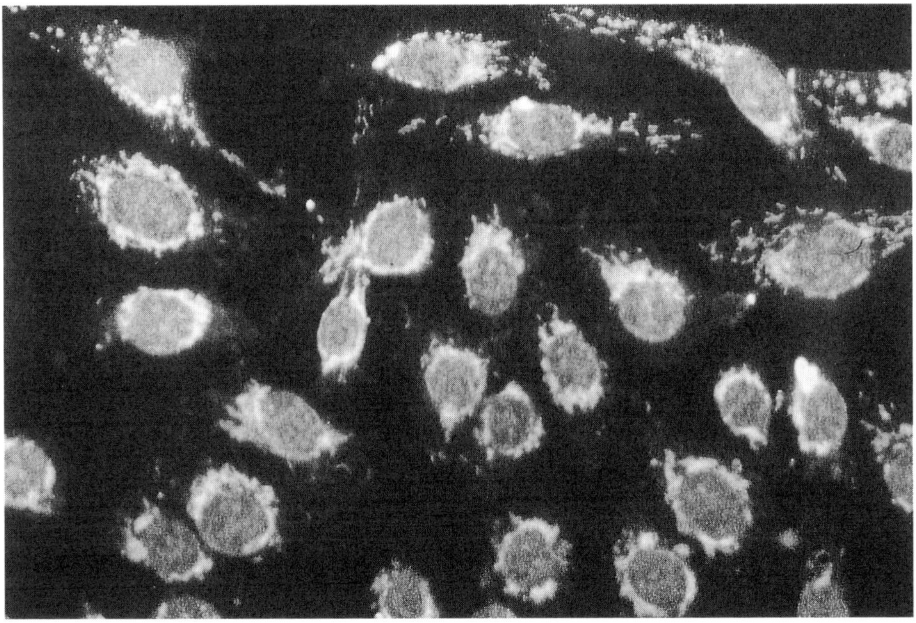

Fig. 7. The same experiment as described in **Fig. 6** with the difference that cells were incubated with 50 μL of virosomes for 15 min.

the mice immunized intranasally with the mumps virus (group H) presented a good IgG response. Analyzing the mucosal immunity, we found that all groups of mice, but those immunized with naked DNA, developed IgA. Only in the nasal washings (NW) of mice immunized intranasally with the mumps virus could we detect IgA at elevated titer (group H).

Three-fifths of mice from group A developed neutralizing antibodies (GMP 1/16) (data not shown). Because not all mice produced neutralizing antibodies, we think that the schedule of vaccination needs to be modified in order to improve the induction of neutralizing antibodies.

Cytokine measurements were performed using splenocytes taken 12 d after immunization. **Table 11** summarizes representative measurements obtained from two separate experiments. Mumps virus antigen-stimulated cells from mice previously vaccinated (intranasally) with DNA-virosomes induced the production of IL-2 and IFN-α. In addition, flu primed mice induced the production of IL-4. Cells taken from mumps virus-immunized animals produced IFN-α, IL-2, IL-4, and IL-10 after in vitro stimulation with mumps antigen. Immunization with DNA-virosomes such as the control immunization with the purified mumps antigens correlated with Th1 phenotype. In addition, considering the ratio between the total level of IgG and the virus-specific IgG1 or IgG2a, the amount of IgG2a isotype was predominant in group A, indicating a Th2 response.

Table 10
The Geometric Mean Titer (GMT) of Humoral IgG, Bronchoalveolar Lavage (BAL) IgA, and Nasal Wash IgA in Mice

Mice	IgG	BAL IgA	NW IgA
Group A	356	8	10
Group B	15	11	10
Group C	12	2	2
Group H	1585	2	20

Table11
Representative Measurements of Cytokine Production in Mice Obtained from Two Separate Experiments

Group	IL-2	IFN-	IL-4	IL-10
A	300	300	150	0
B	150	625	0	0
C	300	100	0	0
H	600	100	150	600

We immunized intranasally groups of mice with (a) naked DNA encoding HN antigen of mumps virus (group C) or (b) with DNA entrapped into virosomes after preimmunization with virosomes (group A) or (c) without preimmunization (group B). A control group (H) was immunized intranasally with live Urabe mumps virus. As shown in **Table 10** the geometric mean titer (GMT) of IgG in the group of mice which had received the preimmunization (A), was higher than that one reported in the groups B and C of mice ***(54,55)***. The group of mice immunized intranasally with naked DNA developed a very low level of IgG, whereas the mice immunized intranasally with the mumps virus (group H) presented a good IgG response. Analyzing the mucosal immunity, we found that all the groups of mice, but those immunized with naked DNA developed IgA. Only in the nasal washings (NW) of mice immunized intranasally with the mumps virus we could detect IgA at elevated titer (group H).

References

1. Gould-Fogerite, S. and Mannino, R. J. (1996) Mucosal and systemic immunization using cochleate and liposome vaccines. *J. Liposom. Res.* **6,** 357–379.
2. Garçon, N. and Friede, M. (1996) Liposomes to induce potent humoral responses to T-independent antigens. *J. Liposom. Res.* **6,** 381–395.
3. Morein, B. and Simons, K. (1985) Subunit vaccines against enveloped viruses: virosomes, micelles and other protein complexes. *Vaccine* **3,** 83–93.
4. Muller, G. M., Shapira, M., and Arnon, R. (1982) Anti-influenza response achieved by immunization with a synthetic conjugate. *Proc. Natl. Acad. Sci. USA* **79,** 569–573.
5. Boudreault, A. and Thibodeau, L. (1985) Mouse response to influenza immunosomes. *Vaccine* **3,** 231–234.

6. Neurath, A. R., Kent, S. B. H., and Strick, N. (1984) Antibodies to hepatitis B surface antigen (HBsAG) elicited by immunization with a synthetic peptide covalently linked to liposomes. *J. Gen. Virol.* **65,** 1009–1014.
7. Lerner, R. A., Green, N., Alexander, H., Liu, F.-T., Sutcliffe, J. G., and Shinnick, T. M. (1981) Chemically synthesized peptides predicted from the nucleotide sequence of the hepatitis B virus genome elicit antibodies reactive with the native envelope protein of Dane particles. *Proc. Natl. Acad. Sci. USA* **78,** 3403–4307.
8. Bhatnagar, P. K., Papas, E., Blum, H. E., Milich, D. R., Nitecki, D., Karels, M. J., and Vyas, G. N. (1982) Immune response to synthetic peptide analogues of hepatitis B surface antigen specific for the A determinant. *Proc. Natl. Acad. Sci. USA* **79,** 4400–4404.
9. Bittle, J. L., Houghton, R. A., Alexander, H., Shinnik, T. M., Sutcliffe, J. G., Lerner, R. A., et al. (1982) Protection against foot and mouth disease by immunization with a chemically synthesized peptide predicted form the viral nucleotide sequence. *Nature* **298,** 30–33.
10. DiMarchi, R., Brooke, G., Gale, C., Cracknell, V., Doel, T., and Mowat, N. (1986) Protection of cattle against foot-and-mouth disease by a synthetic peptide. *Science* **232,** 639–641.
11. Kennedy, R. C., Henkel, R. D., Pauletti, D., Allan, J. S., Lee, T. H., Essex, M., and Dressman, G. R. (1986) Antiserum to a synthetic peptide recognizes the HTLVIII envelope glycoprotein. *Science* **231,** 1556–1559.
12. Miller, L. H., Howard, R. D., Carter, R., Good, M. D., Nussenzweig, V., and Nussenzweig, R. S. (1986) Research toward malaria vaccines. *Science* **234,** 1349–1356.
13. Caryanniotis, G. and Barber, B. H. (1987) Adjuvant-free IgG responses induced with antigen coupled to antibodies against class II MHC. *Nature* **327,** 59–61.
14. Francis, M. J., Fry, C. M., Rowlands, D. J., Brown, F., Bittle, J. L., Houghten, R. A., and Lerner, R. A. (1985) Immunological priming with synthetic peptides of foot-and-mouth disease virus. *J. Gen. Virol.* **66,** 2347–2354.
15. Goodman-Snitkoff, G., Eisele, L. E., Heimer, E. P., Felix, A. M., Andersen, T. T., Fuerst, T. R., and Mannino, R. J. (1990) Defining minimal requirements for antibody production to peptide antigens. *Vaccine* **8,** 257–262.
16. Goodman-Snitkoff, G., Good, M. R., Berzofsky, J. A., and Mannino, R. J. (1991) Role of intrastructural/intermolecular help in immunization with peptide-phospholipid complexes. *J. Immunol.* **147,** 410–415.
17. Mannino, R. J. and Gould-Fogerite, S. (1995) Lipid matrix-based vaccines for mucosal and systemic immunization, in *Vaccine Design: The Subunit and Adjuvant Approach* (Powell, M. F. and Newman, M. J., eds.), Plenum, New York, p. 363.
18. Allen, P. M. (1987) Antigen processing at the molecular level. *Immunol. Today* **8,** 270–273.
19. Gould-Fogerite, S. and Mannino, R. J. (1985) Rotary dialysis: Its application to the production of large liposomes and large proteoliposomes (protein-lipid vesicles) with high encapsulation efficiency and efficient reconstitution of membrane proteins. *Anal. Biochem.* **148,** 15.

20. Gould-Fogerite, S., Mazurkiewicz, J., Lehman, J., Raska, Jr., K., Voelkerding, K., and Mannino, R. J. (1989) Chimerasome-mediated gene transfer in vitro and in vivo. *Gene* **84,** 429–438.
21. Gould-Fogerite, S., Mazurkiewicz, J. E., Bhisitkul, D., and Mannino, R. J. (1987) The reconstitution of biologically active glycoproteins into large liposomes: Use as a delivery vehicle to animal cells, in *Advances in Membrane Biochemistry and Bioenergetics* (Kim, C. H., Diwan, J., Tedeschi, H., and Salerno, J. J., eds.), Plenum, New York, pp. 569–591.
22. Mannino, R. J. and Gould-Fogerite, S. (1988) Liposome mediated gene transfer. *Biotechniques* **6,** 682–690.
23. Miller, M. D., Gould-Fogerite, S., Shen, L., Woods, R. M., Koenig, S., Mannino, R. J., and Letvin, N. L. (1992) Vaccination of rhesus monkeys with synthetic peptide in a fusogenic proteoliposome elicits simian immunodeficiency virus-specific CD8+ cytotoxic T lymphocytes. *J. Exp. Med.* **176,** 1739–1744.
24. Gould-Fogerite, S., Edghill-Smith, Y., Kheiri, M., Wang, Z., Das, K., Feketeova, E., et al. (1994) Lipid matrix-based subunit vaccines: A structure-function approach to oral and parenteral immunization. *AIDS Res. Hum. Retrovirus.* **10,** 99.
25. Allison, A. C. and Gregoriadis, G. (1974) Liposomes as immunological adjuvants. *Nature* **252,** 252–255.
26. Gregoriadis, G. (1990) Immunological adjuvants: a role for liposomes. *Immunol. Today* **11,** 89–97.
27. Glück, R. (1994) Combined vaccines—the european contribution. *Biologicals* **22,** 347–351.
28. Glück, R., Mischler, R., Brantschen, S., Just, M., Althaus, B., and Cryz, S. J. Jr. (1992) Immunopotentiating reconstituted influenza virosome (IRIV) vaccine delivery system for immunization against hepatitis A. *J. Clin. Invest.* **90,** 2491–2495.
29. Gregoriadis, G. (1995) Engineering liposomes for drug delivery: progress and problems. *TIBTECH* **13,** 527–537.
30. Seganti, L., Superti, F., Orsini, N., Gabrielli, R., Divizia M., and Panà, A. (1989) Membrane lipid components interacting with hepatitis A virus. *Microbiologica* **12,** 225–230.
31. Garçon, N. M. and Six, H. R. (1991) Universal Vaccine Carrier. Liposomes that provide T-dependent help to weak antigen. *J. Immunol.* **146/11,** 3697–3702.
32. Tsurudome, M., Glück, R., Graf, R., Falchetto, R., Schaller, U., and Brunner, J. (1992) Lipid interactions of the hemagglutinin HA2NH2-terminal segment during influenza virus-induced membrane fusion. *J. Biol. Chemistry* **267/28,** 20,225–20,232.
33. Durrer, P., Galli, C., Hoenke, S., Corti, C., Glück, R., Vorherr, T., and Brunner, J. (1996) H+ -induced membrane insertion of influenza virus hemagglutinin involves the HA2 amino-terminal fusion peptide but not the coiled coil region. *J. Biol. Chem.* **271/23,** 13,417–13,421.
34. Matlin, K. S., Reggio, H., Helenius, A., and Simmons, K. (1981) Infections entry pathway of influenza virus in a canine kidney cell line. *J. Cell. Biol.* **91,** 601–613.
35. Rott, O., Charreire, J., Mignon-Godefroy, K., and Cash, E. (1995) B cell superstimulatory influenza virus activates peritoneal B cells. *J. Immunology* **155,** 134–142.

36. Rott, O., Charreire, J., Semichon, M., Bismuth, G., and Cash, E. (1995) B cell superstimulatory influenza virus (H2-subtype) induces B cell proliferation by a PKC-activating, Ca2+ -Independent mechansim. *J. Immunology* **154,** 2092–2103.
37. Parker, E. E. and Gould, K. G. (1996) Influenza A virus—a model for viral antigen presentation to cytotoxic T lymphocytes. *Virology* **7,** 61–73.
38. Air, G. M. and Laver, W. G. (1989) The neuraminidase of influenza virus. *Proteins* **6,** 341–356.
39. Muster, T., Ferko, B., Klima, A., Purtscher, M., Trkola, A., Schulz, P., et al. (1995) Mucosal model of immunization against human immunodeficiency virus Type 1 with a chimeric influenza virus. *J. Virology* **69/11,** 6678–6686.
40. Mengiardi, B., Berger, R., Just, M., and Glück, R. (1995) Virosomes as carriers for combined vaccines. *Vaccine* **13,** 1306–1315.
41. Glück, R. (1993) Towards a universal IRIV traveller vaccine. Third Conference on International Travel Medicine, Paris, France, 25–29, April 1993. Abstr. No. 259.
42. Just, M. (1993) Experience with IRIV as carrier for hepatitis A and other antigens. Third Conference on International Travel Medicine, Paris, France, 25–29, April 1993, Abstr. No. 277.
43. Lea, A. P. and Balfour, J. A. (1997) Virosomal hepatitis A vaccine (strain RG-SB): a preliminary review of its immunogenicity protective efficacy and tolerability in at-risk populations. *BioDrugs* **7,** 232–248.
44. Bovier, P., Loutan, L., Farinelly, T., et. al. (1995) Cross-immunogenicity of a booster dose of a virosomal hepatitis A vaccine in healthy travellers after basic immunization with an alum-based hepatitis A vaccine (Abstract). European Conference on Tropical Medicine. Oct. 22–25; Hamburg, Germany.
45. Holzer, B. R., Hatz, C., Schmidt-Sissolak, D., Glück, R., Althaus, B., and Egger, M. (1996) Immunogenicity and adverse effects of inactivated virosome versus alum-adsorbed hepatitis A vaccine: a randomized controlled trial. *Vaccine* **14/10,** 982–986.
46. Poovorawan, Y., Theamboonlers, A., Chumdermpadetsuk, S., Glück, R., and Cryz, S. J., Jr. (1995) Safety, immunogenicity, and kinetics of the immune response to a single dose of virosome-formulated hepatitis A vaccine in Thais. *Vaccine* **13/10,** 891–893.
47. Poovorawan, Y., Tieamboonlers, A., Chumdermpadetsuk, S., Glück, R., and Cryz, S. J. (1994) Control of a hepatitis A outbreak by active immunization of high-risk susceptibles subjects. *J. Infect. Dis.* **169,** 228–229 (Letter to the Editor).
48. Glück, R., Mischler, R., Finkel, B., Que, J. U., Scarpa, B., and Cryz, S. J., Jr. (1994) Immunogenicity of new virosome influenza vaccine in the elderly people. *Lancet* **344,** 160–163.
49. Conne, P., Gauthey, L., Vernet, P., Althaus, B., Que, J. U., Finkel, B., et al. (1997) Immunogenicity of trivalent subunit versus virosome-formulated influenza vaccines in geriatric patients. *Vaccine* **15/15,** 1675–1679.
50. Glück, U., Gebbers, J. O., and Glück, R. (1998) Intranasal application of virosome influenza vaccine. Submitted (*Lancet*).

51. Zurbriggen, R. and Glück, R. (1998) Immunogenicity of IRIV- versus alum-adjuvanted diphtheria and tetanus toxoid vaccines in influenza primed mice. *Vaccine,* in press.
52. Pöltl-Frank, F., Zurbriggen, R., Helg, A., Stuart, F., Robinson, J., Glück, R., and Pluschke, G. Use of reconstituted influenza virus virosomes as an immunopotentiating delivery system for a peptide-based vaccine. In press.
53. Wälti, E. R. and Glück, R. (1998) Delivery to cancer cells of antisense L-myc oligonucleotides incorporated in fusogenic, cationic-lipid-reconstituted influenza-virus envelopes (cationic virosomes). *Int. J. Cancer* **77,** 728–733.
54. Lowell, G. H. (1990) Proteosomes, hydrophobic anchors, iscoms and liposomes for improved presentation of peptide and protein vaccines, in *New Generation Vaccines* (Woodrow, G. C. and Levine, M. M., eds.), Dekker, New York, pp. 141–168.
55. Cusi, M. G. and Glück, R. (1998) Intranasal immunization of mice with mumps DNA entrapped into influenza virosomes. *IBC's 4th Ann. Conf. Genet. Vacc.,* Oct. 25–27, Washington, D.C.
56. Eng, R. S., Pomerantz, R. J., and Friedman, L. S. (1993) Hepatitis A vaccines: past, present and future. *Gastroenterology* **105,** 943–945.
57. Cryz, S., Que, J. U., and Glück, R. (1996) A virosome vaccine antigen delivery system does not stimulate an antiphospholipid antibody response in humans. *Vaccine* **14,** 1381–1383.
58. The European Agency for the Evaluation of Medicinal Products (EMA), Human Medicines Evaluation Unit: Committee for Proprietary Medicinal Products (CPMP), in *Note for Guidance on Harmonisation of Requirements for Influenza Vaccines*; 12 March 1997 (CPMP/BWP/214/96).

10

Cochleates for Induction of Mucosal and Systemic Immune Responses

Susan Gould-Fogerite and Raphael J. Mannino

1. Introduction

1.1. Protective Immune Responses

The vast majority of infectious diseases are caused by pathogens that infect mucosal surfaces or use them as portals of entry. Mucosal immune responses are the first line of defense against these pathogens that are inhaled, ingested, or sexually transmitted. However, some agents may be able to breach these defenses, and go on to cause systemic disease. Therefore, vaccines against these agents may need to induce both mucosal and circulating immune responses for optimal protection ***(1–3)***.

The systemic and mucosal immune systems communicate, but are somewhat compartmentalized ***(1–3)***. In general, induction of immune responses via systemic immunization supports systemic responses. Under appropriate conditions, mucosal introduction of foreign substances (antigens) can induce both mucosal and systemic responses. Following oral delivery, for example, antigens or invading pathogens, which can survive the harsh acid and degradative environments encountered, may be taken up by the specialized microfold or "M" cells in the small intestine and transported to the follicle beneath known as a Peyer's patch. T- and B-cell responses to the antigen occur there, followed by migration of the immune cells to the mesenteric lymph nodes. Activated cells travel via the efferent lymphatics to the thoracic duct, where they enter the circulation and migrate to various effector sites in the gastrointestinal, respiratory, and genitourinary tracts. This "Common Mucosal Immune System" allows the seeding of both systemic and mucosal sites with memory and effector cells ready to respond to the pathogen ***(1–3)***.

From: *Methods in Molecular Medicine, Vol. 42:*
Vaccine Adjuvants: Preparation Methods and Research Protocols
Edited by: D. T. O'Hagan © Humana Press, Inc., Totowa, NJ

There is evidence for both humoral- and cell-mediated responses contributing to the control of viruses, bacteria, and parasites, and having the potential for preventive or therapeutic effects *(3,4)*. Neutralizing antibodies can limit initial infection and pathogen spread *(5–7)*. Cytolytic T-cell responses play an important role in control and recovery from many viral and parasitic infections *(8,9)*. Appropriate T-helper responses are also crucial to protective immunity *(10,11)*.

Current evidence would suggest, therefore, that antibody- and cell-mediated responses, systemically and on mucosal surfaces, would be desirable for optimal protection against most infections.

1.2. Subunit Vaccines

It is becoming increasingly apparent that the natural immune response generated by infection with an organism often does not represent the optimal protective response against that organism *(12)*. Subunit vaccines, consisting of specific components of the pathogen, can be used to direct the immune response to targets that are protective *(13)*. Strain variation of immunologically important sites can be covered by the use of mixtures of peptides, proteins, or nucleic acids that code for them. In addition, less dominant, more highly conserved sites, can be presented more effectively than in the context of the whole organism.

Subunit vaccines are also attractive for reasons of safety. Many infectious organisms are too dangerous to risk even an occasional breakthrough in the process of inactivation used to produce a killed vaccine. Live attenuated vaccines can pose risks of reversion to wild type, as well as causing more severe disease in individuals whose immune system is compromised (e.g., owing to age, malnutrition, treatment with drugs, or infection with viruses, which are immunosuppressive) *(13)*.

The types of immune response generated by natural infection or exposure to the whole organism also may not be optimal for protection. The immune response to a foreign entity is determined by previous exposure to the same or a related structure, the dose and route of introduction, its biochemical composition and physical structure, and the immune status and genetics of the host. With the exception of host genetics and health, the above determinants are all amenable to manipulation and targeting with subunit vaccines. In particular, the use of adjuvants and delivery systems with subunit vaccines is an active and extremely promising area of investigation. Adjuvants and delivery systems can be used not only to augment the strength or duration of response, but also to influence the types of cell mediated and antibody responses induced *(13)*.

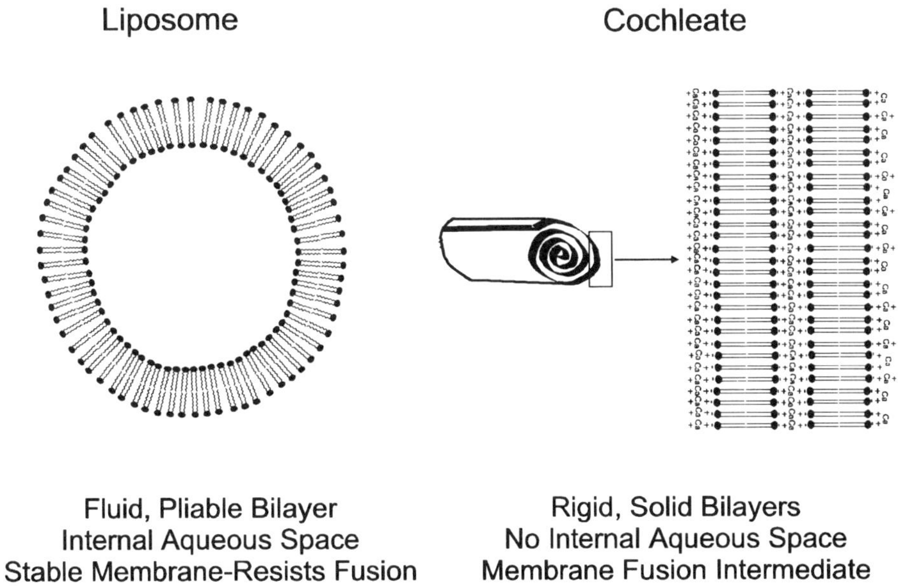

Fig. 1. Schematic representation of liposome and cochleate structures. Liposomes are comprised of internal aqueous space bounded by fluid lipid bilayers. Cochleates are composed of alternating layers of divalent cations (e.g., calcium), and solid lipid bilayer sheets stacked or rolled up in a spiral conformation, with little or no internal aqueous space.

1.3. Cochleate Delivery Vehicles

Cochleate delivery vehicles are unique vaccine carrier and delivery formulations composed of simple, natural materials (phosphatidylserine and calcium) *(14–19)*. Multiple cochleate administrations can be given to the same animal without adverse side effects, as they are nontoxic, noninflammatory, and biodegradable *(14)*. Cochleates are stable phospholipid-calcium precipitates, which are structurally distinct from liposomes (**Fig. 1**). There are substantial and critical differences between the composition and properties of liposomes and cochleates. Liposomes at physiological temperatures are comprised of fluid bilayer membranes with aqueous space contained within the compartments bounded by the lipid bilayers *(20)*. The fluid lipid bilayer is susceptible to attack from harsh environmental conditions, such as extremes of pH, or the presence of enzymes that digest lipid.

Cochleates are prepared through the calcium-induced fusion of liposomes composed of negatively charged phospholipid *(21)*. The binding of the divalent cations to the negatively charged lipid causes the liposomes to collapse

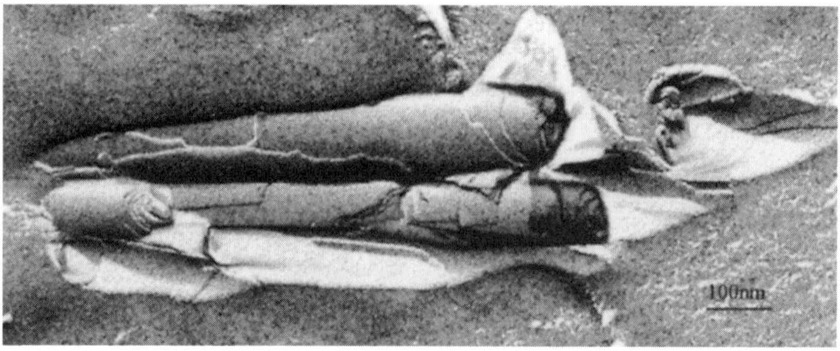

Fig. 2. Electron micrographs of freeze fracture preparations of DNA cochleates. Cochleates are solid, multilayered precipitates of calcium and negatively charged phospholipid. Calcium binding causes collapse and fusion of negatively charged liposomes into large continuous lipid bilayer sheets, which roll up or stack to form scroll-like or stacked sheet structures, excluding water.

into solid sheets that roll up or stack, excluding water (**Fig. 2**) ***(21)***. The multilayered structure provides protection from degradation for associated "encochleated" molecules. Because the entire cochleate structure is a series of solid layers, components within the interior of the cochleate structure remain intact, even though the outer layers of the cochleate may be exposed to harmful environmental conditions or enzymes. Cochleates can be stored as a suspension or lyophilized to a dry powder ***(14–19)***.

Membrane proteins, such as the surface glycoproteins of enveloped viruses, can be integrated into the lipid bilayers of cochleates at high efficiency. Native conformation and biological activities of these proteins are maintained ***(22–24)***. Peptides may be incorporated into cochleates by covalent crosslinking to phospholipid ***(15,16)***. DNA cochleates can be formed by trapping oligonucleotides or high molecular-weight plasmids within or between the lipid bilayers ***(16–18)***.

The protection of encochleated materials and structural stability of the cochleate allows for efficient delivery of proteins and polynucleotides in vivo by various routes. These include mucosal [oral, intragastric (ig), intranasal (in), and intraocular (io)], and parenteral [intramuscular (im), subcutaneous (sc), intraperitoneal (ip), and intradermal (id)], routes of administration (***14–19***, and unpublished).

1.4. Protein Cochleates

Cochleates as carriers for protein and peptide antigens effectively induce antibody- and cell-mediated immune responses. Protection from lethal and

Table 1
Summary of Cochleate Vaccine Studies

Formulations			
Viral Pathogens	Antigens	Routes of administration	
HIV-1	Viral Glycoproteins	Mucosal	Parenteral
Influenza A	Bacterial membrane proteins	Oral	Intramuscular
Parainfluenza	Peptides	Intranasal	Intradermal
Herpes simplex 1 and 2	DNA (polynucleotide) vaccines	Intraocular	Subcutaneous

Immune Responses			
Antibody		Proliferation	Cytotoxicity
Serum	Intestinal	Spleen	Spleen
Saliva	Fecal	Peyer's patches	Intestinal intraepithelial lymphocytes (iIELs)
Bronchial	Vaginal	Mesenteric lymph nodes	
		Inguinal lymph nodes	

Protection from Virus Challenge			
Cochleate vaccine	Route of immunization	Route of challenge	Protection from
Influenza A (protein)	Intramuscular, intranasal, oral	Intranasal	Replication
Herpes simplex 1 (DNA)	Intragastric or intramuscular	Intravaginal	Lethal dose
Herpes simplex 2 (DNA)	Intramuscular 1^0, intragastric, or intramuscular 2^0	Footpad	Neurological symptoms

infectious dose challenge with viruses administered parenterally and mucosally has also been achieved (*see* **Table 1** for summary) (***14–19***, and manuscripts in preparation). For example, cochleate vaccines containing the glycoproteins and lipids from the envelope of influenza virus were given to mice by gradually dispensing liquid into the mouth and allowing it to be swallowed (***14***, and in preparation). This study demonstrated that high circulating antibody titers could be achieved by simply drinking cochleate vaccines containing influenza virus glycoproteins. The response was boosted by repeated administration and was dose related to the amount of glycoprotein used. Hemagglutination inhibition titers indicated maintenance of the native viral glycoprotein conformation and induction of neutralizing antibodies following cochleate formulation and oral administration. Strong spleen cell proliferative responses were also generated (***14***, and in preparation).

In order to determine whether oral administration of this subunit vaccine afforded protective immunity in the respiratory tract, mice were immunized with cochleates and then were challenged by intranasal application (while awake) of influenza virus at one week after the final boost. Three days after viral challenge, the mice were sacrificed and the lungs and trachea were cultured to detect virus. The oral vaccine provided a high degree of protection from viral replication in the trachea and lungs. All the mice that received the four highest doses of vaccine (12.5 to 100 μg) were negative for virus upon culture. The 3- and 6-μg dose groups had reduced viral burdens in the lungs when compared to the controls (***14***, and in preparation).

In contrast to these results, in analogous experiments utilizing influenza glycoproteins in polylactide polyglycolide microspheres, oral delivery did not stimulate significant antibody responses. Intramuscular priming was required to obtain significant circulating or mucosal responses, and reduction of viral burdens in the respiratory tract, rather than protection from infection, was obtained ***(25)***. Hemagglutination inhibition titers generated by microspheres were also significantly lower, whereas corresponding enzyme-linked immunosorbent assay (ELISA) titers were high. This probably indicates a loss of native hemagglutinin (HA) glycoprotein conformation on exposure to the organic solvents involved in their formulation ***(25)***. The physiologically gentle conditions and lack of antigen exposure to organic solvents is one of the advantages of cochleate vaccine formulation.

In studies performed in our laboratories, the effects of lipid composition and liposome vs cochleate structure on immune responses to influenza glycoproteins were compared ***(17)***. Liposomes and cochleates containing synthetic dioleyol phosphatidylserine (PS), having two 18-carbon acyl chains, each with one unsaturated bond, and liposomes containing synthetic dimyristal phosphatidylglycerol (PG), with two 14-carbon saturated (no double bond) acyl chains, were prepared. Although PG has a negatively charged head group, liposomes containing the dimyristal PG did not collapse or form cochleates upon exposure to calcium, but instead retained their liposomal structure.

Mice were immunized orally or intramuscularly at 0 and 3 wk. At short time-points (week 1 and week 4), all three vaccines stimulated comparable levels of both IgG_1 and IgG_2a antibodies following im immunization. This antibody subtype distribution indicates the induction of both T-helper cell type 1 and type 2 responses (supporting IgG_2a and IgG_1, respectively). This has been confirmed by other experiments with cochleates in the influenza system and with proteins from other viruses, by antibody and cytokine (IL-4 and IFN-gamma elispot and cultured supernatant) assays. The pattern seen is for somewhat higher IgG_1 responses than IgG_2a, both increasing with subsequent immunizations. ELISA titers range from hundreds to millions, depending on the antigen, the dose, and immunization regimen. Interestingly, the ratio of IgG_1 to IgG_2a, after several immunizations with a given antigen, does not appear to be significantly different when comparing oral vs im immunization (***14,15,17***, and manuscripts in preparation). Other studies indicate that cochleate responses are slower to develop (particularly after oral delivery) and remain high longer than liposomes, supporting the possibility of slower release or availability (***14*** and unpublished observations).

Following oral administration, both PS liposomes and PS cochleates induced serum IgA antibodies, which were detectable at the first time-point, and increased at the second. The PG liposomes, however, did not stimulate production of IgA antibodies at either time-point. None of the formulations stimulated production of IgA when given intramuscularly. This difference of oral from intramuscular is consistent with induction of the immune response at a mucosal surface. In other studies, the amount of serum IgA was shown to be proportional to the number of oral (and not im) immunizations. In addition, oral immunization supports induction of salivary IgA responses, whereas im does not (***14,16***, and in preparation). Salivary IgG levels, in contrast, may be induced by either route, and tend to reflect serum levels, probably as a result of transudation (***14,16***, and in preparation). Oral or in delivery of protein or peptide cochleates has also been shown to stimulate production of other mucosal antibodies such as bronchial or vaginal wash, and fecal (***15*** and unpublished).

We initially hypothesized that the PS cochleates would work much better than the PS liposomes following oral delivery. However, IgG_1 and IgG_2a were measurable in the 4-wk samples for both PS formulations (and at 1 wk if measuring total IgG). In contrast, the PG liposomes failed to induce any IgG_2a, and only a very low amount of IgG_1 at week 4. The induction of fairly strong circulating antibody titers following oral immunization with the PS liposomes was significant and unexpected. Most protein based vaccines work very poorly or not at all when given orally, require priming by another route, or inclusion of mucosal adjuvants (which are often toxic) ***(1,2,25)***.

Obtaining these results led us to investigate the calcium concentrations in mouse saliva and stomach fluids. These were found to be more than sufficient (several millimolar) to collapse PS liposomes into cochleates. In addition, acid pH tends to stabilize and favor formation of cochleate structure. Therefore, the PS liposomes probably were converted to cochleates in vivo, and thereby protected from degradation in the stomach. The PG liposomes, which do not convert to cochleates in the presence of calcium, induced fairly strong responses when given intramuscularly, but failed to stimulate IgA or IgG_2a, and induced only a very low level of IgG_1 when given orally. This would be consistent with their degradation in the stomach. Very little protein probably remained intact, to be taken up by the Peyer's patches in the small intestine for induction of mucosal and systemic responses. This study supports the hypothesis that protection of proteins within the cochleate structure is important for immunogenicity following oral administration.

Peptides can also be strongly immunogenic when associated with cochleates. The V3 loop, a 32 amino acid loop from the surface glycoprotein of human immunodeficiency virus (HIV-1), was covalently crosslinked to phosphatidylethanolamine and incorporated into cochleates. Oral immunization (by drinking) induced serum, saliva, and fecal antibody responses. Cellular responses included proliferation of splenic, Peyers patch, and mesenteric lymph node cells, as well as cytolytic activity in intestinal intraepithelial lymphocytes (iIELs) (***16*** and in preparation). Intramuscular immunization induced serum antibodies, antigen specific proliferation of inguinal lymph node and splenocytes, and cytolytic activity by spleen cells (***16*** and in preparation).

1.5. DNA Cochleates

Cochleates are also highly effective carriers for DNA vaccines (***16–19***, and in preparation). Cochleates have been used to mediate the in vivo delivery and expression of a plasmid coding for the *env*, *tat*, and *rev* genes of HIV-1 (***16,17***, and in preparation). Induction of *gp160* (*env*) specific splenocyte proliferation and cytotoxic lymphocyte activity was observed following oral, as well as im, administration of DNA-cochleate formulations. The cochleates induced superior responses compared to naked DNA or DNA encapsulated in fusogenic proteoliposomes ***(17)***. Strong cytolytic and proliferative responses were induced to a single im injection of 3 or 17 μg encochleated DNA. Whereas 50 μg naked DNA generated little or no cytolytic or proliferative activity. Oral delivery, by swallowing cochleates at 0 and 4 wk, led to responses that were equivalent to those achieved intramuscularly. In contrast, a larger dose of naked DNA swallowed yielded no measurable proliferative or cytolytic responses (***16,17***, and in preparation). These results (and the ability to induce serum, fecal, and vaginal antibody responses) have been confirmed and extended in other viral systems in other laboratories (***16–18***, and manuscripts in preparation).

1.6. Adjuvants

Cochleates may be formulated with or coadministered with adjuvants, including protein, lipid, chemical, and DNA-based systems. The immune response to the cochleate associated antigen can be enhanced and modified by copresentation with adjuvants. These applications are currently being investigated (unpublished).

1.7. Summary

The above observations have been confirmed and extended in numerous studies in viral and bacterial systems using proteins, peptides, and DNA. The ability of cochleates to induce antibody- and cell-mediated responses, systemically and on mucosal surfaces, makes them desirable candidates for development of preventive and therapeutic vaccines. Current work focuses on the development of cochleates as safe and efficient protein- and nucleotide-based vaccines for the induction of mucosal and systemic immunity in humans and animals. Applications in gene therapy and drug delivery are also being developed *(26,27)*.

2. Materials

1. Lipids: Synthetic phosphatidylserine (1,2-Dipalmitoyl-sn-Glycero-3-Phospho-L-Serine) in chloroform and cholesterol in chloroform, in glass ampules, under nitrogen, were purchased from Avanti Polar Lipids in Birmingham, AL, and stored at –20°C. Organic solvents were purchased from Avanti or Fisher Scientific Company, Fairlawn, NJ.
2. Thick-walled polycarbonate ultracentrifuge tubes (10-mL capacity) from Beckman Instruments, Palo Alto, CA, were used for pelleting cochleates for quantitation of encochleated materials.
3. n-octyl-β-D-glucopyranoside (OCG), and chemicals for buffers, protein, and phosphate determinations were obtained from Sigma Chemical Company, St. Louis, MO.
4. Citrate buffer: 150 m*M* NaCl, 1.2 m*M* citric acid, 29 m*M* sodium citrate, 0.27 m*M* disodium edetic acid (EDTA), (pH 6.4).
5. Extraction buffer: 2 *M* NaCl, 0.02 *M* sodium phosphate (pH 7.4).
6. TES buffer: 2 m*M* TES (N-tris[hydroxymethyl]methyl-2-aminoethanesulfonic acid), 2 m*M* L-histidine, 100 m*M* NaCl (pH 7.4).
7. Dialysis tubing: Spectrapor 4 (10-mm diameter, 12,000–14,000 MW cutoff) was used for detergent removal in LC and DC methods (**Subheadings 3.2.** and **3.3.**). See note below for preparation and use of dialysis tubing. Alternative methods for detergent removal, such as ultrafiltration, may be used.
8. Bath sonicator: A Model G112SP1G bath-type sonicator from Laboratory Supplies Company, Hicksville, NY, was used for sonication of liposomes for trapping method. Alternative methods for production of small liposomes can be used (e.g., dialysis, ultrafiltration, homogenization, microfluidization).

3. Methods

3.1. Principles of Use

Macromolecules and drugs associate with cochleates according to their physical properties. Hydrophobic and electrostatic forces can be involved. The multilayered particulate structure of the cochleates determines their biodistribution, ability to protect and stabilize associated molecules, and the kinetics of release.

The efficiency of delivery of DNA, and the ability to induce CD8+ cytotoxic T-lymphocytes (CTL) responses with protein cochleates, may be caused by the fusion of cochleates with cell membranes in vivo. Many naturally

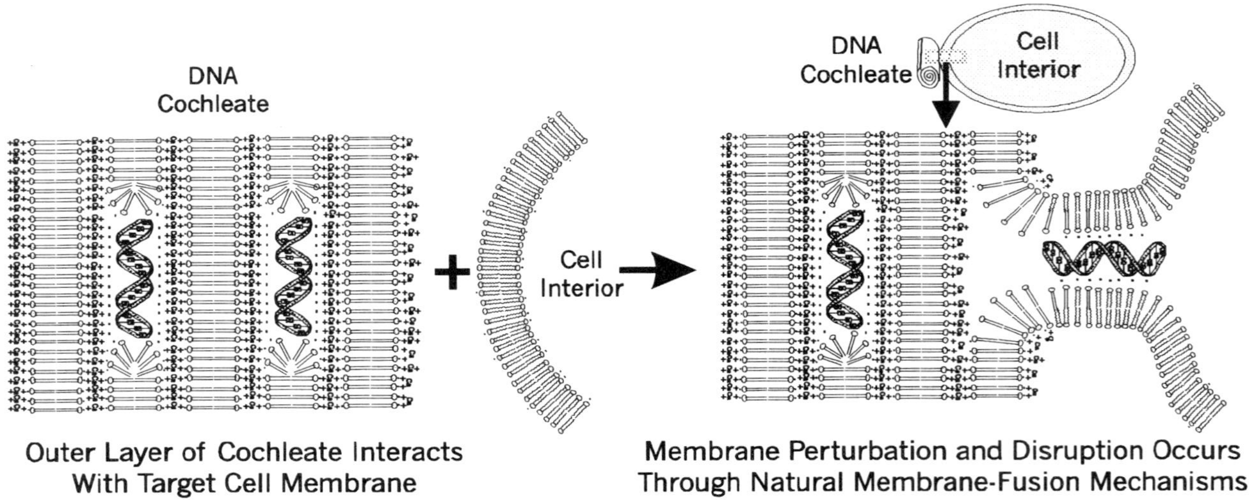

Fig. 3. Schematic representation of hypothetical fusion mechanism of a DNA cochleate with a cell. Cochleates may mimic natural fusion mechanisms involving calcium binding to negatively charged phospholipids in cell membranes.

occurring membrane fusion events involve membrane perturbations resulting from the interaction of calcium with negatively charged phospholipids (generally phosphatidylserine and phosphatidylglycerol) *(28)*. Cochleates can therefore be envisioned as membrane fusion intermediates (**Fig. 3**). Cochleates made with trace amounts of fluorescent lipids have been shown to bind and gradually transfer lipids to the plasma membrane and interior membranes of white blood cells (primary and cell lines) in vitro. In contrast, cochleates do not appear to fuse with red blood cells and are not hemolytic *(27)*.

3.2. LC Dialysis Method

This method for encochleation involves the removal of detergent from a *solution* of lipid and material to be encochleated, *followed by* addition of calcium. This method is particularly suited to the formulation of vaccines containing membrane proteins with intact transmembrane regions (*see* **Notes 1, 5, 6** below for more details and references), or peptides with hydrophobic tails (*see* **Note 7** below and **ref.** *29*).

1. Material to be encochleated is added to (or purified in) a solution containing a detergent in a high-salt buffer (e.g., 2% Octyl β-D glucopyranoside in extraction buffer).
2. Lipids (e.g., phosphatidylserine and cholesterol) are dried to a thin film in a supercleaned (*see* **Note 3**) glass tube by blowing nitrogen in while rotating at a 45° angle by hand or in a rotary evaporator flushed with nitrogen. Alternatively, lipid in powdered form is added to a polypropylene tube.
3. Buffer containing the material to be encochleated is added, nitrogen gas is blown in gently to replace air, and the lipid is suspended by agitation (vortex at least 7 min).
4. Incubate in ice bath 1 h.
5. Filter sterilize (0.22 μm filter) and transfer to dialysis bags. The detergent is removed by dialysis against TES buffer, resulting in the formation of small lipid vesicles. Other methods of detergent removal may be used (e.g., ultrafiltration).
6. Calcium is added by dialysis against TES buffer with 3 m*M* calcium chloride, then 6 m*M* calcium chloride, resulting in the formation of sheets of calcium-chelated phospholipid bilayers. Alternatively, liposomes may be removed from the bag or ultrafiltration unit, and calcium may be added directly in small aliquots, or continuously by injection using a pump.
7. The sheets roll up or stack to form cochleates containing the material of interest.
8. Cochleates are removed from the bags with a 1-mL pipet. Using the same pipet, the inside of the bag is rinsed with a small volume of TES 6 m*M* calcium buffer, to obtain higher recovery.
9. Store at 4°C under nitrogen, as a solution or lyophilized, protected from light.

3.3. DC Dialysis Method

This method for encochleation involves the removal of detergent from a solution of lipid and material to be encochleated by dialysis against a buffer containing calcium. This method has been applied to the formulation of vaccines containing membrane proteins (although protein recovery is lower than the LC method), and DNA plasmids.

1. Material to be encochleated is added to (or purified in) a solution containing a detergent in a high salt buffer (e.g., 2% Octyl β D glucopyranoside in extraction buffer).
2. Lipids (e.g., phosphatidylserine and cholesterol) are dried to a thin film in a super-cleaned glass tube by blowing nitrogen in while rotating at a 45° angle by hand or in a rotary evaporator flushed with nitrogen. Alternatively, lipid in powdered form is added to a polypropylene tube.
3. Buffer containing the material to be encochleated is added, nitrogen gas is blown in gently to replace air, and the lipid is suspended by agitation (vortex at least 7 min).
4. Filter sterilize if the sample is protein, but not if DNA plasmids are to be encochleated.
5. Transfer to dialysis bags.
6. The detergent is removed and calcium is added by dialysis against TES buffer with 3 m*M* calcium, then 6 m*M* calcium, resulting in the formation of sheets of calcium-chelated phospholipid bilayers.
7. The sheets roll up or stack to form cochleates containing the material of interest.
8. Cochleates are removed from the bags with a 1-mL pipet. Using the same pipet, the inside of the bag is rinsed with a small volume of TES 6 m*M* calcium buffer, to obtain higher recovery.
9. Store at 4°C as a solution or lyophilized, protected from light.

3.4. Trapping Methods

Trapping methods for encochleation involve the addition of calcium to a suspension of lipid and material to be encochleated. Variations of this method have been applied to DNA plasmids, oligonucleotides, soluble proteins, and amphipathic drugs *(27)*. Efficiency of encochleation of DNA is affected by ionic conditions and presence of calcium chelators.

1. Lipid (and material to be encochleated, if it is soluble in organic solvent) is dried to a thin film in a super-cleaned glass tube by blowing nitrogen in while rotating at a 45° angle by hand or in a rotary evaporator flushed with nitrogen. Alternatively, lipid in powdered form is added to a polypropylene tube.
2. Buffer is added, and the lipid is suspended by agitation (vortex at least 7 min) If starting from a lipid film in a glass tube, scrape any remaining lipid from the sides with a plastic, endotoxin-free pipet, vortex additional 1 min, and transfer the sample to a polypropylene tube. Blow nitrogen in, cap tightly, and wrap parafilm around cap and top of tube. Bath sonicate for a total of 5 min (1 min at a time). Bath sonicator should be precooled. Add clean water to sonicator to about full. Add approximately 5 mL of detergent (e.g., 7x glass washing detergent) to

increase efficiency of sonication. Add ice to fill. Remove ice prior to sonicating. Height of water should be adjusted to obtain maximal sonication (high pitch and splashing). Tube should be dunked up and down during sonication, as maximal sonication occurs at surface of bath. Ear protection should be worn.

3. Aqueous soluble material to be encochleated (e.g., DNA plasmid) is added to the liposome suspension in small aliquots (e.g., dropwise or 10-μL aliquots) with mixing by shaking gently by hand.
4. The addition of calcium in small (e.g., 10-μL aliquots) with mixing by hand results in the formation of sheets of calcium-chelated phospholipid bilayers.
5. The sheets roll up or stack to form cochleates containing the material of interest.
6. Store at 4°C under nitrogen, as a solution or lyophilized, protected from light.

3.5. Pelleting and Resuspension

Although it is not necessary, cochleates may be separated from unencochleated material by ultracentrifugation. Cochleates can then be resuspended to the exact concentrations (higher or lower than initial formulation) needed for immunization.

1. Distribute cochleates into sterile (rinse with ethanol, then three times with TES 6 m*M* calcium buffer) thick-walled polycarbonate tubes.
2. Ultracentrifuge 60 min, (60,000*g*), 5°C, in a TI 75 or comparable rotor.
3. Carefully remove supernatants. Pool and retain for analysis.
4. Resuspend cochleate pellets by vortexing in small volumes of TES 6 m*M* calcium buffer (pH 7.4), pooling in a single tube and rinsing sequentially to obtain quantitative transfer.
5. Measure cochleate associated material and correct to desired volume.

3.6. Quantitation of Cochleate Associated DNA

Following pelleting of cochleates, removal of supernatant and resuspension in TES 6 m*M* calcium buffer, aliquots may be taken for conversion to liposomes. Cochleate-associated DNA can be quantified and visualized by densitometric scanning of ethidium bromide (EthBr)-stained agarose gels. It is necessary to convert to liposomes first, as DNA in cochleates is not available for quantitation or visualization.

1. Transfer three 10-μL aliquots of resuspended cochleates (e.g., at 10 mg/mL) into each of three microfuge tubes. Vortex immediately prior to taking each sample, as cochleates settle.
2. Add 10 μL of TES buffer (pH 7.4) to each tube.
3. Add 150 m*M* EDTA (pH 9.5) in 5-μL aliquots (vortex after each addition), until sample becomes slightly alkaline (e.g., 10 μL). Monitor pH by removing 0.5-μL aliquots and depositing on pH paper (preferably pH 6.0–8.0 range with 0.1 U distinction).

4. Add 150 m*M* EDTA (pH 7.4) in 5-µL aliquots, until cochleates are converted to liposomes (e.g., 10 µL). Suspension turns from white particulate to opalescent. Check by light microscopy (x1000), oil immersion, phase contrast to confirm conversion of cochleate crystals to liposomes. Measure volume with a micropipetor.
5. Add 20 µL liposomes, 20 µL of 20% OCG, 80 µL 1X TE buffer, and 28 µL of 5X loading buffer to a microfuge tube. Vortex to mix and dissolve liposomes.
6. Add 10 or 20 µL of dissolved samples to individual wells (3 wells each) of a 1% agarose gel (0.5 µg EthBr/mL of 1X TAE (Sigma) running buffer, 10 min at 100 V, then approximately 2 h 30 min at 75 V.
7. Make standard curve with known amounts of starting material plasmid on same gel (e.g., from 0.031–2.0 µg). Dilute in buffer, lipid, and OCG like cochleate.
8. Determine concentration of unknowns by comparison with standard curve following densitometric scanning (e.g., using Bio-Rad (Richmond, CA) Fluor-S Multimager with Multianalyst software).

3.7. Quantitation of Cochleate-Associated Proteins

Following conversion to liposomes, cochleate associated protein can be quantified by the Modified Lowry Method of Peterson *(30)* and visualized by polyacrylamide gel electrophoresis (PAGE). It is necessary to convert to liposomes first, as proteins in cochleates are not available for quantitation or visualization.

1. Transfer 100 µL of cochleate suspension into each of three thick-walled polycarbonate tubes.
2. Dilute cochleates with 2.0 mL of TES 6 m*M* calcium buffer (pH 7.4).
3. Pellet by ultracentrifugation for 60 min (60,000*g*), 5°C, in a TI 75 or comparable rotor.
4. Carefully remove supernatants and retain for analysis.
5. Add 50 µL of TES buffer (pH 7.4). Vortex to resuspend.
6. Add 150 m*M* EDTA (pH 9.5) in 5-µL aliquots until solution is slightly basic. Monitor pH by removing 0.5-µL aliquots and depositing on pH paper (preferably pH 6.0–8.0 range with 0.1 U distinction).
7. Add 150 m*M* EDTA (pH 7.4) in 10-µL aliquots, until cochleates are converted to liposomes. Suspension turns from white particulate to opalescent. Check by light microscopy (×1000, oil immersion, phase contrast) to confirm conversion of cochleate crystals to liposomes. Measure volume and correct to 100 µL.
8. Determine protein concentration by running several volumes of each liposome aliquot in the Modified Lowry assay. Modified Lowry is the preferred method. In other methods, intact liposomes will cause light scattering, liposomes may convert back to cochleates (because of divalent cation concentrations), lipids may cause color development, and EDTA may inhibit color development.

4. Notes

1. Most cochleate formulations used for immunogenicity studies have utilized a 9:1 weight ratio of phosphatidylserine to cholesterol. Other negatively charged

lipids may be used as the predominant lipid and other lipids may be included. Cholesterol may be omitted. All the effects of these variations on cochleate structure and immunogenicity have not been defined and continue to be investigated.

2. The dioleoyl form of phosphatidylserine is unsaturated. Precautions to avoid oxidation, particularly when in organic solvent or dried down as a thin film, should be taken. Lipids should be stored at –20°C, and exposure to light and oxygen (keep under nitrogen) should be minimized. PS may be purchased as a powder, eliminating the need for organic solvents. The highest quality PS should be purchased and integrity maintained, as contaminants or oxidation products will affect structure and activity.
3. High quality borosilicate glass tubes can be utilized to dry lipids to a thin film using a stream of nitrogen. These tubes should be "super-cleaned" by brush washing with detergent, then bath sonication while filled with detergent solution, rinsing thoroughly, and sonicating while filled with water. Then rinse with methanol, then chloroform, followed by air-drying in a biosafety hood. This is to remove any chemical contaminants, or small particulate material that may promote oxidation of the lipid. Tubes are then covered with aluminum foil and baked at 250°C for 30 min or 180°C for 4 h to destroy endotoxin. Polypropylene tubes can be used for powdered lipid.
4. As with all research involving immunogenicity studies, endotoxin contamination should be avoided. All glassware is washed and rinsed thoroughly, then baked to sterilize and destroy endotoxin. Endotoxin-free pipets, tips, reagents, and water should also be utilized. DNA plasmids will be contaminated with large amounts of endotoxin unless specifically purified from it. Endotoxin has strong adjuvanting activity, which will lead to spurious and variable results. We routinely use the Qiagen EndoFree giga kits to purify plasmids, and the BioWhittaker (Walkersville, MD) kinetic LAL assay to assess endotoxin levels in reagents.
5. Dialysis: Spectrapor 4 (6-mm dry diameter, 12,000–14,000 MW cutoff). Dialysis tubing was boiled twice with Na_2CO_3, rinsed, then boiled twice with distilled H_2O. Wearing sterile gloves, appropriate length pieces (approx 25 cm) were cut, tied with two knots at one end, and autoclaved in distilled H_2O prior to use. Pieces were removed under sterile conditions, samples added with a 1-mL pipet, closed by tying two knots, and placed in a sterile, baked, graduated cylinder. Buffers and stirring bar should be sterilized by autoclaving. Rate of detergent removal can affect structures and efficiencies obtained. The first dialysis should be slow. For example, overnight against a ratio of 1 to 20 dialysate to buffer (e.g., 5–100 mL). Subsequent dialysis is faster. For example, 5 mL against 250 mL, changing at 4-h intervals (or overnight). For LC method, approximately six changes of TES, two of TES 3 m*M* calcium, two of TES 6 m*M* calcium. For DC method, six of TES 3m*M* calcium, two of TES 6 m*M* calcium. Other methods of detergent removal may be used.
6. Membrane proteins can be isolated from viral envelopes as previously described ***(14,31)***. The nonionic detergent, OCG, has been used extensively to promote reconstitution of membrane proteins into cochleates. OCG maintains native con-

formation and is easily removed by dialysis. We have routinely used OCG concentrations of 2% (20 mg/mL) at a detergent to lipid weight ratio of 6:1. We have found that high salt concentrations, (e.g., 2*M* NaCl), helps avoid protein aggregation and promotes high-quality recovery into cochleates. These conditions are also useful for isolating and solubilizing recombinant or purified viral or bacterial membrane proteins. We typically have utilized protein to lipid ratios of from 1:4 to 1:12 for membrane proteins. Trapping of soluble proteins has been accomplished at weight ratios of protein to lipid from 1:1 to 1:50.

7. Peptides containing a terminal cysteine may be linked to phosphatidylethanolamine using a heterobifunctional crosslinker (succinimidyl-4-*p*-maleimidophenyl) butyrate [SMPB, Pierce]) as previously described ***(29)***. This allows high-efficiency association of the peptides with cochleates and effective immunological presentation.
8. DNA may be encochleated by the trapping or DC methods. We have typically used a 1:10 weight ratio DNA to lipid, with DNA concentration between 0.33 to 3.0 mg/mL. DNA in citrate buffer, water, or TE, at a 1:2 volume ratio with Extraction buffer, has typically been used. Ionic strength, pH, the presence of various ionic species, and chelating agents, affect encochleation. These parameters are currently under investigation to define optimal conditions for DNA encochleation.
9. Hydrophilic proteins and drugs, and amphipathic molecules can be associated with cochleates by the trapping method. Ionic conditions and pH can be modified to obtain optimal encochleation.

Acknowledgments

We would like to thank Dr. Yvette Edghill-Smith, Dr. Eleonora Feketeova, Dr. Masoumeh T. Kheiri, Ruying Lu, Zheng Wang, and Dr. Fan Zhang, for contributions to the work on immune responses to cochleate vaccines; Dr. Daniel Brois and Dr. Zi Wei Chen for cochleate mediated gene expression; Anthony Scolpino and Dr. Leila Zarif for cochleate interactions with drugs and cells; and Joan Hudock for administrative support. The freeze fracture electron micrograph in **Fig. 2** was done in collaboration with Dr. Brigitte Papahadjopoulos-Sternberg.

References

1. McGhee, J. R., Mestecky, J., Dertzbaugh, M. T., Eldridge, J. H., Hirasawa, M., and Kiyono, H. (1992) The mucosal immune system: from fundamental concepts to vaccine development. *Vaccine* **10,** 75–88.
2. Walker, R. I. (1994) New strategies for using mucosal vaccination to achieve more effective immunization. *Vaccine* **12,** 387–396.
3. (Ogra, P., Mestecky, J., Lamm, M., Strober, W., McGhee, J. R., and Bienenstock, J., eds.) (1998) *Mucosal Immunology*, 2nd Edition. Marcel Dekker, New York.

4. (Levine, M. M., Woodrow, G. C., Kaper, J. B., and Cobon, G. S., eds.) (1997) *New Generation Vaccines*, 2nd Edition. Marcel Dekker, New York.
5. Wilson, J. A. and Cox, N. J. (1990) Structural basis of immune recognition of influenza virus hemagglutinin. *Ann. Rev. Immunol.* **8,** 737–771.
6. Michetti, P., Mahan, M. J., Slauch, J. M., Mekalanos, J. J., and Neutra, M. R. (1992) Monoclonal secretory immunogloboulin A protects mice against oral challenge with the invasive pathogen salmonella typhimurium. *Infect. Immun.* **60,** 1786–1792.
7. Bruck, C., Thiriart, C., Fabry, L., Francotte, M., Pala, P., vanOpstal, D., et al. (1994) HIV-1 neutralizing antibody titers induced by vaccination correlate with protection from infection and decreased virus load in chimpanzees. *Vaccine* **12,** 141–48.
8. McMichael, A. J., Gotch, F. M., Noble, G. R., and Beare, P. A. S. (1983) Cytotoxic T-cell immunity to influenza. *N. Engl. J. Med.* **309,** 13–17.
9. Safrit, J. T., Andrews, C. A., Zhu, T., Ho, D. D., and Koup, R. A. (1994) Characterization of human immunodeficiency virus type 1-specific cytotoxic T lymphocyte clones isolated during acute seroconversion: Recognition of autologous virus sequences within a conserved immunodominant epitope. *J. Exp. Med.* **179,** 463–72.
10. Doherty, P. C., Allen, W., Eichelberger, M., et al. (1992) Roles of αβ and γδ T cell subsets in viral immunity. *Annu. Rev. Immunol.* **10,** 123–151.
11. Shearer, G. M. and Clerici, M. (1997) Vaccine strategies: selective elicitation of cellular or humoral immunity? *Trends Biotechnol.* **3,** 106–109.
12. Marrack, P. and Kappler, J. (1994) Subversion of the immune system by pathogens. *Cell* **76,** 323–328.
13. (Powell, M. F. and Newman, M. J., eds.) (1995) *Vaccine Design: The Subunit and Adjuvant Approach.* Plenum, New York.
14. Mannino, R. J. and Gould-Fogerite, S. (1995) Lipid matrix-based vaccines for mucosal and systemic immunization, in *Vaccine Design: The Subunit and Adjuvant Approach* (Powell, M. F. and Newman, M. J., eds.), Plenum, New York, pp. 363–387.
15. Gould-Fogerite, S. and Mannino, R. J. (1996) Mucosal and systemic immunization using cochleate and liposome vaccines. *J. Lipo. Res.* **6,** 357–379.
16. Mannino, R. J. and Gould-Fogerite, S. (1997) Antigen cochleate preparations for oral and systemic vaccination, in *New Generation Vaccines* (Levine, M. M., Woodrow, G. C., Kaper, J. B., and Cobon, G. S., eds.), 2nd Edition, Marcel Dekker, New York, pp. 229–237.
17. Gould-Fogerite, S., Kheiri, M. T., Zhang, F., Wang, Z., Scolpino, A., Feketeova, E., et al. (1998) Targeting immune response induction with cochleate and liposome-based vaccines. *Adv. Drug Del. Rev.* **32,** 273–287.
18. Gould-Fogerite, S. (1998) Cochleate vaccines for mucosal and systemic immunization, in *The Proceedings of the Onzieme Colloque Des Cent Gardes*. Elsevier Science, Shannon, Ireland, pp. 215–220.
19. Michalek, S. M., O'Hagen, D. T., Gould-Fogerite, S., Osterhaus A. D. M. E., and Rimmelzwaan, G. F. (1998) Antigen delivery systems: nonliving microparticles,

liposomes, cochleates, and ISCOMS, in *Mucosal Immunology*, 2nd Edition (Ogra, P., et al., eds.), Marcel Dekker, New York, pp. 759–778.
20. Gregoriadis, G. (1996) Liposome vaccines. *J. Lipo. Res.* **6,** 1–642.
21. Papahadjopoulos, D., Vail, W. J., Jacobson, K., and Poste, G. (1975) Cochleate lipid cylinders: formation by fusion of unilamellar lipid vesicles. *Biochim. Biophys. Acta* **394,** 483–490.
22. Gould-Fogerite, S. and Mannino, R. J. (1985) Rotary dialysis: Its application to the production of large liposomes and large proteoliposomes (protein-lipid vesicles) with high encapsulation efficiency and efficient reconstitution of membrane proteins. *Anal. Biochem.* **148,** 15–25.
23. Gould-Fogerite, S., Mazurkiewicz, J. E., Bhisitkul, D., and Mannino, R. J. (1987) The reconstitution of biologically active glycoproteins into large liposomes: Use as a delivery vehicle to animal cells, in *Advances in Membrane Biochemistry and Bioenergetics* (Kim, C. H., Diwan, J., Tedeschi, H., and Salerno, J. J., eds.), Plenum, New York, pp. 569–586.
24. Gould-Fogerite, S., Mazurkiewicz, J., Lehman, J., Raska, Jr., K., Voelkerding, K., and Mannino, R. J. (1989) Chimerasome-mediated gene transfer in vitro and in vivo. *Gene,* **84,** 429–438.
25. Moldoveanu, Z., Novak, M., Huang, W-Q., Gilley, R. M., Staas, J. K., Schafter, D., et al. (1993) Oral immunization with influenza virus in biodegradable microspheres. *J. Infect. Dis.* **167,** 84–90.
26. Zarif, L., Brois, D., Chen, Z. W., Zhang, F., Gould-Fogerite, S., and Mannino, R. J. (1997) Utilization of cochleates for the delivery of genetic material in vivo, in *Cancer Gene Therapy* (Mazarakis, H. and Swart, S. J., eds.), IBC Library Series, Southborough, UK, pp. 77–89.
27. Zarif, L. and Mannino, R. J. (2000) Cochleates: lipid based vehicles for gene delivery-Concept, achievements, and future development, in *Cancer Gene Therapy: Past Achievements and Future Challenges* (Habib, N., ed.), Plenum, London, pp. 83–94.
28. Creutz, C. E. (1992) The annexins and exocytosis. *Science* **258,** 924–931.
29. Goodman-Snitkoff, G., Good, M. F., Berzofsky, J. A., and Mannino, R. J. (1991) Role of Intrastructural/Intermolecular help in immunization with peptide-phospholipid complexes. *J. Immunol.* **147,** 410–415.
30. Peterson, G. L. (1977) Modified Lowry procedure for protein determination. *Anal. Biochem.* **83,** 346–356.
31. Gould-Fogerite, S. and Mannino, R. J. (1992) Targeted fusogenic liposomes: functional reconstitution of membrane proteins into large unilamellar vesicles via protein-cochleate intermediates, in *Liposome Technology*: 2nd Edition (Gregoriadis, G., ed.), CRC, Boca Raton, FL. vol. III, ch. 17, pp. 262–275.

11

Virus-like Particles As Vaccine Adjuvants

Sarah C. Gilbert

1. Introduction

Adjuvants are available to promote the generation of antibodies to an antigen following immunization. However, many of these adjuvants do not enhance priming of cytotoxic T lymphocytes (CTL). The reason for this lies in the existence of two alternative antigen processing pathways, leading to stimulation of $CD4^+$ T cells, and, in turn, to the generation of antibodies, or stimulation of $CD8^+$ CTL. In general, exogenous proteins enter the antigen presenting cell (APC) by endocytosis. Peptides produced by proteolytic degradation of these proteins bind to major histocompatibility complex (MHC) Class II molecules that travel to the surface of the cell before stimulating $CD4^+$ T cells. Peptides derived from cytoplasmic proteins are translocated into the endoplasmic reticulum and bind to MHC Class I molecules. When these reach the surface of the APC, they prime $CD8^+$ CTL. Thus to generate a CTL response following immunization, it is necessary to feed peptides into the correct processing pathway. This can be done by expressing the antigen inside the APC, using a DNA vaccine or recombinant virus. DNA vaccines can be produced easily, but there are still concerns over the long-term safety of this new type of vaccine, and the $CD8^+$ T-cell response may only be moderate *(1)*. Recombinant viruses are more difficult to prepare, and there are safety concerns over the use of some viruses as vaccines. However, recombinant virus-like particles (VLPs) are a safe and highly immunogenic alternative. These small particles consisting of one or more viral coat proteins can act as an adjuvant by carrying peptide sequences inside the APC and feeding into the "endogenous" processing pathway *(2,3)*, a phenomemon known as "cross-priming." No additional adjuvant is needed. If

From: *Methods in Molecular Medicine, Vol. 42:*
Vaccine Adjuvants: Preparation Methods and Research Protocols
Edited by: D. T. O'Hagan © Humana Press, Inc., Totowa, NJ

VLPs are administered with alum, CTL priming does not take place, although the antibody response to the VLPs is enhanced *(4,5)*.

The effect of other adjuvants on CTL induction with Ty-VLPs has also been studied *(5)*. Mice immunized with recombinant Ty-VLPs mixed with aqueous adjuvants (Detox, γ-inulin, galactosaminylmuramyl dipeptide, or Chemivax) generated CTL responses, but at levels lower than in the "no adjuvant" group. Other adjuvants (alhydrogel, algamulin, or SAF-MF) completely abrogated CTL responses, although formulation of the Ty-VLPs with a very low level of alum (sufficient to bind 6% of the TyVLP protein) enhanced the CTL response.

Recombinant VLPs are safe and well tolerated. They do not contain any nucleic acids, and are produced by the overexpression of one or more viral proteins in the absence of the rest of the viral genome. They are therefore noninfective, and are produced using an expression system (*Saccharomyces cerevisiae*) that can easily be handled in the laboratory and is completely safe to use.

Many viral coat proteins have been used to produce VLPs. In some cases it is of interest to induce an immune response against epitopes contained with the particle-forming protein itself. The widely used vaccine against hepatitis B consists of VLPs, and studies have been carried out using VLPs to immunize against HIV *(6)*, Norwalk virus *(7)*, and rotavirus *(8)*. However, some VLP-forming proteins will tolerate the addition of peptide sequences without losing the ability to form particles, and then act as an adjuvant for the additional sequence. Some, such as the hepatitis B core antigen *(9)* and the cowpea mosaic virus *(10)*, can only carry a small number of amino acids, but there are several systems for producing VLPs carrying long N- or C-terminal extensions.

A number of chimeric particles have been constructed using the NS1 protein of bluetongue virus expressed in recombinant baculovirus *(11)*. Up to 116 amino acids were inserted at the C-terminus, resulting in the formation of tubules with the foreign sequence exposed on the surface. When insect cells were coinfected with three different recombinant baculovirus constructs, hybrid tubules containing the foreign sequence from all three were produced, proving this to be a flexible system. Chimeric VLPs have also been produced using papillomavirus proteins *(12)*. Up to 43 kDa can be fused to the L2 minor capsid protein, which is then coexpressed with the L1 major capsid protein, resulting in the formation of hybrid particles carrying the foreign sequence. However, as the VLPs consist mainly of the nonrecombinant L1, the dose of foreign sequence per VLP is reduced.

Ty-VLPs are formed from a single protein species derived from the p1 protein of the TyA retrotransposon found in *S. cerevisiae.* The p1 protein can be expressed from a multicopy plasmid in *S. cerevisiae*, resulting in the formation of hollow, spherical 30-nm particles in the cytoplasm of the yeast. VLPs still assemble when only the first 381 amino acids of the p1 sequence are expressed, and foreign sequences of up to 42 kDa can be fused to the C-terminus without preventing particle formation ***(13)***. In one study, strings of epitopes were synthesized, linked together and fused to TyA p1. The longest epitope string tested contained 229 amino acids, and VLP yield was not reduced by the presence of the foreign sequence ***(14)***. As Ty-VLPs are produced in *S. cerevisiae*, it is highly likely that the protein particles have mannose residues attached.

It is thought that this contributes to the adjuvant effect by enhancing uptake of Ty-VLPs into APCs, although the mechanism of uptake has not been studied in detail.

In a study designed to compare CTL induction using 10 different vaccine/adjuvant combinations, only lipopetides and Ty-VLPs carrying a foreign epitope consistently primed CTL responses in all immunized animals ***(15)***. After a single subcutaneous (sc) dose of 100 µg Ty-VLPs carrying a CTL epitope, net-specific lysis ranged from 42 to 62% when assayed at an effector: target (E: T) ratio of 40: 1. Reducing the dose to 20 µg resulted in net-specific lysis levels of 25 to 42% at the same E: T ratio. Mucosal immunization of macaques with a Ty-VLP carrying simian immunodeficiency virus (SIV) p27 resulted in induction of MHC Class I restricted $CD8^+$ CTL responses ***(16)***. In this study, short-term cell lines were grown from peripheral blood mononuclear cells (PBMCs) following repeated immunization with Ty-VLPs carrying the SIV p27 sequence. Between 33 and 42% of cell lines were positive for SIV p27-specific lysis, whereas no positive lines were present in animals that had been immunized with Ty-VLPs lacking the SIV p27 sequence. High titre neutralizing antibodies to HIV V3 were produced when recombinant Ty-VLPs were injected with alum ***(17)***. Clinical trials have been carried out with Ty-VLPs carrying HIV sequences, with and without alum. The vaccine was safe and well tolerated. Antibodies and lymphoproliferative responses were generated when alum was used ***(18,19)***, and CTL were primed when alum was omitted ***(20)***.

It may sometimes be desirable to induce either T-cell responses or antibodies against the same protein sequence. This can be done with recombinant Ty-VLPs by immunizing with or without alum. However, if only an antibody response is required, this is probably best achieved by a simpler approach such as immunizing with protein mixed with an adjuvant.

This chapter describes the production of recombinant Ty-VLPs. Some sequences have been found to prevent particle formation, or reduce the expression of the recombinant protein to a level that makes purification difficult. However, the majority of sequences that have been tested resulted in particle formation. In order to produce Ty-VLPs, DNA encoding the desired sequence is fused in frame to the C-terminus of the truncated TyA *p1* gene, which is controled by a galactose inducible promoter. *S. cerevisiae* is then transformed with the new construct, together with a second plasmid that improves VLP yield after galactose induction. The transformed yeast is then grown to high cell density and Ty-VLP production is induced by the addition of galactose. The yeast cells are harvested and lysed to release the Ty-VLPs, which are purified by density gradient centrifugation using sucrose. The protocol, which can easily be carried out in a laboratory, produces Ty-VLPs of a quantity and purity suitable for animal immunisation or in vitro studies. If material for clinical trials is required, the production process can be scaled up and carried out in a GMP facility.

2. Materials

2.1. Plasmids and Yeast Strain

Plasmid pOGS40 contains a C-terminal truncated *p1* gene (amino acids 1-381) in a multicopy yeast plasmid (**Fig. 1**). A *Bam*HI site immediately 5′ to the stop codon allows additional coding sequence to be inserted. Plasmids pOGS 40, 41, and 42 have the *Bam*HI site in reading frames 1, 2, and 3, respectively, but are otherwise identical. These three plasmids contain the yeast *LEU2* marker that will transform a *leu2* auxotroph to leucine independence.

The *p1* gene is under the control of the strong, galactose-inducible PAL promoter. In the absence of galactose in the yeast cell, the GAL80 protein binds to the GAL4 protein. When galactose is present, GAL4 is released and binds to an upstream activation sequence in the PAL promoter, thereby activating transcription. However, the amount of GAL4 protein present in the yeast cell is low, and limits the induction of transcription from a multicopy plasmid containing a galactose-inducible promoter. Plasmid pUG41S contains the *GAL4* gene under the control of a galactose-inducible promoter, and the *URA3* marker. When a yeast cell is transformed with this plasmid as well as pOGS40, the amount of GAL4 protein available to activate transcription after galactose induction is increased, resulting in the production of larger amounts of the p1 fusion protein, which then assembles into Ty-VLPs.

The yeast strain for Ty-VLP production must be auxotrophic for leucine and uracil (*leu2*, *ura3*). It is also advantageous if it has mutations in intracellular proteases, which could otherwise degrade the Ty-VLPs during the purification process. Yeast strain MC2 is a suitable strain, but is also auxotrophic for tryptophan. Therefore, after transformation with pUG41S and a derivative of pOGS40, tryptophan must be included in the selective medium.

The plasmids described above and the yeast strain MC2 may be obtained from Dr. Guy Layton, British Biotechnology Ltd., Watlington Road, Cowley, Oxford OX4 5LY, U.K.

A

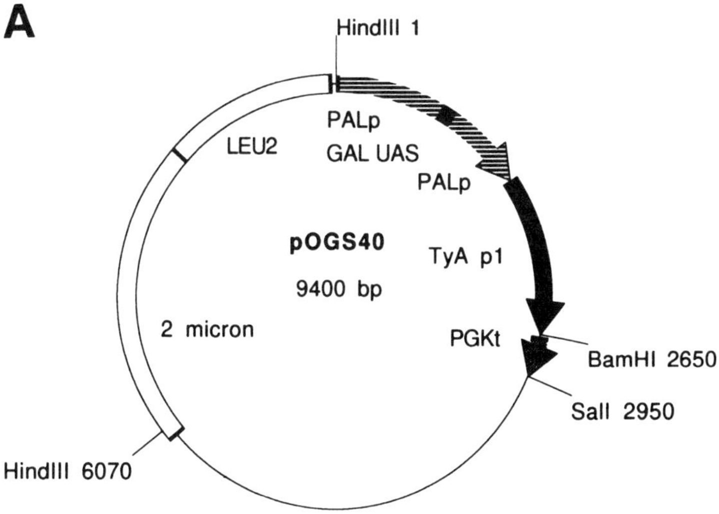

B

Sequence around the *Bam*HI site in pOGS40

```
              BamHI
AAA GCC GGA TCC GGG AAA TAA
 K   A   G   S   G   K  Stop
```

Oligonucleotides to ligate into *Bam*HI site

```
5'GA TCC AAG GGA AAC GAC AAG TCC TTG TAC G 3'
     3'G TTC CCT TTG CTG TTC AGG AAC ATG CTA G 5'
      S   K   P   N   D   K   S   L   Y   G
```

Fig. 1. **(A)** Plasmid map of pOGS40. **(B)** the DNA sequence around the *Bam*HI site at the 3′ end of the TyA *p1* gene, and an example of a pair of oligonucleotides designed to ligate into the *Bam*HI site, encoding the HLA-B35 CTL epitope KPNDKSLY from the liver stage antigen 1 gene of *Plasmodium falciparum*.

2.2. Yeast Transformation

1. YEPD medium: yeast extract 10 g/L, peptone 20 g/L, glucose 20 g/L, autoclaved.
2. Sterile distilled water.
3. 40% polyethylene glycol 3000 solution, autoclaved.
4. Selection plates: 6.7 g/L yeast nitrogen base (YNB), 10 g/L glucose, 20 g/L agar, 1*M* sorbitol. Autoclave and cool to 50°C. Filter sterilize a 1% solution of tryptophan and add 2 mL/L. Swirl to mix and pour plates.

5. 20% sucrose, autoclaved.
6. Bio-Rad Gene Pulser (Richmond, CA) electroporation apparatus and 0.2-cm gap cuvets.

2.3. Growth of Yeast to Induce Ty-VLP Production

1. Growth medium: 6.7 g/L YNB, 10 g/L glucose, autoclaved. Add 2 mL/L 1% tryptophan, filter sterilized, just before use.
2. Induction medium: 6.7 g/L YNB, 3 g/L glucose, 10 g/L galactose, autoclaved, with tryptophan added just before use, as above.
3. TEN buffer: 100 m*M* Tris pH7.4, 10 m*M* EDTA, 1.4*M* NaCl. Autoclave and chill before use.

2.4. Yeast Cell Disruption

1. Glass beads, 40 mesh (BDH, London, England), autoclaved.

2.5. Purification of Ty-VLPs

1. 60% sucrose in TEN buffer, autoclaved.
2. 35% sucrose in TEN buffer, autoclaved.
3. Prepared dialysis tubing.

2.6. Assessment of Ty-VLP Yield and Purity

1. Sodium dodecyl sulfate-polyacrylamide gel electrophoresis (SDS-PAGE) minigel apparatus and reagents.
2. Denaturing sample buffer.
3. Coomassie stain and destain.

3. Methods

3.1. Preparation of Plasmids

1. To make Ty-VLPs expressing additional amino acid sequences, the required sequence is added at the *Bam*HI site of pOGS 40, 41, or 42. This sequence may consist of single B- or T-cell epitopes, strings of epitopes joined together, or whole antigens. If defined epitopes are to be used, the DNA sequence coding for the epitope should be synthesized as oligonucleotides. These should be designed to fuse in frame to one of the pOGS vectors (*see* **Fig. 1**). No stop codon is necessary as this is present after the *Bam*HI site in the vectors. If the epitope is derived from an organism with a codon usage very different from that of yeast, the insert should be designed using yeast codon bias.
2. It is then necessary to check for the possibility of the formation of secondary structures within the oligos, and alter the sequence if necessary (*see* **Note 1**). It is preferable to synthesize oligos for both the top and bottom strand of the insert. They should be purified after synthesis (high-pressure liquid chromatography [HPLC] or gel purification) and 5′ phosphate groups should be added. The oligos are then annealed by heating 5 pmol of each in 20 µL water to 95°C, and allowing

them to cool slowly. Five μL of this mixture is then ligated to 0.1 μg of the appropriate pOGS vector, which has been digested with *Bam*HI and phosphatased to prevent religation of the vector. Competent cells of *Escherichia coli* are then transformed with the ligation mix, and plasmids prepared by standard methods.

3. For very small inserts, it is not possible to determine the orientation by restriction digests, so the plasmid must be sequenced (*see* **Note 2**). All oligo inserts need to be sequenced to confirm that the newly synthesized sequence does not contain errors.
4. The maximum length for oligo synthesis is around 80 bases if a reasonable yield is to be obtained. For an insert of greater than 30 amino acids, design two oligos for the top strand and two for the bottom, with an overlap of eight basepairs in the center. If epitope strings of more than 60 amino acids are required, it is preferable to construct a series of cassettes containing three or four epitopes in each, with a *Bgl*II site at the 5′ end and a *Bam*HI site at the 3′ end. Each cassette can be assembled in a cloning vector and sequenced. The first cassette is then introduced at the *Bam*HI site of pOGS40, leaving a single *Bam*HI site at the 3′ end for the addition of further cassettes.

3.2. Yeast Transformation

There are several methods by which yeast cells may be transformed. The method given below, electroporation, needs little technical expertise, but requires the use of an electroporation apparatus. Other methods for yeast transformation (lithium acetate, sphaeroplasting) are given in ***(21)***.

1. Grow yeast MC2 in YEPD (50 mL in a 250-mL conical flask). Monitor cell density by removing a sample aseptically, diluting the sample 1 in 10 with water and measuring OD_{600} in a spectrophotometer, using water as a blank. The cells are ready to use when the OD_{600} of the diluted sample is between 0.4 and 0.6 (*see* **Note 3**).
2. Harvest by centrifugation in sterile 50-mL Falcon tubes in a benchtop centrifuge, 10 min at 1900*g*, 4°C.
3. Resuspend the pellet in 50 mL ice-cold sterile distilled water, pellet cells again. Repeat this wash step twice more.
4. Resuspend the cells in 5 mL ice-cold sterile distilled water. Chill on ice.
5. Add the two plasmids for cotransfection (pOGS40 derivative and pUG41S) to an electroporation cuvet. Use 5 μg of each plasmid in a total volume of 10 μL sterile distilled water. Chill on ice.
6. Add 100 μL yeast cells and 50 μL 40% PEG 3000 solution to the cuvet containing the DNA. Mix, incubate on ice for 10 min.
7. Set the following values on the gene pulser apparatus: resistance 1000, capacitance 25, voltage 0.8. Dry the cuvet and pulse.
8. Add 0.5 mL 20% sucrose to the cuvet, mix and transfer the contents to a sterile Eppendorf tube.
9. Plate out all the yeast cells on selection plates, spreading approximately 200 μL per plate. Allow the surface of the plates to dry, then incubate at 30°C. Colonies should appear within 1 wk. (*See* **Note 4**).

10. When transformants appear, streak each one on a fresh selection plate (sorbitol need not be included at this stage) and incubate for 2–3 d. For short-term storage, these plates can be sealed with parafilm and held at 4°C. For longer term storage of transformants, prepare glycerol stocks (**Note 5**).

3.3. Growth of Yeast to Induce Ty-VLP Production

1. Inoculate 50 mL of growth medium in a 250-mL conical flask with a loopful of cells grown from a single transformant, or a glycerol stock.
2. Incubate at 30°C in a shaking incubator for at least 24 h.
3. Remove a sample of the culture aseptically. Dilute 100 µL of the cells with 900 µL water and measure the OD_{600} in a spectrophotometer, using water as a blank. The OD_{600} of the diluted sample should be at least 0.2. If it is below this, return the flask to the incubator and continue monitoring (*see* **Note 6**).
4. Inoculate 500 mL of induction medium in a 2-L conical flask with the 50-mL culture. Incubate at 30°C with shaking for 18 h. Monitor OD_{600}. If it is less than 0.2, continue to incubate the culture for another 6 h.
5. Harvest the induced culture by centrifugation at 4°C, for example 15 min at 5000*g* in a Beckman (Fullerton, CA) J-6MC centrifuge with JS4.2 rotor. Discard the supernatant and resuspend the cells in 50 mL chilled TEN buffer. Transfer to a 50-mL Falcon tube and pellet the cells in a benchtop centrifuge, 5 min at 1900*g*, 4°C.
6. Repeat the wash step once more, and discard the supernatant. The cells can be frozen at –70°C at this point for assay at a later date if required.

3.4. Yeast Cell Disruption

1. Resuspend the cell pellet in 2 mL ice-cold TEN buffer and add 6 g sterile glass beads.
2. Vortex vigorously for 5 min (*see* **Note 7**).
3. Centrifuge the homogenate for 5 min at 1900*g*, 4°C in a benchtop centrifuge. Remove the supernatant to a 50-mL Falcon tube, on ice.
4. Add another 2 mL of TEN buffer to the pellet and vortex vigorously for 5 min. Centrifuge and add the supernatant to that collected in **step 3**.
5. Add 1 mL of TEN buffer to the pellet; vortex, centrifuge, and add the supernatant to that collected in **steps 3** and **4**.
6. Centrifuge the supernatant for 20 min at 13,000*g*, 4°C, for example in a Beckman J2-MC centrifuge with JA12 rotor.
7. Carefully transfer the supernatant (clarified lysate) to a clean tube and keep on ice. Retain a sample of the supernatant for SDS-PAGE analysis.

3.5. Purification of Ty-VLPs

1. Add 2.75 mL of the clarified lysate to a 3.2-mL polycarbonate ultracentrifuge tube. Set a Gilson P200 pipet to 250 µL, and carefully underlay 250 µL of 60% sucrose in TEN buffer at the bottom of the tube (*see* **Note 8**).
2. Prepare a balance tube and centrifuge at 417,000*g* for 17 min at 4°C, in a Beckman Optima TL benchtop ultracentrifuge with TLA 100.4 rotor. Acceleration and deceleration rates should be set to midrange *(5)*.

3. The Ty-VLPs will accumulate just above the 60% sucrose layer, and it may be possible to see a milky band in the tube at this point. Remove the supernatant above this and discard. If no milky band is visible, it will still be possible to distinguish the interface between the sucrose and the supernatant. Remove the supernatant leaving 2 to 3 mm above the interface.
4. Resuspend the material remaining in the tube in 1 mL ice-cold TEN buffer.
5. Add 1.5 mL of 35% sucrose in TEN to a clean centrifuge tube. Underlay with 250 µL 60% sucrose in TEN as before. Slowly layer the resuspended material from **step 4** on top of the 35% sucrose.
6. Prepare a balance tube and centrifuge at 417,000*g* for 40 min at 4°C.
7. Repeat **step 3**. Resuspend the remaining material in 1 mL ice-cold TEN buffer. Retain a sample for SDS-PAGE analysis.
8. Remove the sucrose from the Ty-VLPs by overnight dialysis in TEN buffer, at 4°C. Measure the protein concentration using, for example, the Bio-Rad protein assay kit. Aliquot and freeze samples for storage at –70°C (*see* **Note 9**).

3.6. Assessment of Ty-VLP Yield and Purity

1. Prepare a 10% SDS-PAGE minigel.
2. Prepare the samples for analysis in denaturing loading buffer. Boil the samples for 2 min. This causes the Ty-VLPs to dissociate into protein monomers which can easily be visualized after SDS-PAGE. Samples should include the clarified lysate (diluted 1 in 10) and the final preparation, with size standards covering the range 6–175 kDa. It is also helpful to include Ty-VLPs prepared from yeast cotransformed with the pOGS40 vector and pUG41S, as a positive control for galactose induction and VLP preparation.
3. Run the SDS-PAGE gel, loading 2, 5, and 10 µL of each sample. Stain the gel with Coomassie.
4. Ty-VLP momomers should be clearly visible on the destained gel, although the yield obtained with fusions to the p1 sequence may be less than that obtained using the pOGS40 vector alone. TyA from pOGS40 has an apparent molecular weight of around 65 kDa (**Fig. 2**). If no Ty-VLPs are present, but a band of the expected size is found in the clarified lysate, the fusion of the additional sequence has interfered with particle formation.

3.7. Scale Up of Purification

The purification method described above yields around 1 mg of purified Ty-VLPs per 500-mL culture, if the additional sequence does not result in a decreased expression level. As only 50 to 100 µg is required to immunize a mouse, and the method can easily be carried out with four 500-mL cultures at the same time, this will provide sufficient Ty-VLPs for many experiments.

If larger amounts are required the same procedure can be scaled up by using a full size ultracentrifuge for the density gradient centrifugation. Purity can be improved by size exclusion chromatography after density gradient centrifuga-

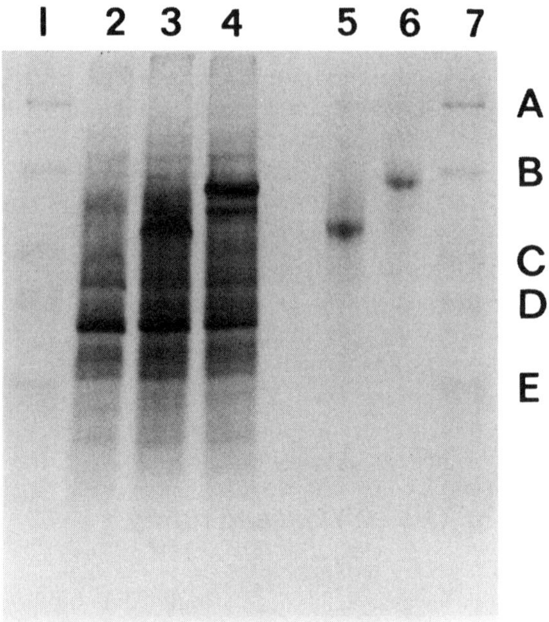

Fig. 2. Coomassie-stained SDS-PAGE gel showing purified and unpurified Ty-VLPs. Lanes 1 and 7: molecular-weight markers **(A)** 175 kDa; **(B)** 83 kDa; **(C)** 62 kDa; **(D)** 47.5 kDa; **(E)** 32.5 kDa. Lanes 2–4: total yeast soluble protein after galactose induction. Lane 2: untransformed yeast. Lane 3: yeast transformed with pOGS40 and pUG41S. Lane 4: pOGS40 with 229 amino acid C-terminal fusion and pUG41S. Lanes 5 and 6: Ty-VLP monomers after sucrose gradient purification. Lane 5: pOGS40; lane 6: pOGS40 with 229 amino acid C-terminal fusion.

tion, and if necessary the preparation can be concentrated by ultrafiltration *(13)*. This method can be used to produce Ty-VLPs suitable for immunization of humans.

3.8. Assessment of Immunogenicity in Mice

Ty-VLPs injected without adjuvant prime a cytotoxic T-cell response to the epitopes carried on the particles. They may be administered via the sc, im, in, iv, or ip routes at a dose of 20 to 100 µg *(22)*. Two weeks after immunization, splenocytes are prepared and tested in a chromium release lysis assay or IFN-γ ELISPOT assay *(1)*. Ty-VLPs can be used to load target cells for a chromium release assay *(15)*. An example of the results of a chromium release lysis assay is shown in **Fig. 3**.

Subcutaneous injection of Ty-VLPs with alum prevents the induction of a CTL response, but enhances antibody production *(5)*.

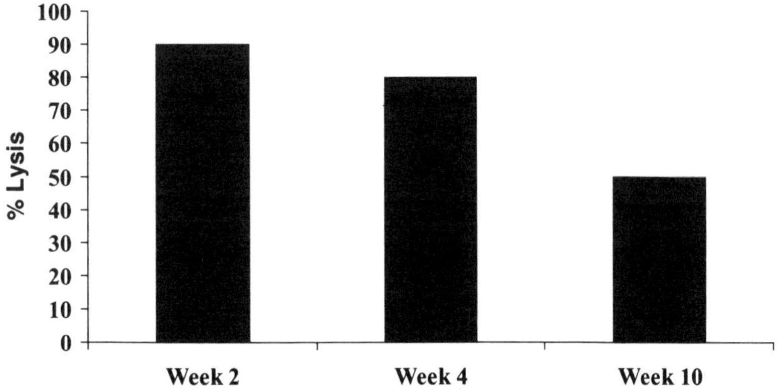

Fig. 3. CTL response in mice. Balb/c mice were immunized with a single sc injection of 100 µg Ty-VLPs carrying a single CTL epitope from the CS gene of *Plasmodium berghei* (SYIPSAEKI). Spleens were taken at week 2, 4, or 10 after immunization. No adjuvant was used, and the assay was carried out after in vitro restimulation for 1 wk with the appropriate peptide, using peptide-loaded target cells at an effector: target ratio of 40:1.

4. Notes

1. If the oligo that has been designed contains sequences that can pair internally to form large secondary structures (hairpins) it is not likely that the insert will anneal as desired when the oligos are ligated into the vector. There are many computer packages that can check this, such as those designed to look at RNA secondary structures, or PCR primer design packages. If a strong secondary structure could be formed, it is necessary to change bases within the sequence to prevent secondary structure formation without changing the amino acid sequence.
2. Suitable primers to sequence inserts in the pOGS plasmids are GAA GAA TGA TTC TCG CAG CTA (anneals to 3′ end of p1 protein) and AGA AAA AAA TTG ATC TAT CG (anneals to the 5′ end of the transcription terminator).
3. Grow a 10-mL culture inoculated with a loopful of yeast cells taken from a YEPD plate in YEPD overnight. The next morning set up a series of 50-mL flasks of YEPD, inoculating with a range of volumes (0.05 to 1.0 mL) from the overnight culture. Incubate all the flasks and monitor OD_{600} after 3 to 6 h, by which time one of the flasks should contain cells at an appropriate density to prepare for electroporation.
4. Cotransformation with two plasmids is a very inefficient process and few transformants are expected to grow. The DNA used for transformation should be highly pure, preferably prepared using Qiagen (Chatsworth, CA) columns. Carrying out several replicates with each pair of plasmids can increase chances of success.
5. Grow each transformant in 50 mL growth medium, to late log or early stationary phase (OD_{600} of 1 in 10 dilution between 0.2 and 0.6). Centrifuge and resuspend in 5 mL growth medium containing 15% glycerol. Aliquot 1 mL per vial and freeze on dry ice. Store at –70°C. To use, thaw in warm water and transfer to growth medium.

6. Some cultures are slow to grow, and the initial growth phase can take up to 3 d.
7. It is essential to break all the yeast cells open. Press the tube hard onto the vortex mixer, holding the tube at an angle. Check for cell breakage by examining the cells under a phase contrast microscope. Intact cells appear bright, broken cells are dark.
8. The 60% sucrose solution is very viscous, so fill the pipet tip and dispense the solution very slowly. The pipet tip should be placed at the bottom of the centrifuge tube before starting to dispense the sucrose.
9. Ty-VLPs should not be repeatedly frozen and thawed, as this disrupts the particle structure resulting in loss of immunogenicity. It is therefore most convenient to divide the sample into 100-µg aliquots before freezing.

References

1. Schneider, J., Gilbert, S. C., Blanchard, T. J., Hanke, T., Robson, K. J., Hannan, C. M., et al. (1998) Enhanced immunogenicity for CD8+ T cell induction and complete protective efficacy of malaria DNA vaccination by boosting with modified vaccinia virus Ankara. *Nat. Med.* **4,** 397–402.
2. Schirmbeck, R., Melber, K., and Reimann, J. (1995) Hepatitis B virus small surface antigen particles are processed in a novel endosomal pathway for major histocompatibility complex class I-restriced epitope presentation. *Eur. J. Immunol.* **25,** 1063–1070.
3. Schirmbeck, R., Deml, L., Melber, K., Wolf, H., Wagner, R., and Reimann, J. (1995) Priming of class I-restricted cytotoxic T lymphocytes by vaccination with recombinant protein antigens. *Vaccine* **13,** 857–865.
4. Schirmbeck, R., Melber, K., Kurober, A., Janowicz, J., and Reimann, J. (1994) Immunization with soluble hepatitis B virus surface protein elicits murine H-2 Class I-restricted CD8+ cytotoxic T lymphocyte resonses in vivo. *J. Immunol.* **152,** 1110–1119.
5. Harris, S., Woodrow, S. A., Gearing, A. J. H., Adams, S. A., Kingsman, A. J., and Layton, G. T. (1996) The effects of adjuvants on CTL induction by V3 : Ty-virus-like-particles (V3-VLPs) in mice. *Vaccine* **14,** 971–976.
6. Kelleher, A. D., Roggensack, M., Jaramillo, A. B., Smith, D. E., Walker, A., Gow, I., et al. (1998) Safety and immunogenicity of a candidate therapeutic vaccine, p24 virus-like aprticle, combined with zidovudine, in asymptomatic subjects. *AIDS* **12,** 175–185.
7. Ball, J. M., Hardy, M. E., Atmat, R. L., Conner, M. E., and Estes, M. K. (1998) Oral immunisation with recombinant Norwalk virus-like particles induces a systemic and mucosal immune response in mice. *J. Virol.* **72,** 1345–1353.
8. O'Neal, C. M., Crawford, S. E., Estes, M. K., and Conner, M. E. (1997) Rotavirus virus-like particles administered mucosally induce protective immunity. *J. Virol.* **71,** 8707–8717.
9. Sharma, A., Rao, Z., Fry, E., Booth, T., Jones, E. Y., Rowlands, D. J., et al. (1997) Specific interactions between human integrin alpha v beta 3 and chimeric hepatitis B virus core particles bearing the receptor-binding epitope of foot-and-mouth disease virus. *Virology* **239,** 150–157.

10. Dalsgaard, K., Uttenthal, A., Jones, T. D., Xu, F., Merryweather, A., Hamilton, W. D., et al. (1997) Plant-derived vaccine protects target animals against a viral disease. *Nat. Biotechnol.* **15,** 248–252.
11. Mikhailov, M., Monastyrskaya, K., Bakker, T., and Roy, P. (1996) A new form of particulate single and multiple immunogen delivery system based on recombinant bluetongue virus-derived tubules. *Virology* **217,** 323–331.
12. Greenstone, H. L., Nieland, J. D., de Visser, K. E., De Bruijn, M. L., Kirnbauer, R., Roden, R. B., et al. (1998) Chimeric papillomavirus virus-like particles elicit antitumor immunity against the E7 oncoprotein in an HPV16 tumor model. *Proc. Natl. Acad. Sci. USA* **95,** 1800–1805.
13. Burns, N. R., Gilmour, E. M., Kingsman, S. M., Kingsman, A. J., and Adams, S. E. (1994) Production and Purification of Hybrid Ty-VLPs. *Molec. Biotechnol.* **1,** 137–145.
14. Gilbert, S. C., Plebanski, M., Harris, S. J., Allsopp, C. E., Thomas, R., Layton, G. T., and Hill, A. V. (1997) A protein particle vaccine containing multiple malaria epitopes. *Nat. Biotechnol.* **15,** 1280–1284.
15. Allsopp, C. E., Plebanski, M., Gilbert, S., Sinden, R. E., Harris, S., Frankel, G., et al. (1996) Comparison of numerous delivery systems for the induction of cytotoxic T lymphocytes by immunization. *Eur. J. Immunol.* **26,** 1951–1959.
16. Klavinskis, L. S., Bergmeier, L. A., Gao, L., Mitchell, E., Ward, R. G., Layton, G., et al. (1996) Mucosal or targeted lymph node immunization of macaques with a particulate SIVp27 protein elicits virus-specific CTL in the genito-rectal mucosa and draining lymph nodes. *J. Immunol.* **157,** 2521–2527.
17. Griffiths, J. C., Berrie, E. L., Holdsworth, L. N., Moore, J. P., Harris, S. J., Senior, J. M., et al. (1991) Induction of high-titer neutralizing antibodies, using hybrid human immunodeficiency virus V3-Ty virus-like particles in a clinically relevant adjuvant. *J. Virol.* **65,** 450–456.
18. Weber, J., Cheinsong Popov, R., Callow, D., Adams, S., Patou, G., Hodgkin, K., et al. (1995) Immunogenicity of the yeast recombinant p17/p24:Ty virus-like particles (p24-VLP) in healthy volunteers. *Vaccine* **13,** 831–834.
19. Martin, S. J., Vyakarnam, A., Cheingsong Popov, R., Callow, D., Jones, K. L., Senior, J. M., et al. (1993) Immunization of human HIV-seronegative volunteers with recombinant p17/p24:Ty virus-like particles elicits HIV-1 p24-specific cellular and humoral immune responses. *AIDS* **7,** 1315–1323.
20. Gilbert, S. C. and Hill, A. V. S. (1997) Protein particle vaccines against malaria. *Parasitol. Today* **13,** 302–306.
21. Lundblad, V. (1997) *Saccharomyces cerevisiae*, in *Current Protocols in Molecular Biology*. Wiley, New York.
22. Layton, G. T., Harris, S. J., Myhan, J., West, D., Gotch, F., Hill Perkins, M., et al. (1996) Induction of single and dual cytotoxic T-lymphocyte responses to viral proteins in mice using recombinant hybrid Ty-virus-like particles. *Immunology* **87,** 171–178.

12

The Adjuvant MF59: *A 10-Year Perspective*

Gary Ott, Ramachandran Radhakrishnan, Jia-Hwa Fang, and Maninder Hora

1. Introduction

Over the last decade, advances in subunit vaccine technology, achieved in many cases with recombinant DNA techniques, have created a dramatic increase in demand for vaccine adjuvants which can help to ellicit protective responses from subunit antigens which, in general, are poorly immunogenic when administered in the absence of an adjuvant *(1)*. The purpose of this chapter is to summarize our extensive experience with the oil-in-water emulsion adjuvant MF59 and to emphasize to the reader that MF59 is no longer a research formulation, but a functional commercial adjuvant. Here we provide information on good manufacturing processes (GMP), and methods of characterization for postproduction release and demonstration of long-term stability of MF59, as well as representative data to demonstrate the consistency of the product. We also provide information on the in vitro and in vivo performance of MF59 in combination with various vaccine antigens, which we have gathered during the decade of development, which has resulted in formulation of MF59 in the Fluad® vaccine, that marks the first European approval of a nonalum adjuvant for human use.

1.1. Mechanistic Approaches to Adjuvant Design

A variety of approaches have been utilized in searching for adjuvants that would be useful for clinical application to human disease prevention. Both alum, the principal adjuvant licensed for use in conjunction with human vaccines, and polylactide-coglycolide (PLG) microspheres have been reported to provide a depot that release antigen over an extended period of time *(2)*. A

From: *Methods in Molecular Medicine, Vol. 42: Vaccine Adjuvants: Preparation Methods and Research Protocols*
Edited by: D. T. O'Hagan © Humana Press, Inc., Totowa, NJ

number of molecular immunostimulators including muramyl peptides *(3)*, lipid A derivatives *(4)*, saponins *(5)*, and bacterial toxins *(6)* have been used in combination with subunit antigens for both systemic and mucosal immunization. Many of the adjuvant formulations recently under development, including syntex adjuvant formulation (SAF) *(8)* and the SmithKline-Beecham (SKB) emulsions *(9)*, liposomes *(10)*, immunostimulating complex (ISCOMS) *(11)*, and virus-like particles (VLPs) (Dupuis, M., personal communication), function as delivery systems that enhance transport of either antigen or molecular immunostimulators to antigen presenting cells. The emulsion adjuvant MF59 does not contain any known immunostimulatory molecules nor has any association between antigen and the emulsion droplets been shown to be critical for adjuvant activity. The administration of this particulate immunostimulator has been shown to result in the recruitment of antigen-presenting cells (APCs) to the site of injection *(12)*, and to increased uptake of soluble antigen by the APCs *(13)*.

1.2. Adjuvant Potency

The success of any vaccine/adjuvant formulation is dependent upon fulfillment of several requirements. The most important of these are potency, tolerable reactogenicity, and pharmaceutical feasibility. In order to be protective, the antigen/adjuvant formulation must have a specific potency for generation of the appropriate immune function. It is useful to classify adjuvants in terms of their performance regarding the correlation of immunity historically established for a variety of disease models. The generation of neutralizing antibody, present in serum or at mucosal surfaces, has frequently been correlated with protection *(1)*. The presence of specific antibody subtypes and the demonstration of antibody-dependent cellular cytotoxicity are likely to be associated with protection in some cases. Generation of cellular immunity, most particularly, cytotoxic T-lymphocytes (CTLs), has been thought to be contributory to protection in other cases. Finally, generation of specific cytokine profiles or generation of other soluble factors, including chemokines, has been considered to be potentially critical for protection in yet other systems. MF59 has been demonstrated to generate antibody titers determined by both enzyme-linked immunosorbent assay (ELISA) and neutralization assays, which are significantly greater than those obtained with aluminum salts for an extensive list of subunit antigens. Recognizing that cytokine profiles obtained after immunization are dependent on a number of variables, we would characterize MF59 as a Th-2 directing adjuvant. Finally, because CTLs have been obtained with some antigens by the very active subcutaneous (sc) route in mice, we do not characterize MF59 as a potent adjuvant for CTL generation.

1.3. Adjuvant Reactogenicity

Limiting reactogenicity of adjuvanted vaccines to a tolerable level for widespread administration to humans has been a critical problem in transition from animal models to the clinic. The first priority in formulation of MF59 was to ensure safety, thus a very conservative formulation based upon low-risk components has been utilized. Clinical testing with both influenza and herpes simplex virus (HSV) vaccines in more than 18,000 subjects have demonstrated minimal reactogenicity of these formulations and the adjuvant has been approved for both commercial use and for further testing in both infants and pregnant women.

1.4. Pharmaceutical Feasibility

The advanced state of development of MF59 offers the potential user significant advantages. MF59s manufactured under GMP conditions at a scale commensurate with commercial use as part of an adjuvanted influenza vaccine (Fluad). Extensive characterization of raw materials, development of a reproducible manufacturing process and derivation of suitable conditions for long-term stability have been achieved during the product development cycle. MF59 has shown excellent compatibility with a variety of subunit antigens, all of which have been formulated by a simple mixing of the antigen with the adjuvant. This simple approach allows final formulation to be performed in the clinic and reduces the need for extensive stability studies on early-phase candidate vaccines. On selected vaccines, storage stability in the presence of MF59 has also been established demonstrating the feasibility of long-term compatibility of antigens with MF59 on a case-by-case basis.

2. Materials

The second generation MF59 emulsion with enhanced stability characteristics has been designated as MF59C.1 and consists of the following components.

1. Squalene (2,6,10,15,19,23-hexamethyl-2,6,10,14,18,22-tetracosahexaene).
2. Polysorbate 80.
3. Sorbitan trioleate.
4. Trisodium citrate dihydrate.
5. Citric acid monohydrate.
6. Water-for-injection (WFI).

3. Methods

3.1. Manufacturing Process for 50l-Scale Production of MF59

Methods for laboratory-scale production of MF59 previously described ***(14)***, allow preparation of as little as 10 mL of emulsion with the Microfluidizer

110S. Here we describe the manufacturing process for sterile clinical grade MF59C.1 having defined release specifications and demonstrated long-term stability. The 50l scale manufacturing process for MF59C.1 is shown in **Fig. 1**. Briefly, polysorbate 80 is dissolved in WFI and combined with aqueous sodium citrate–citric acid buffer solution. Separately, sorbitan trioleate is dissolved in squalene. These two solutions are combined together and processed in an inline homogenizer to yield a coarse emulsion. The coarse emulsion is fed into a microfluidizer, where it is further processed to obtain a stable submicron emulsion. The coarse emulsion is passed through the interaction chamber of the microfluidizer repeatedly until the desired particle size is obtained. The bulk emulsion is filtered through a 0.22-μm filter under nitrogen to remove large droplets, yielding MF59C.1 adjuvant emulsion bulk that is filled into glass bottles. For vaccine antigens that have demonstrated long-term stability in the presence of MF59 for shelf storage, the antigen and MF59 are combined and sterile-filtered through a 0.22-μm membrane. The combined "single-vial" vaccine is filled into single-dose containers. For vaccine antigens, where long-term stability has not been demonstrated, the adjuvant is supplied as a separate vial. In such cases, the MF59 bulk is filter-sterilized, filled, and packaged in final single-dose vials.

3.2. In Process Assays for MF59C.1

The manufacturing process yields an MF59C.1 product in a reproducible and consistent manner. **Figure 2** presents the combined particle size data from seven representative lots to demonstrate the efficient and repeatable reduction of mean particle size of MF59C.1 during each pass of the microfluidizer in the process. In addition to the mean particle size, we monitor the number of large particles, i.e., particles >1.2 μm in size, per milliliter of the adjuvant emulsion. Emulsions are thermodynamically unstable systems and are subject to flocculation (reversible aggregation of oil particles) and coalescence (irreversible aggregation of oil particles to form large particles and eventual, irrevocable separation of oil, and aqueous phases) during storage. For manufacturing of stable emulsions, a key objective is to keep the number of large particles down to a minimum because large particles act as nucleation sites for further aggregation during storage potentially leading to phase separation. **Figure 3** shows data from seven representative lots of MF59C.1 for reduction in the number of large particles during the manufacturing process. After the microfluidization step, filtration of the emulsion through a 0.22-μm membrane removes 99.5% of particles >1.2 μm in size. The bulk emulsion contains less than 0.1% of total particles that are >1.2 μm.

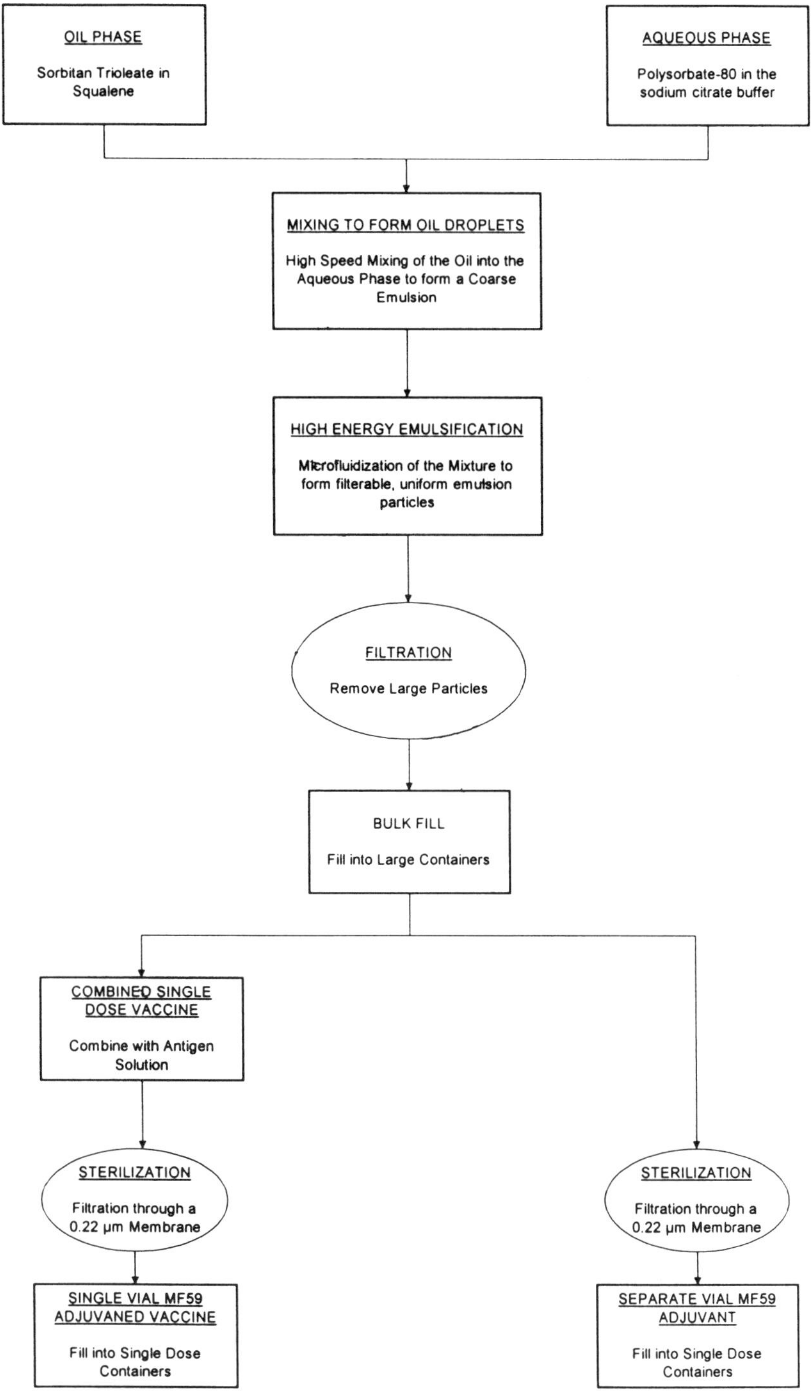

Fig. 1. MF59 manufacturing process.

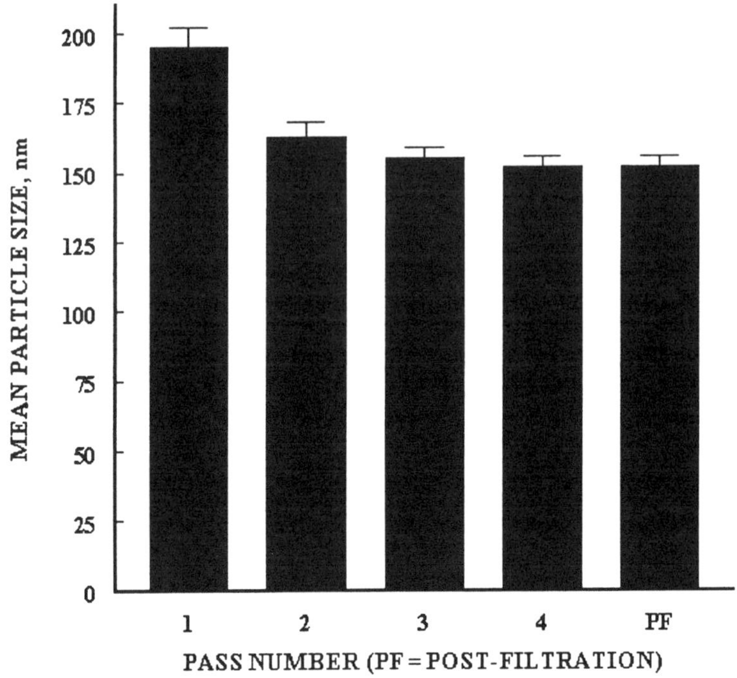

Fig. 2. Mean particle size profiles of MF59 during microfluidization.

3.3. Release Assays for MF59C.1

MF59C.1 is a well-defined emulsion produced to preestablished release specifications. The emulsion bulk and final single-dose adjuvant are analyzed using a battery of assays in accordance with Chiron's standard operating procedures. Key assays include visual appearance, pH, mean particle size, and number of large particles per milliliter for quality, squalene, polysorbate 80, and sorbitan trioleate concentrations by high-performance liquid chromatography (HPLC) procedures for content and, endotoxin and bioburden content for safety. Visually, MF59C.1 is a milky white, homogenous liquid that is free of extraneous particles. Under stress conditions, such as prolonged exposure to high temperatures or freezing, large oil globules are formed. Storage of MF59C.1 under such conditions must, therefore, be avoided. MF59C.1 is buffered with the sodium citrate–citric acid buffer to pH 6.5. As during the process, mean particle size of MF59C.1 and the number of large particles per milliliter are important quality parameters for the bulk and final adjuvant emulsions. The mean particle size of MF59C.1 is approximately 150 nm and an upper specification of 1×10^7 particles ≥ 1.2 µm is observed. The quantities of squalene, polysorbate 80, and sorbitan trioleate must be within an acceptable

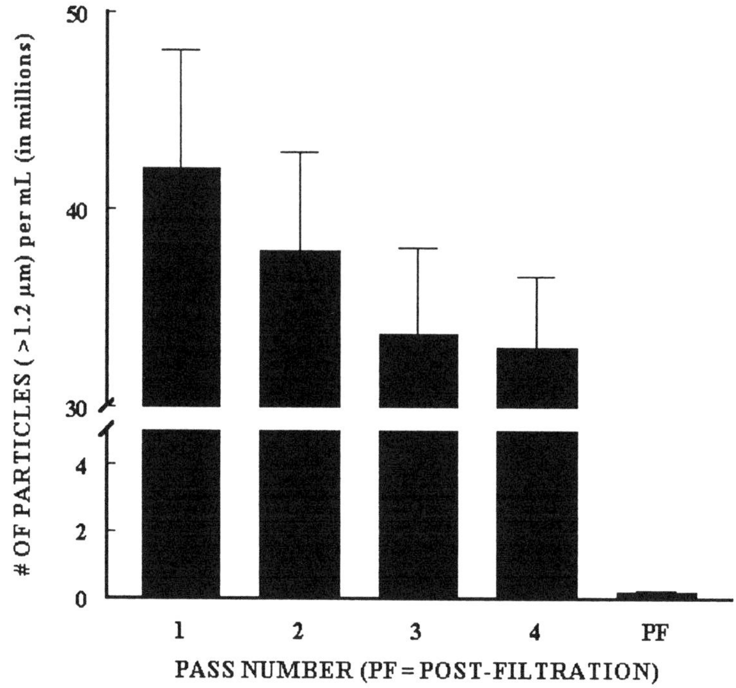

Fig. 3. Number of ≥1.2 µm particles in MF59 bulk.

range around the nominal concentration values of 39, 4.7, and 4.7 mg/mL, respectively.

3.4. Stability Assays for MF59C.1

MF59C.1 is stable at 2–8°C for three years when stored in glass bottles protected from direct light. Physically, the emulsion is stable except for slight flocculation seen after it is placed at 2–8°C for a few weeks. Studies have demonstrated that MF59C.1 in its original particle size profile is obtained by inverting the closed container a few times. The pH, mean particle size, and squalene concentrations of MF59C.1 remain unchanged from initial values throughout the three-year shelf-life at 2–8°C. Finally, the number of large particles per milliliter of the adjuvant remains below its upper specification during the shelf-life period. Stability data from representative MF59C.1 lots are displayed in **Figs. 4** and **5**.

3.5. Final Vaccine Formulation

3.5.1. Vaccine Formats

A variety of antigens including HSV-2 gB/gD, HBV, HIV *gp120* and/or *p24*, CMV gB, and influenza hemagglutinin (HA) have been formulated with

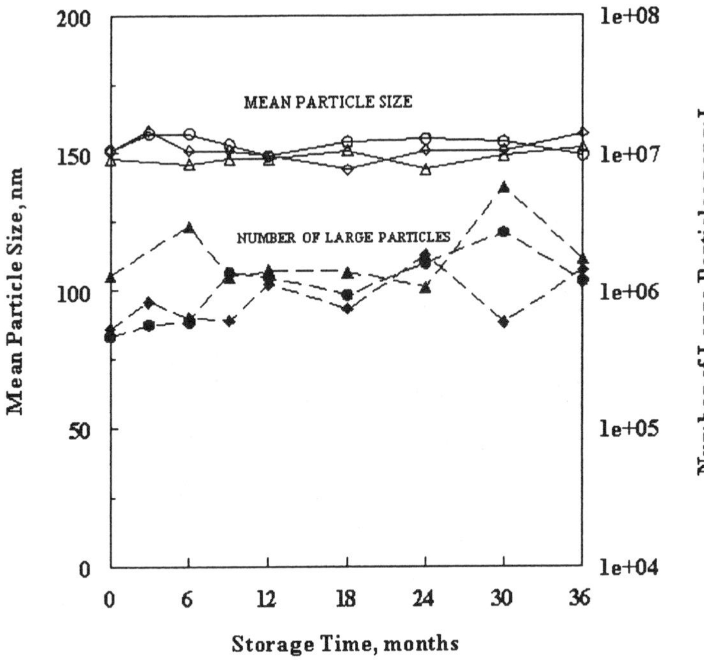

Fig. 4. Long-term particle size stability of the three representative MF59C.1 bulk lots at 2–8°C.

the adjuvant emulsion MF59C.1 in one of two formats: either in single containers or in separate vials (admixed prior to administration and therefore referred to as dual vial vaccines). The antigens tested fall into three distinct classes of proteins:

1. soluble antigens: either monomeric low-molecular-weight type (e.g., HSV2 gD, 43 kDa) or high-molecular-weight aggregate (e.g., CMV gB 800 kDa aggregates);
2. hydrophobic: integral membrane protein with an intrinsic ability to self-associate forming protein micelles or to associate with lipid bilayers or emulsions (e.g., influenza HA);
3. particulate antigens: the protein is naturally associated to form defined structures optionally with lipids embedded as an integral part of the structure [e.g., hepatitis B surface antigen (HBsAg)].

Antigens of all three types have been successfully formulated into single-vial vaccines after sufficient formulation optimization. These single-container vaccines showed different stability behaviors depending on the nature of the antigen and the susceptibility of the antigen to interact with the adjuvant. **Table 1** summarizes much of the stability data obtained for MF59 vaccine formulations

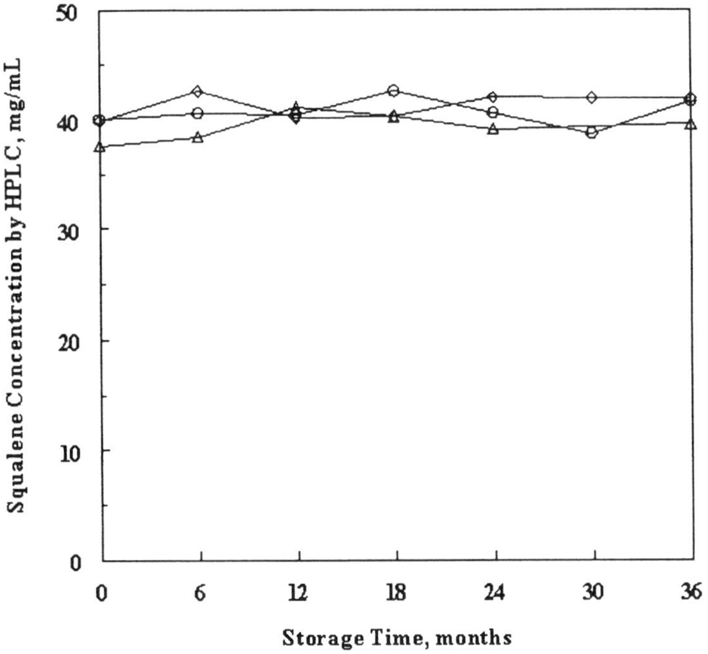

Fig. 5. Long-term stability of squalene in three representative MF59C.1 bulk lots at 2–8°C.

at Chiron Corporation. Only two of the antigens, HIV *gp120* and CMV gB, were not suitable for single-vial formulation. HIV *gp120* has been shown to undergo time-dependent conformational changes in single-container formulations. Such changes are evident by a loss in CD4 binding, a measurement, considered an in vitro surrogate potency assay. At this point, it is not clear if the polysorbate 80 in the adjuvant bound to the V3 loop of *gp120* or the adjuvant (or oxidized MF59) triggered reactions occurred in a functional domain of the antigen to cause a loss in activity. The conformational changes observed could account for the changes in the immunological responses to the single-container vaccines. In order to meet rapid timelines, dual-vial formulations were developed as candidate vaccines for advanced clinical trials. Recombinant CMV gB has shown the propensity to exist as an equilibrium mixture of various high molecular weight aggregates. Single-vial formulations of CMV gB with MF59 have shown a change in the composition of the antigen presumably because of the surfactant-induced disaggregation of the antigen. In addition, incubations of the single-container vaccines at >25°C led to pronounced crosslinking of the adjuvant with the antigen. A major portion of this reaction appeared to be unrelated to disulfide crosslinking of the protein. Mechanisti-

Table 1
Summary of Formulation Experience with MF59

Antigen	Source	Physico-chemical characteristics	Vaccine format	Comments
HSV gD2	CHO-cell line	Soluble 43 kDa.	Single-container with MF59 and gB2.	Stable formulation for two years at 2–8°C.
HIV gB2	CHO-cell line	Soluble 190 kDa dimer.	Single-container formulation with MF59 and gD2.	Excipients protect formulation.
HIV gp120	CHO-cell line	Soluble 120 kDa monomer.	Single-container formulation.	Unstable; CD4 binding decreases with time. Third immunization with single vial formulation gave neutalizing titers comparable to second immunization with dual vial vaccine.
HIV gp120		Soluble 120 kDa monomer.	Dual-vial vaccine.	Stable for 18-mo storage at 2–8°C by ELISA and neutralization responses.
HIV p24	CHO-cell line	Soluble 24 kDa.	Dual-vial vaccine.	Stable.
CMV gB	CHO-cell line	Soluble multimeric antigen.	Dual-vial vaccine.	Stable.
		Soluble multimeric antigen.	Single-container formulation.	Change in aggregation state of antigen and immunogenicity.
Flu HA	Chicken eggs	Hydrophobic integral membrane protein. Soluble trimeric noncovalently linked monomeric antigens of 77 kDa each.	Single-container formulation.	Altered SRID pattern with time. Antigen probably aggregates or integrates into emulsion. Animal immunogenicity not affected very much.
HBV	CHO-cell line	Soluble 30 kDa.	Dual-vial vaccine.	Stable and highly immunogenic in animals and humans.

		Soluble 30 kDa.	Single-container formulation with MF59.	Highly immunogenic. Probably interacts with MF59 resulting in slight delipidation and oxidized lipid induced antigen changes.
HPV E7	*E. coli*	Soluble disulfide-linked oligomers, 11 kDa, early transforming protein.	Dual vial.	Addition of thioglycerol and polysorbate 80 prevented antigen aggregation and provided sufficient stability. Antigen was stored at <–60°C for early clinical studies.
HPV L1	Yeast	Major capsid protein, 55 kDa, self assembles to 50 nm capsids or VLP, insoluble at low-ionic strength.	Dual vial.	Antigen has been stored at <–60°C for early clinical studies.
HCV Core	*E. coli*	Highly hydrophobic 192 residue protein.	Dual vial.	Core primarily undergoes disulfide induced cross-linking. Excipients have to balance the combinational vaccine with E2. This antigen has been stored. at –60°C for use in early clinical studies.
HCV E2	CHO	β-sheet protein (64–67%).		Antigen reacts with thioglycerol and shows least binding in NOB (Neutralization of Binding) assay. Polysorbate/EDTA containing formulations are sufficiently stable. This antigen has demonstrated sufficient stability at <–60°C and used in Phase I clinical trials.

Table 2
Summary of Preclinical Experience with MF59[a]

Antigen	Mouse	Guinea Pig	Rabbit	Goat	Baboon
HIV gp120					26
HSV gD2		34		9	5
HBV Surface Ag	13	18	2	7	42
Influenza HA[b]	35	25	5	122	
Hib/CRM197					7
MenC/CRM197	6				6

[a]Ratio of titer obtained with MF59/titer obtained with alum.
[b]Ratio of titer obtained with MF59/titer obtained with Influenza HA alone.

cally, oxidized surfactant and/or squalene may have generated reactive species such as malondialdehyde capable of generating nonreducible covalent crosslinks with the protein. In view of these experimental results, dual-vial formulations were further developed for clinical evaluations of this vaccine. In all other cases, single-vial formulations stable for several years were derived. For early phase testing where formulation optimization is impractical, antigens for the dual-vial vaccines are provided either frozen (especially for early clinical trials) or as a liquid at 2–8°C. Antigens are typically combined with the adjuvant, MF59C.1, by gentle mechanical mixing to provide single-container vaccines. The stabilities of the dual-container vaccines were governed by the intrinsic storage stabilities of the antigens and MF59 and short-term compatabilities of the vaccines generated upon mixing. In general, the antigen formulations were stable to storage for at least two years at 2–8°C. As discussed earlier, the buffered adjuvant was also quite stable to storage and the vaccines generated from these components were stable for at least for one workday, i.e., eight hours at ambient temperatures that facilitated administrations in clinical studies.

3.6. The Use of MF59 as a Vaccine Adjuvant

The MF59 emulsion adjuvant was developed with the objective of generating a broad spectrum of recombinant vaccines for human use. The specific aim was to elicit neutralizing titers in humans significantly greater than those obtainable with the alum adjuvants in common usage. An extensive body of preclinical efficacy data has been obtained based on ELISA titers obtained with a variety of subunit antigens in a spectrum of animal model systems. A summary of this data is shown in **Table 2**. Data are presented as the ratio of serum ELISA titers obtained with MF59 to that obtained with alum formulated

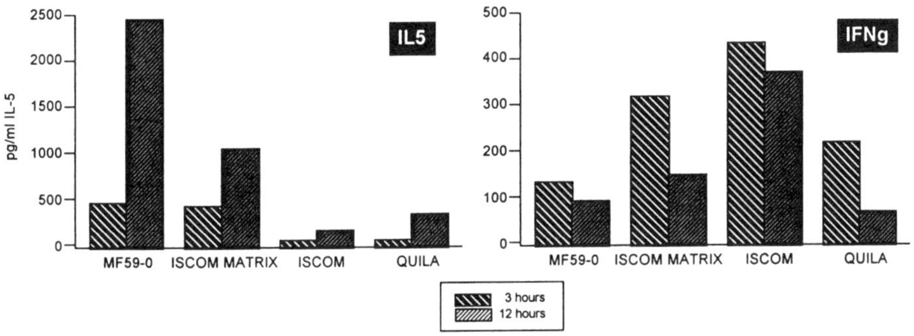

Fig. 6. In vivo cytokine response to HIV envelope proteins and adjuvants.

vaccine. (In one case (*), where alum vaccines have been shown to be ineffective, the ratio of titers obtained with MF59 to that obtained with antigen alone is presented.) The principal conclusion to be drawn from this data is that MF59 is a significantly more potent adjuvant than the aluminum salts for most of the antigens tested in a variety of animal models. The enhancement of titer typically falls in the range from 5 to 40X. Most of the antigens used for development of MF59 were soluble recombinant truncates of viral surface glycoproteins (HIV *gp120*, HSV gD2, CMV gB, HCV E2). Significant activity has been demonstrated with glycoconjugate antigens (Hib, MenC) ***(15)***. MF59 has shown dramatic effects with two particulate antigens influenza HA ***(14)*** and (HBsAg) ***(16)***. No systematic trends have yet been established for antigenic characteristics that determine the degree of efficacy of MF59, though some very poorly soluble antigens have not shown good titers in this system (data not shown). Data in **Table 2** also demonstrate that MF59 is effective across a spectrum of animal models typically used for preclinical testing. So far, no species tested has been unresponsive to MF59, which should be an excellent candidate for formulation of a variety of veterinary vaccines.

Because MF59 is clearly effective for generation of serum antibody titers and CD4 T-cell response (data not shown), these responses are only protective against a subset of the pathogens for which novel or improved vaccines would be of utility. Two attributes of a number of vaccines formulated with MF59 may be of significance in design of additional adjuvanted vaccines. The cytokine balance associated with immunization has been shown to be important to protection in several instances. **Figure 6** shows typical serum cytokine data obtained at either 3 or 12 h after a third intramuscular (im) immunization with MF59/HIV *gp120* or *gp120* with several Quil A-containing formulations. Immunizations with formulations containing MF59 result in greater serum concentration of interluken-5 (IL-5) and smaller concentrations of interferon

Table 3
Cytotoxic T-cell Activity Induced in Mice with Whole Recombinant Proteins Combined with MF59

	Effector target ratio	% Specificity cytotoxicity against target cells loaded with: Specific epitope peptide	Irrelevant peptide
HSV gB2	50	81	8
	10	62	7
	2	34	4
HIV-1 p24 gag	50	53	5
	10	34	2
	2	16	2
HIV-1 gp120	50	91	3
	10	77	1
	2	57	1

(IFN-γ) than those obtained with Quil A containing systems. While we are aware that the Th-1/Th-2 balance represented by the IFN-γ/IL-5 ratio obtained upon immunization is a multivariate function, depending upon antigen identity and dose, adjuvant identity, genetics of the animal immunized and route of administration, we would characterize MF59 as a Th-2 directed adjuvant. The ratio of immunoglobulin (Ig) isotypes (IgG_1/IgG_2a), which frequently correlates with cytokine ratio, is a significant factor in complement-mediated cytotoxicity. Immunization with both HIV and HSV antigens in combination with MF59 results in high ratios of IgG_1/IgG_2a that are consistent with our characterization of MF59 as a Th-2 adjuvant. In contrast, we have shown that it possible to generate CTL with several antigens when formulated with MF59 (**Table 3**). However, the mouse system we have used, base of the tail sc administration of antigen to mice, is the most permissive system for generation of CTL in routine use. So far, attempts to extend the data set into the somewhat more restrictive im mouse mode have not been successful. Limited work in primates (data not shown) has not shown reproducible production of CTL activity. We conclude that the MF59C formulation is most appropriate for application where antibody is the desired end point (e.g., antihormone therapies) or Th-2 cytokines and CD4 T cells are advantageous (e.g., *Helicobacter pylori*) including situations where CTL are not essential or may be dangerous.

3.7. Assurance of Clinical Safety

The most critical concern in the development of postalum adjuvants has been the demonstration of safety for the large populations who receive the

Table 4
Summary of Subjects Receiving MF59 and Vaccine Antigens through March 1999 in Chiron-Sponsored Programs

Vaccine	Seronegatives	Seropositives
Herpes simplex		
gD2, gB2,gD2/gB2	1854	209
gD2/gB2dTM	359	0
Human immunodeficiency		
gp120 SF2	810	55
gp120 Thai E	96	0
gp120SF2/gp120 Thai E	383	0
p24	30	0
Env 2-3	32	58
Influenza		
Fluad	0	12,044
Influ	0	31
Cytomegalovirus		
gB	634	67
Hepatitis B		
HbsAg+preS2	187	0
Hepatitis C		
E2	36	0
Subtotal Vaccine Antigens with MF59		
	4421	12,464
Placebo	1373	173
Grand TOTAL		18,431

vaccine. Adjuvants, by definition, increase immunological responsiveness, which may result in immune reactivity to epitopes other than those necessary for protection as well as giving rise to side effects associated with generation of the response. The MF59 formulation has been restricted to components that are not individually immunostimulatory. The principal component, squalene, is a naturally occurring intermediate in cholesterol synthesis that is widely distributed in nature and is the primary component of shark liver oil. The MF59 emulsion is immunostimulatory and the safety of each vaccine formulated with the adjuvant must be demonstrated under controlled clinical conditions. Chiron has tested MF59 under such controlled clinical conditions with an extensive set of well-characterized antigens in more than 18,000 subjects (**Table 4**). These clinical cohorts have been screened and carefully monitored postvaccination. The results have been published in detail for trials with HIV ***(16)***, HSV ***(17–19)***, CMV ***(20)***, and influenza ***(21–22)*** antigen-containing MF59 vaccines. The MF59 vaccines tested have been shown to be generally safe and immunogenic. Chiron's influenza vaccine, Fluad, was approved by the Italian regulatory authorities in 1997. Since its introduction, more than 500,000 doses of Fluad have been commercially distributed. In accordance with current regulatory practices, Chiron continues to monitor safety data. The safety of Fluad, as demonstrated in a Phase IV trial, was excellent and similar to that of a licensed influenza vaccine that did not contain any adjuvant.

4. Notes

1. In situations where high antibody titers are desired in combination with Th-1 cytokines and higher IgG_2a/IgG_1 ratios, we have shown that combinations of MF59 with PLG microspheres are useful. Development of MF59-based formulations, which generate Th-1 cytokine profiles and CTL, is ongoing.
2. Fluorescently labeled MF59 (3,3′-dioctadecylindocarbcyanine (CM DiI) has been successfully used to track adjuvant in vivo ***(13)***. The adjuvant is taken up by Mac 1+ antigen-presenting cells in the muscle where it induces enhanced local uptake of antigen. Labeled cells have been shown to migrate to the draining lymph node where they express the markers associated with active dendritic cells.
3. Chiron Corporation routinely makes limited volume samples of clinical grade MF59 available for evaluation of preclinical vaccine formulations. In order to obtain MF59 for testing, it is necessary to submit a brief written summary of the proposed experiments and to agree to the terms of a standard materials transfer agreement, which will be transmitted upon receipt of the proposal summary. The process is typically accomplished within four weeks. We reserve the right to impose additional terms in situations where Chiron Corporation has commercial interest. For further information or materials, please contact the first author, G. Ott.

References

1. Powell, M. and Newman, M. (1995) Design considerations for subunit vaccines, in *Vaccine Design the Subunit and Adjuvant Approach* (Powell, M. and Newman, M., eds.), Plenum, New York, pp. 1–28.
2. Gupta, R., Rost, B., Relyveld, E., and Siber, G. (1995) Adjuvant properties of aluminum and calcium compounds, in *Vaccine Design the Subunit and Adjuvant Approach* (Powell, M. and Newman, M., eds.), Plenum, New York, pp. 229–248.
3. O'Hagan, D., Ott, G., and Van Nest, G. (1997) Recent advances in vaccine adjuvants: the development of MF59 emulsion and polymeric microparticles. *Molec. Med. Today* **3,** 69–75.
4. Ullrich, J. and Myers, K. (1995) Monophosphoryl lipid A as an adjuvant: past experiences and new directions, in *Vaccine Design the Subunit and Adjuvant Approach* (Powell, M. and Newman, M., eds.), Plenum, New York, pp. 495–524.
5. Kensil, C., Soltysik, S., Patelu, M., and Marciani, D. (1992) Structure/function relationships in adjuvants from Quillajasaponaria molina, in *Vaccines* (Brown, F., Channock, G., Ginsberg, H., and Lerner, R. A., eds.), Cold Spring Harbor Laboratory, vol. 72, pp. 35–40.

6. Spangler, B. (1992) Structure and function of cholera toxin and the related escherichia coli heat-labile enterotoxin. *Microbiolog. Rev.* **56,** 622–647.
7. Allison, A. and Byers, N. E. (1986) An adjuvant formulation resulting in the formation of antibodies of isotype and cell-mediated immunity. *J. Immunol. Meth.* **95,** 157–168.
8. Stoute, J., Slaoui, M., Gray-Heppner, D., Momin, P., Kester, K., Desmon, P., et al. (1997) A preliminary evaluation of a recombinant circumsporozoite vaccine against plasmodium falciparum malaria. *N. Eng. J. Med.* **336,** 86–91.
9. Gluck, R., Mischler, R., Finkel, B., Que, J., Scarpa, B., and Cryz, S. (1994) Immunogenicity of a new virsome influenza vaccine in elderly people. *Lancet* **344,** 160–163.
10. Morein, B., Sundquist, B., Hoglund, S., Dalsgaard, K., and Osterhaus, A. (1984) Iscom a novel structure for antigenic presentation of membrane proteins from enveloped viruses. *Nature* **308,** 457–460.
11. Wagner, R., Fliessbach, H., Wanner, G., Motz, M., Niedrig, M. Deby, G., et al. (1992) Studies on processing, particle formation and immunogenicity of the HIV-1 gag product: a possible component of an HIV vaccine. *Arch. Virol.* **127,** 117–137.
12. Dupuis, M., Murphy, T., Higgins, D., Ugozzoli, M., Van Nest, G., Ott, G., et al. (1998) Dendritic cells internalize vaccine adjuvant after intramuscular injection. *Cell Immunol.* **186,** 18–27.
13. Ott, G. Barchfeld, G., and Van Nest, G. (1995) Enhancement of humoral response against human influenza vaccine with the simple submicron oil/water emulsion MF59. *Vaccine* **13,** 1557–1562.
14. Traquina, P., Morandi, M., Contorni, M., and Van Nest, G. (1996) MF59 enhances the antibody response to recombinant hepatitis B surface antigen vaccine in primates. *J. Inf. Dis.* **174**, 1168–1175.
15. Granoff, D., McHugh, Y., Raff, H., Mokatrin, A. and Van Nest, G. (1997) MF59 adjuvant enhances antibody responses of infant baboons immunized with hemophilus influenzae type B and neisseria meningitidis group C oligosaccharide-CRM 197 conjugate vaccine. *Inf. Immun.* **65,** 1710–1715.
16. Kahn, J., Sinangil, F., Baenziger, J., Murcar, N., Wynne, D., Coleman, R., et al. (1994) Clinical and immunologic responses to human immunodeficiency virus (HIV) type I_{SF2} gp120 subunit vaccine combined with MF59 adjuvant with or without muramyl tripeptide dipalmitoyl phosphatidyl ethanolamine in non-HIV-infected human volunteers. *J. Inf. Dis.* **170,** 1288–1291.
17. Langenberg, A., Burke, R., Adair, S., Sekulovich, R., Tigges, M., Dekker, C., and Corey, L. (1995) A recombinant glycoprotein vaccine for herpes simplex type 2: safety and efficacy. *Ann. Int. Med.* **122,** 889–898.
18. Ashley, R., Crisostomo, F., Doss, M., Sekulovich, R., Burke, R., Shaughnessy, M., et al. (1998) Cervical antibody responses to a herpes simplex type 2 glycoprotein subunit vaccine. *J. Inf. Dis.* **178,** 1–7.
19. Strauss, S., Wald, A., Kost, R., McKenzie, R., Langenberg, A., Hohman, P., et al. (1997) Immunotherapy of recurrent genital herpes with recombinant herpes

simplex virus type 2 glycoproteins D and B: results of a placebo-controlled vaccine trial. *J. Inf. Dis.* **176,** 1129–1134.

20. Wang, J. B., Adler, S. P., Hempfling, S., Burke, R. L., Duliege, A. M., Starr, S. E., et al. (1996) Mucosal antibodies to human cytomegalovirus glycoprotein B occur following both natural infection and immunization with human cytomegalovirus vaccines. *J. Inf. Dis.* **174,** 387–392.
21. Minutello, M., Senatore, F., Cecchinelli, G., Bianchi, M., Andreani, T., Podda, A., et al. (1999) Safety and immunogenicity of an inactivated subunit influenza virus vaccine combined with MF59 adjuvant emulsion in elderly subjects, immunized for three consecutive influenza seasons. *Vaccine* **17,** 99–104.
22. De Donato, S., Granoff, D., Minutello, M., Lecchi, G., Faccini, M., Agnello, M., et al. (1999) Safety and immunogenicity of MF59-adjuvanted influenza vaccine in the elderly. *Vaccine* **17,** 3094–3101.

13

Preparation of the Syntex Adjuvant Formulation (SAF, SAF-m, SAF-1)

Deborah M. Lidgate

1. Introduction

The Syntex adjuvant formulation (SAF) is an effective adjuvant composed of a muramyl dipeptide derivative (threonyl-MDP) in an oil-in-water (o/w) emulsion vehicle. Threonyl-MDP (N-acetyl muramyl-L-threonyl-D-isoglutamine) was identified as a superior adjuvant to muramyl dipeptide (N-acetyl muramyl-L-alanyl-D-isoglutamine, MDP) demonstrating a lack of side effects (pyrogenicity, uveitis, adjuvant-induced arthritis) and increased adjuvant activity *(1–3)*. The SAF emulsion vehicle contains Pluronic® L121 (poloxamer 401) that has exhibited adjuvant activity in its own right *(4–7)*. Many investigators have utilized the SAF adjuvant with a variety of antigens such as influenza *(8)* and malaria *(9)*. Whereas SAF has shown versatility with a variety of antigens (eliciting both cell-mediated and humoral immune responses), it may be most effective with antigens that are amphipathic *(10)*. An amphipathic antigen would be retained at the surface of the oil droplet through hydrogen bonding with pluronic (also retained at the surface of the oil droplet) and hydrophobic association between the hydrophobic region of the antigen with that of pluronic and squalane, the oil portion of the SAF emulsion. Antigen retention at the oil droplet may lead to an enhanced immune response through more efficient antigen presentation *(3,10)*. SAF, or a suitable equivalent (*see* **Note 1**), provides an excellent tool for vaccine research.

1.1. Emulsion Theory

To form an emulsion, such as the one used in this formulation, the interfacial tension (between the oil and the water phases) needs to be reduced. As this

From: *Methods in Molecular Medicine, Vol. 42: Vaccine Adjuvants: Preparation Methods and Research Protocols*
Edited by: D. T. O'Hagan © Humana Press, Inc., Totowa, NJ

interfacial tension decreases, the interfacial contact, or area, increases. This increase in interfacial area leads to increased free energy of the system and results in thermodynamic instability. Emulsion instability can be lessened by the choice and amount of emulsifier, the dispersed droplet size, the density differences between the internal and external phases, the viscosity of the external phase, and the manufacturing technique.

Typically, emulsion physical instability is evident by either creaming (or sedimenting, depending on density differences) and/or coalescence. Creaming occurs when the two phases of the emulsion have different specific gravities and/or when the dispersed droplets are initially large (and are not responsive to Brownian movement). If coalescence does not occur simultaneously, the emulsion can be redispersed with gentle mixing. Adjusting the specific gravity of one or both phases, reducing the droplet size, and/or increasing the viscosity of the continuous phase can minimize creaming.

Coalescence occurs when the interfacial film ruptures between two droplets of the internal phase. Larger droplets have a greater tendency to coalesce. Often, coalescence is irreversible, unless an emulsifier is chosen to facilitate reemulsification on shaking. Reducing the tendency of emulsion creaming, increasing the charge on the droplets, and increasing the viscosity of the continuous phase can minimize coalescence.

Emulsifiers promote stabilization of dispersed droplets by reducing interfacial free energy and creating physical or electrostatic barriers to droplet coalescence ***(11)***. Nonionic emulsifiers orient at the interface and produce relatively bulky structures, which lead to steric avoidance of the dispersed droplets. Anionic or cationic emulsifiers induce formation of an electrical double layer by attracting counterions; the double-layer repulsive forces cause droplets to repel one another when they approach.

Emulsifiers are typically categorized with an HLB number (hydrophile-lipophile balance). The HLB expresses the relative simultaneous attraction for water and oil. Chemical composition and extent of ionization determine the HLB. The emulsifier HLB contributes to the type of emulsion formed: a low HLB promotes water-in-oil (w/o) emulsions, a high HLB promotes o/w emulsions.

1.2. Manufacturing Considerations

Emulsion manufacturing equipment must supply appropriate shear force to adequately disperse the emulsion's internal phase and avoid coalescence and potential physical deterioration of the emulsion. The manufacturing equipment can facilitate better orientation of the emulsifier at the oil–water interface, thus providing a barrier to coalescence. The equipment should also produce an emulsion with a uniform droplet size.

The typical equipment used to manufacture emulsions includes propeller mixers, turbine rotors and stators, colloid mills, homogenizers, and sonicators. The mechanical forces encountered with these mixers involve shear, impact, and/or cavitation.

For manufacture of the SAF emulsion a Microfluidizer® (providing all three mechanical forces) was selected for its ability to reproducibly provide an elegant, physically stable emulsion with consistent particle size ***(12,13)***. Emulsion formation occurs in a Microfluidizer as two fluidized streams interact at high velocities within an interaction chamber. The Microfluidizer is air or nitrogen driven and can operate at internal pressures in excess of 20,000 psi with a throughput of 300–500 mL/min. After several passes through the Microfluidizer, the SAF emulsion had an average particle size (*see* **Notes 2** and **3**) of approximately 165 nm, with a range of approximately 80–300 nm. With this droplet-size range, the final emulsion was successfully filtered through a 0.22-μm filter, rendering a sterile product.

It should be noted that SAF was also manufactured using alternate mixing methods. Early in the development of SAF, all formulation components were mixed in a test tube using a vortex mixer. Scale-up studies involved the use of blade mixers and homogenizer mixers. Emulsion from all types of manufacturing processes showed equivalent biological efficacy ***(13)***. The Microfluidizer was selected, as noted above, because of the superior physical stability and appearance of the resulting emulsion. In addition to biological efficacy, the physical appearance was an important commercial consideration. Regarding nomenclature, SAF prepared via the Microfluidizer was designated SAF-m; SAF prepared via an alternate mixing method was designated SAF-1.

2. Materials

2.1. SAF Components and Chemistry

1. Threonyl-muramyl dipeptide (threonyl-MDP), Syntex (Palo Alto, CA). Threonyl-MDP is comprised of a muramyl sugar derivative and two nonaromatic amino acids linked by amide bonds. Its solubility is greater than 600 mg/mL in aqueous solution over a wide pH range. Its solubility in nonpolar solvents, such as chloroform, methylene chloride, and hexane, is less than 3 μg/mL. The apparent octanol/water and methylene chloride/water partition coefficients were found to be 0.0044 and 0.00017, respectively. The degradation rate of threonyl-MDP in aqueous solution was determined as a function of pH and temperature. Based on the degradation rate plot, the maximum stability is expected at pH 4.5, and a 2-yr shelf-life is predicted for a threonyl-MDP solution formulated at a pH of 4.5 and stored at 25°C. At physiological pH, the predicted shelf-life of threonyl-MDP in aqueous solution at room temperature is less than 40 d; at 5°C, a shelf-life of 2 yr may be possible.

2. Squalane, NF, Robeco Chemicals or other vendors. Squalane (2,6,10,15,19,23-hexamethyltetracosane) is free-flowing oil with a molecular weight of 422.8 and a density of approximately 0.811. Squalane is chemically saturated and is obtained by complete hydrogenation of squalene, found in shark liver oil. Squalane is metabolizable oil that has been used in pharmaceutical and cosmetic products. The squalane used in the SAF formulation conforms to National Formulary (NF) requirements.
3. Poloxamer 401 (Pluronic L121), BASF Corporation (Mount Olive, NJ). Pluronic L121 is a block copolymer of ethylene oxide and propylene oxide. This particular nonionic surfactant contains 10% by weight of the hydrophilic ethylene oxide group. The average molecular weight for Pluronic L121 is 4400; it is liquid at room temperature and has an HLB close to 1.0. This low HLB value puts it in a class of water-insoluble surfactants known as spreading agents. Spreading agents do not stabilize emulsions; they adhere preferentially to hydrophobic surfaces in contact with aqueous media. Because of their distinct hydrophilic and hydrophobic portions, they promote interaction with macromolecules (such as antigens) at the oil–water interface of the emulsion. Researchers suggest that this characteristic of Pluronic L121 contributes to the adjuvant activity by increasing the concentration of antigen presented to cells of the immune system *(3)*.
4. Polysorbate 80, NF, Ruger Chemicals or alternate vendor. Polysorbate 80 (Tween®-80) is extensively used in foods, cosmetics and pharmaceuticals. The polysorbate 80 used in the SAF formulation conforms to the NF requirements. Polysorbate 80 has an HLB in the range of 12–16; it is therefore very soluble in aqueous media. Polysorbate 80 serves as an emulsifier in the formulation and helps stabilize the emulsion over longer-term storage.
5. Sodium chloride, USP.
6. Potassium chloride, USP.
7. Potassium phosphate monobasic, NF.
8. Sodium phosphate dibasic, anhydrous, USP.

   Phosphate-buffered saline (PBS) comprises the continuous, aqueous, phase of the emulsion formulation. The salts listed here, sodium chloride, potassium chloride, potassium phosphate monobasic, and sodium phosphate dibasic, anhydrous, are used to prepare PBS. With these salts, the formulation is isotonic with a pH of approximately 7.4. These buffer salts can be obtained from various vendors.
9. Microfluidizer M110Y, Microfluidics Corporation (Newton, MA). The M110Y model has a pump that provides sufficiently high internal operating pressures to achieve reduced droplet size, thus enabling sterile filtration.
10. 0.22-µm sterilizing filter, such as a Millipak 60 (from Millipore) or suitable equivalent.

3. Methods

3.1. Formulation

The SAF emulsion formulation was typically manufactured as a twofold concentrate. Prior to use, the emulsion was diluted with a twofold concentrate

Table 1
Components of the 2X SAF Emulsion Concentrate

Ingredient	Formulation manufactured as a 2X concentrate (%w/v)
Poloxamer 401	5.0
Polysorbate 80, NF	0.4
Squalane, NF	10.0
Sodium chloride, USP	0.736
Potassium chloride, USP	0.0184
Potassium phosphate monobasic, NF	0.0184
Sodium phosphate dibasic, anhydrous, USP	0.11
Water for injection, USP q.s.	100.0

of threonyl-MDP and antigen. The threonyl-MDP was formulated in an isotonic buffered solution at a pH that was optimal for its stability. The emulsion formulation, as manufactured, is provided in **Table 1** (*see* **Notes 4–6**). After development of the SAF formulation, several modifications were evaluated for their impact on the biological efficacy, physical appearance, and physical stability. The following changes proved successful: (a) reduction of the pluronic concentration, *see* **Note 7**; (b) substitution of tetronic 1501 for pluronic, *see* **Note 8**; and (c) substitution of synthetic squalane for natural squalane, *see* **Note 9**. Whereas these changes were not incorporated into the formulation, they are viable options and could be successfully implemented.

Once SAF was manufactured via the Microfluidizer, the resulting product appeared as a white fluid emulsion. SAF-m remained physically stable for prolonged periods of time (>2 yr) when stored at or below 30°C (*see* **Notes 10** and **11**).

3.2. Details of SAF Manufacture

A stepwise procedure for manufacture of 1000 mL of SAF-m emulsion is provided below. This example can be scaled within a 100–5000 mL range.

1. In a 1-L volumetric flask, add the following components: 7.36 g sodium chloride, USP; 0.184 g potassium chloride, USP; 0.184 g potassium phosphate monobasic, NF; 1.1 g sodium phosphate dibasic, anhydrous, USP.
2. To the volumetric flask, add approximately 700 mL of water for injection, USP. With mixing, dissolve all the salts in the volumetric flask.
3. To the volumetric flask, add 4.0 g of polysorbate 80, USP. With gentle mixing, allow the polysorbate 80 to completely dissolve (avoid foaming with aggressive mixing).
4. To the volumetric flask, add 50.0 g of poloxamer 401. With gentle mixing, allow this excipient to completely hydrate and disperse.

5. To the volumetric flask, add 100 g of squalane, NF.
6. Bring the mixture to 1000 mL with water for injection, USP.
7. Using a magnetic stir bar, at a speed sufficient to create a vortex, mix the components together.
8. Prepare the Microfluidizer M110Y by flushing with 2–5 L of ethanol followed by 5–15 liters of sterile water for injection.
9. Pass the emulsion mixture prepared in **step 8** through the Microfluidizer four times (*see* **Notes 12–15**).
10. Under a laminar flow hood, filter the emulsion through a 0.22-µm filter (such as a Millipak 60 cartridge filter) using positive nitrogen pressure. Collect the filtered emulsion in a sterile container.
11. Package the emulsion as appropriate. (Both glass and plastic vials were found compatible with the SAF emulsion.)

4. Notes

1. At this time, there is no availability of threonyl-MDP. This material had been manufactured by or for Syntex or its licensees. This compound is no longer being synthesized. A description of threonyl-MDP and related analogs can be found in U.S. Patent 4,082,735, authored by Jones, G. H., Moffett, J. H., and Nestor, J. J. The literature also suggests other MDP analogs of potential interest ***(14)***. Any inquiries regarding threonyl-MDP should be directed to Dr. Gary Ott of Chiron (Emeryville, CA, telephone: 510-923-2964).
2. Droplet-size analysis can be performed by several techniques. To confirm or validate the results of any one method, it is recommended that a second method be employed. For example, particle size analyzers utilizing laser (such as a Brinkmann or Malvern) are convenient to use and provide fairly reproducible results. To confirm the results of these types of instruments, a microscope technique (such as a light microscope) would be a suitable second method.
3. When measuring droplet size of SAF emulsion, an aliquot of emulsion will need substantial dilution. To preserve the droplet size of the emulsion, the best dilution vehicle is the continuous phase of the emulsion (i.e., a solution containing the salts of the PBS portion of the SAF emulsion).
4. The SAF emulsion listed in **Table 1** is referred to as the 2X concentrate. It should be noted that the components of the PBS are not concentrated; they are present in the proper amount to make an isotonic solution. Typically, the 2X-concentrated SAF is diluted with a concentrated antigen and threonyl-MDP solution also formulated in a 1X salt-buffer solution (or alternate isotonic-buffered solution).
5. After dilution, the SAF emulsion contained 2.5% poloxamer 401, 0.2% polysorbate 80, and 5.0% squalane with threonyl-MDP and antigen in PBS.
6. Other SAF emulsion concentrates can be prepared (1.5X, 3X, 4X, and so on) depending on the volume of antigen required for a specific vaccine. To prepare an alternate concentrate, simply adjust the amounts of squalane, polysorbate 80, and poloxamer 401, accordingly.

7. The concentration of poloxamer 401 in the SAF emulsion can be reduced by half. A modified 2X concentrate of SAF emulsion containing 2.5% poloxamer 401 was prepared. The physical appearance and stability of this modified emulsion was consistent with the original SAF. Likewise, the biological responses were identical to the original SAF emulsion (antibody titers, log2, in guinea pigs vaccinated with ovalbumin were determined at week 6, postvaccination; the results were: 6.5 ± 0.2 for the reduced poloxamer 401 formulation vs 6.9 ± 0.3 for the original formulation. Cell-mediated immunity was determined by delayed hypersensitivity skin reactions in the same guinea pigs, measured in mm at week 6, postvaccination: 18.1 ± 0.7 for reduced poloxamer 401 SAF vs 19.4 ± 1.1 for the original SAF).
8. Tetronic®1501, a tetrafunctional block copolymer, was substituted for poloxamer 401 in the formulation. At a 2X concentration of 5.0%, the physical characteristics of the formulation were identical to the original SAF emulsion. Biological responses were also identical to the original SAF emulsion (antibody titers, as described in **Note 7**, were: 7.1 ± 0.1 for the tetronic formulation vs 6.9 ± 0.3 for the original pluronic formulation. Cell-mediated immunity was determined by delayed hypersensitivity skin reactions, as described in **Note 7**, with the following results: 16.8 ± 0.6 for tetronic SAF vs 19.4 ± 1.1 for the original SAF).
9. A final modification to the formulation is worth mentioning. Robeco, the manufacturer of squalane (which is naturally derived from shark liver oil) was evaluating a synthetic version of squalane (Robane® SXL). This synthetic version was directly substituted in the formulation with satisfactory results from a physical and biological standpoint. Antibody titers of mice immunized with influenza B hemagglutinin were determined at weeks 3, 5, and 9 postvaccination; the values reported here are enzyme-linked immunosorbent assay (ELISA) titers expressed as $\log_3$ of the serum dilution giving an optical density reading of 0.5 absorbance units. The results are provided below.

	Antibody Titers		
	Week 3[a]	Week 5[a]	Week 9
SAF with naturally derived squalane	8.4	9.4	8.9 ± 0.7
SAF with synthetic squalane	8.7	9.5	8.6 ± 0.9

[a]Values were determined from pooled sera of groups of immunized mice.

10. Physical stability of the final product (SAF-m) was found to be acceptable when stored below 30°C. A modest amount of creaming was observed over prolonged storage periods (yr). With shaking, the emulsion appeared homogenous. The actual change in droplet size over time was not measured in our laboratories. It is expected, though, that particle size will increase with time.
11. Storage temperatures will impact the physical stability of the emulsion. Elevated temperatures are detrimental to an emulsion. SAF was typically stored at or below 25°C. Storage at 5°C and –20°C were also found to be acceptable (as determined

by observation of the physical condition of the emulsion and the antibody and cell-mediated biological responses).

12. As noted in the text, alternate mixing equipment can be utilized. In our laboratory, the following procedures were successfully used (*see* **ref. *13***): (a) Greerco homogenizer mixer, at approximately 4750 rpm for 30 min; (b) blade mixing, using a gate blade, at approximately 740 rpm for 40 min; and (c) vigorous vortex mixing until all visible solids had dispersed. During manufacture, especially if using a homogenizer, it is important to keep the emulsion cool (preferably below 30°C).
13. The initial physical appearance of a SAF-1 emulsion may look acceptable. Depending on the chosen manufacturing method, the physical appearance may decline rapidly (min). The rate of physical deterioration generally relates to the equipment's ability to effectively reduce particle size. Typically SAF-1 manufactured via all alternate methods described in **Note 12** showed extensive creaming (a heavy white layer, composed of squalane-surfactant droplets, at the top of the emulsion). Fortunately, coalescence (characterized by a layer of pure squalane at the top of the emulsion) was not observed. With vigorous shaking, the creamed-emulsion could be restored to a more uniform appearance prior to animal vaccination.
14. When using a Microfluidizer to manufacture SAF, the high-energy mixing forces encountered in the Microfluidizer leads to heat generation that readily transfers to the emulsion product. Uncontrolled, the temperature of the emulsion could exceed 60°C. At this temperature, squalane will coalesce. The temperature of the product must be maintained below 30°C. This can be achieved by surrounding the interaction chamber with ice and passing the emulsion through a cooling coil also surrounded with ice.
15. The number of times the emulsion is processed through the Microfluidizer is critical to droplet size of the final emulsion. During the first four processing cycles through the Microfluidizer, the droplet size decreases to approximately 165 nm. Further processing does not decrease the mean droplet size. However, further processing will decrease the distribution of droplet size (one processing cycle gave a mean droplet size of 187 nm with a range of 115–1000 nm; four cycles gave a mean of 164 nm with a range of 118–315 nm; and seven cycles gave a mean of 165 nm with a range of 81–270 nm).

References

1. Allison, A. C. (1994) Adjuvants and immune enhancement. *Intl. J. Technol. Assess. Health Care* **10,** 107–120.
2. Waters, R. V., Terrell, T. G., and Jones, G. H., (1986) Uveitis induction in the rabbit by muramyl dipeptides. *Infect. Immun.* **51,** 816–825.
3. Allison, A. C. and Byars, N. E. (1992) Syntex adjuvant formulation. *Res. Immunol.* **143,** 519–525.
4. Hunter, R., Strickland, F., and Kezdy, F. (1981) The adjuvant activity of nonionic block polymer surfactants. I. The role of hydrophile-lipophile balance. *J. Immunol.* **127,** 1244–1250.

5. Hunter, R. L. and Bennett, B. (1984) The adjuvant activity of nonionic block polymer surfactants. II. Antibody formation and inflammation related to the structure of triblock and octablock copolymers. *J. Immunol.* **133,** 3167–3175.
6. Hunter, R. L. and Bennett, B. (1986) The adjuvant activity of nonionic block polymer surfactants. III. Characterization of selected biologically active surfaces. *Scand. J. Immunol.* **23,** 287–300.
7. Hunter, R., Olsen, M., and Buynitzky, S. (1991) The adjuvant activity of nonionic block copolymers. IV. Effect of molecular weight and formulation on titre and isotype of antibody. *Vaccine* **9,** 250.
8. Hjorth, R. N., Bonde, G. M., Piner, E. D., Goldberg, K. M., and Levner, M. H. (1997) The effect of Syntex adjuvant formulation (SAF-m) on humoral immunity to the influenza virus in the mouse. *Vaccine* **15,** 541–546.
9. Pye, D., Vandenberg, K. L., Dyer, S. L., Irving, D. O., Goss, N. H., Woodrow, G. C., et al. (1997) Selection of an adjuvant for vaccination with the malaria antigen, MSA-2. *Vaccine* **15,** 1017–1023.
10. Allison, A. C. and Byars, N. E. (1990) Adjuvant formulations and their mode of action. *Immunology* **2,** 369–374.
11. Boyd, J., Parkinson, C., and Sherman, P. (1972) Factors affecting emulsion stability, and the HLB concept. *J. Colloid Interface Sci.* **41,** 359–370.
12. Lidgate, D. M., Trattner, T., Shultz, R. M., and Maskiewicz, R. (1992) Sterile filtration of a parenteral emulsion. *Pharm. Res.* **9,** 860–863.
13. Lidgate, D. M., Fu, R. C., Byars, N. E., Foster, L. C., and Fleitman, J. S. (1989) Formulation of vaccine adjuvant muramyldipeptides. III. Processing optimization, characterization, and bioactivity of an emulsion vehicle. *Pharm. Res.* **6,** 748–752.
14. Gupta, R. K., Relyveld, E. H., Lindblad, E. B., Bizzini, B., Ben-Efraim, S., and Gupta, C. K. (1993) Adjuvants—a balance between toxicity and adjuvanticity. *Vaccine* **11,** 293–306.

14

The ISCOM™ Technology

Karin Lövgren-Bengtsson and Bror Morein

1. Introduction

Classical adjuvant formulations, such as Freund's adjuvants and aluminium salts, are blended with antigens to formulate an emulsion, or the antigens are adsorbed onto a three-dimensional gel containing adjuvant *(1)*. The ISCOM™ (immunostimulating complex, Iscotec AB, Uppsala, Sweden) is a complex consisting of lipids, saponins, and antigens, which form spontaneously when the right constituents are allowed to interact at correct stoichiometry.

ISCOMs are typically 40-nm cage-like structures that combine a multimeric presentation of antigen with a built-in saponin adjuvant *(2)*, e.g., semipurified preparations, such as Quil-A™ (Superfos AS) *(3)* or suitable purified fractions thereof.

The physical three-dimensional structure of the ISCOM is built up from 10–12 nm subunits formed by Quillaja saponins and cholesterol *(4–6)*. In the presence of phospholipids, hydrophobic and amphipathic antigens, or antigen-made hydrophobic by any of the modifications described in **Subheading 3.**, are incorporated into ISCOMs by hydrophobic interactions during the assembly of the ISCOM subunits *(7)*.

1.1. ISCOM Technology

The classical procedure for ISCOM formation is to mix antigens and saponin with detergent-solubilized cholesterol and phospholipid *(8)*. ISCOMs are formed when detergent is removed by dialysis, ultrafiltration, or ultracentrifugation *(9–11)*. However, not all antigens spontaneously incorporate into ISCOMs using standard procedures even if they are hydrophobic; also, many

From: *Methods in Molecular Medicine, Vol. 42:*
Vaccine Adjuvants: Preparation Methods and Research Protocols
Edited by: D. T. O'Hagan © Humana Press, Inc., Totowa, NJ

antigens are too hydrophilic to incorporate. Alternative methods for incorporation of such antigens are described in **Subheadings 3.3.** and **3.4.**

1.1.1. Composition of ISCOMs

Whichever method is used for incorporation/binding of antigens into ISCOMs, the goal is the same: to prepare a highly immunogenic particle of low toxicity that contains an exposed antigen with retained antigenicity. Also, the degree of antigen incorporation is important to analyze because it affects the overall composition, antigen presentation, and targeting of the ISCOM. The coadministration of antigen and adjuvant in the same particle is considered to play a major role for the strong immunogenicity of ISCOMs.

The composition of "the ideal ISCOM" is, of course, dependent upon several factors such as the immunogenicity of incorporated antigens, grade and purity of Quillaja saponin, the species to be immunized, and the antigen dose to be used for immunization. An increased ratio of Quillaja saponin to protein can increase the immunogenicity in such a way that a 1-μg dose of antigen in ISCOMs with a high proportion of Quil A is as immunogenic as a 10-μg dose of antigen in ISCOMs with a low proportion of Quil-A ***(12)***. However, the ratio of Quil-A and antigen in ISCOMs must be properly balanced to avoid side effects caused by too high a dose of Quil-A (*see* **Subheadings 1.1.2.** and **3.5.**).

1.1.2. Immune Modulatory Properties of ISCOMs

ISCOM-associated antigen is rapidly removed from the site of injection and transported to draining lymph nodes (LN). In the draining LN, a potent but transient response of antigen-driven proliferation of T cells producing interleukin 2 (IL-2) and interferon (IFN)-γ is recorded at days 4–8 after immunization. A similar, but lower, response is later (from days 8–11 and onward) detected in the spleen ***(13)***.

The immune enhancement of ISCOMs is characterized as increased major histocompatibility complex (MHC) class II expression on antigen-presenting cells (APCs) ***(14,15)***, antigen-driven proliferation of lymphocytes secreting IL-2 and high amounts of IFN-γ ***(10,16,17)***, and generation of potent long-lasting antibody responses ***(18–22)***, involving all immunoglobulin isotypes and immunoglobulin G (IgG) subclasses ***(19,23,24)***. ISCOMs stimulate APCs to produce IL-1 ***(25–27)***, IL-6 ***(26,28)***, and IL-12 ***(29)*** and induce T-helper cells of both Th1 and Th2 type ***(16,23,30)*** and the cell-mediated immune response includes CD8+ class I restricted cytotoxic T cells ***(31,32)***. Interestingly, human immunodeficiency virus-type 1 (HIV-1) ISCOMs were shown to induce β-chemokines, MIP-1α, MIP-1β, and regulated upon activation, normal T cell expressed and secreted (RANTES) ***(33)***. ISCOMs are potent inducers of antibody responses in serum, as well as in local and distant mucosal surfaces after intranasal administration (in) ***(19,31,34–36)***.

The same dose ranges as those mentioned for free Quil-A are generally valid for ISCOMs, although the dose of Quil-A in ISCOMs required for a potent immune response is lower by far. One of the main advantages of ISCOM formulations is that the dose of antigen required may be as low as one-tenth of that required with other adjuvant formulations ***(10)***. Consequently, the dose of Quil-A is also reduced compared with the use of free Quil-A.

As with other adjuvants, the dose of saponin in ISCOM and ISCOM-matrix™ should be adjusted to the antigen and the animal species. Attention must also be focused on the purity of the saponins, because crude saponin preparations may require considerably higher doses. As a guideline, Dalsgaard et al. ***(37)*** gave the following dose recommendations for free Quil-A (a semipurified and characterized preparation of adjuvant active saponins): 10 μg for use in mice, 50 μg in guinea pigs, 200 μg in rabbits, 500 μg in pigs, and 1000 μg in cattle.

1.2. Iscomatrix™ Technology

Iscomatrix™ (Iscotec AB, AdVet AB) is an adjuvant formulation that is closely related to ISCOM. The ISCOM-matrix is a particle with identical composition, shape, and appearance as the ISCOM, except that it lacks incorporated antigens ***(7)***. ISCOM-matrix is simply mixed with antigens. Because association of antigen and adjuvant into the same particle offers an advantage over nonassociated formulations ***(12,36,38)***, ISCOMs are generally more immunogenic than ISCOM-matrix formulations. A major advantage of using the ISCOM-matrix, compared with using free saponin, is that the hemolytic activity of saponins in ISCOM-matrix is abolished or drastically reduced ***(5,39)***. The saponins are bound to cholesterol in the complex and therefore do not bind to tissue cholesterol at the site of injection and thereby lytic activity and local reactions are avoided ***(39)*** and (Sundquist, Iscotec AB, personal communication). Compared to that of ISCOMs, less information is available concerning the mechanism of adjuvant activity of ISCOM-matrix ***(12,38,40)***. Some antigens, particularly basic antigens with high isoelectric points, do adsorb to ISCOM-matrix. In these cases, the preparations should rather classify as ISCOMs and the mechanism would most likely be identical to that of classically prepared ISCOMs (unpublished observations).

For antigens that do not adsorb to or incorporate into ISCOMs, ISCOM-matrix can be used as a carrier to which hydrophilic antigens are conjugated to form ISCOMs. ISCOM-matrix used for conjugation of antigens must contain a constituent with an exposed functional group suitable for conjugation, e.g., phosphatidyl ethanol amine (PE) ***(41,42)***. We found ISCOM-matrix preparations consisting of cholesterol and egg-PC with 20–50% of the egg-PC exchanged for egg-PE, dioleyl-PE, or dimyristoyl-PE suitable.

1.2.1. Immune Modulatory Properties of ISCOM-Matrix

The IgG subclass distribution of antigen-specific serum antibodies in mice immunized with antigens mixed with ISCOM-matrix roughly parallel that in mice immunized with ISCOMs. Likewise, spleen cells from mice immunized with ISCOM-matrix adjuvanted antigen produce high levels of IL-2 and IFN-γ after antigen restimulation in vitro ***(12)***. Another prominent feature of ISCOMs, the activation of cytotoxic T-lymphocytes (CTL), is reported also after immunization with ISCOM-matrix formulations ***(38)***. However, these CTL responses were substantially weaker (about threefold) than those induced by ISCOMs.

ISCOM-matrix formulations may lack the superior antigen-presenting ability of ISCOMs because the antigen is not physically associated with the ISCOM-matrix. However, if the antigen is associated with the ISCOM-matrix, e.g., by electrostatic interactions, the adjuvant activity approaches that of ISCOMs (unpublished observations). ISCOM-matrix, like saponins in general, is a potent and useful adjuvant for particulate antigens, but inferior with monomeric antigens ***(43–48)***.

Following parenteral administration, ISCOM-matrix formulations are often potent enhancers of antibody responses. After intranasal immunization, moderate IgA responses are detected in the lungs but, compared to immunization with ISCOMs, lower IgA titers are induced in remote mucosa of the intestinal and genital tracts ***(36)***.

The dose recommendations for Quillaja saponins are likely to be valid also for ISCOM-matrix.

2. Materials

1. Protein antigen: The handling of the antigen before incorporation is important. The antigens most suited for ISCOM formulation are hydrophobic or amphipathic. Such antigens must be purified in the presence of a detergent to prevent micelle or aggregate formation because pure protein micelles or aggregates are very difficult to dissociate to make their hydrophobic part accessible for hydrophobic interactions. There are many examples where antigens that theoretically should incorporate well, in fact do not, as a result of such aggregates.

   Some hydrophobic antigens are poorly soluble, even in detergents. Such antigens can be solubilized in, e.g., dimethyl sulfoxide (DMSO), urea, ethylene glycol (EG), or guanidine hydrochloride (GuaHCl), thereafter, lipid in detergent stock solution and saponin is added. Dialysis or ultrafiltration is performed against decreasing concentration of the solubilizer (DMSO, urea, EG, or GuaHCl) followed by a physiological buffer, e.g., phosphate-buffered saline (PBS).

Hydrophilic antigens do not incorporate into ISCOMs. To make ISCOMs that contain hydrophilic antigens, hydrophobic regions must be introduced, e.g., by binding lipids to them ***(34,49–52)*** or exposed, e.g., by low pH treatment ***(53)***. At first glance, one may think that such a treatment will irreversibly denature the antigens, and for some antigens this is true. In practice, low pH treatment was often shown less denaturing than random chemical modification (Lövgren-Bengtsson, K., Morein, B., Ekström, J., Åkerblom, L., and Villacres-Eriksson, M., unpublished observations).

2. Quillaja saponin: The basis for ISCOM formation is the interaction of Quillaja saponins with cholesterol. Not all saponins in a crude or semipurified extract form "classical" 40-nm ISCOMs, even though some type of complexes or macromolecular structures are often formed when Quillaja saponins ***(5)*** or other saponins ***(54)*** are incubated with cholesterol. There are preparations of Quillaja saponins commercially available that are tested and selected for ISCOM-forming ability: Quil-A, Spikoside (AdVet AB), and Iscoprep™ 703 (Iscotec AB).

   A 100-mg/mL stock solution of Quil-A, Spikoside, or Iscoprep 703 is prepared in sterile distilled water. Keep aliquots frozen at –20°C.

3. Lipids: Cholesterol (CHOL) is indispensable for ISCOM formation because the unique affinity of Quillaja saponins for cholesterol is the cause of the complex formation. Phospholipids (PL) are often used as a supplementary lipid, even though other lipids can replace them. The choice of phospholipid has always been an open question and there have been few arguments to favor one over another. We have routinely used phosphatidyl choline from egg (egg-PC).

   Lately, it has been noticed that phospholipids may have immunomodulatory effects in liposomes ***(55–57)*** and preliminary findings have also indicated that ISCOMs made with different phospholipids may differ in terms of immunogenicity and toxicity (***38***, Åkerblom, L. and Morein, B., unpublished).

   The choice of phospholipid/lipid can also be used to influence the surface charge and solubility of the ISCOM particle.

   PC/CHOL stock solution: Dissolve 100 mg/mL each of cholesterol and phosphatidyl choline in 10 mL 20% MEGA-10 (or β-octylglucoside). The lipids dissolve slowly at 30–60°C while being stirred. Stock solutions of individual and other lipids are made accordingly. Lipids supplied in solvent solution are dried onto a glass vial using N_2 prior to the addition of detergent.

   Keep aliquots of the stock solutions frozen at –20°C. A small amount of adioactive lipid, e.g., ^{3}H-cholesterol added to the lipid stock solutions can be useful for detection and rapid quantification.

4. Detergents: The detergent used for preparation of lipid mixtures and for solubilization of antigens is preferably nonionic because it must be harmless to the antigen and have a sufficiently high critical micellar concentration (cmc) if a dialysis or ultrafiltration method will be used. Examples of suitable detergents are MEGA-10 and octylglucoside.

Table 1
Heterobifunctional Crosslinking Reagents and Activated Lipids for Conjugation

Name	Reaction toward	Supplier	Described in subheading(s)
EDC 1-Ethyl-3-(dimethylaminopropyl)carbodiimide	-COOH $-NH_2$	Pierce Chemical Co., Rockford, IL	3.4.2.
SPDP *N*-succinimidyl-3-(2-pyridyldithio)propionate	$-NH_2$ -SH	Pierce Chemical Co.	3.3.1., 3.3.2., 3.3.5., 3.3.6.
MBS *m*-Maleimidobenzoyl-*N*-hydroxysuccinimide ester	$-NH_2$ -SH	Pierce Chemical Co.	3.3.3., 3.3.7.
PDPH (3-(2-pyridyldithio) propionyl hydrazide)	-COH -SH	Pierce Chemical Co.	3.3.8.
MPBH (4-(4-N-maleimidophenyl)butyric acid hydrazid)	-COH -SH	Pierce Chemical Co.	3.3.8
PDP-DPPE N-((2-Pyridyldithio)propionyl)-1,2-dipalmitoyl-*sn*-glycero-3-phosphoethanolamine	-SH	Nothern Lipids Inc., Vancouver, Canada	3.4.3.
MBP-DPPE N-(4-*p*-Maleimidophenyl)butyryl)-1,2-dipalmitoyl-*sn*-glycero-3-phosphoethanolamine	-SH	Nothern Lipids Inc.	3.4.3.
MB-DPPE N-(3-Maleimidobenzoyl)1,2-dipalmitoyl-*sn*-glycero-3-phosphoethanolamine	-SH	Nothern Lipids Inc.	3.4.3.
NPS (N-palmitoyloxysuccinimide)	$-NH_2$	Sigma, St. Louis, MO	3.4.1.
NOS (N-oleoyloxysuccinimide)	$-NH_2$	Sigma	3.4.1.

Make a 20% (w/w) stock solution by adding 8 mL distilled water to 2 g of detergent. Dissolve by gentle heating (30–50°C). During storage of MEGA-10 at room temperature, MEGA-10 crystallizes. Redissolve crystals of MEGA-10 by gentle heating prior to use. To avoid crystallization, all MEGA-10 containing solutions should preferably be stored at –20°C.

5. Buffers: The choice of buffer is not critical for the methodology. The buffer should be chosen to maximize the solubility of all ingredients, most importantly, the antigen. In most cases, a PBS (e.g., 10 m*M* phosphate, 150 m*M* NaCl, pH 6.8–7.4) buffer will do. Owing to instability of Quillaja saponins at high pH (>8) prolonged incubations in buffers with a pH >8 should be avoided. Once the ISCOMs or ISCOM-matrix are formed, the Quillaja saponins are much more stable, even at elevated pH (Sundquist and Rönnberg, Iscotec AB, personal communication).

Table 2
Chemical Modification of ISCOM-Matrix (Aminogroup Reactions)

Reagent	Generation of	Reactive toward	Described in subheading
SPDP	2-pyridyldisulfide	-SH	3.3.1.
SPDP/DTT	-SH	maleimide or 2-pyridyldisulfide	3.3.2.
MBS	maleimide	-SH	3.3.3.

Table 3
Antigen Modification

Functional group	Reagent	Reactive group	Reactive towards	Described in subheading
$-NH_2$	SPDP	2-pyridyldisulfide	-SH	3.3.5.
	SPDP/DTT	-SH	maleimide	3.3.6.
	MBS	maleimide	-SH	3.3.7
Disulfide	DTT	-SH	maleimide or 2-pyridyldisulfide	3.3.4.
Carbohydrate	$NaIO_4$	-CHO	hydrazide	3.3.8
	$NaIO_4$/PDPH	2-pyridyldisulfide	-SH	3.3.8
	$NaIO_4$/PDPH/DTT	-SH	maleimide or 2-pyridyldisulfide	3.3.8
Carbohydrate	$NaIO_4$	-CHO	-hydrazide	3.3.8.
	$NaIO_4$/MPBH	maleimide	-SH	3.3.8.

6. Special chemicals: Heterobifunctional crosslinking reagents and lipids for chemical conjugation. There is an increasing number of useful reagents available. Some of them, including those employed in the examples below, are listed in **Table 1**. Their use for chemical modification of ISCOM-matrix and antigens are summarized in **Tables 2** and **3**, respectively.
7. Dialysis tubing: MWCO (molecular-weight cutoff) 12–14.000 for standard preparations, a lower molecular-weight cutoff can be used for smaller antigens.
8. Equipment: There is no need for any sophisticated equipment for small-scale non-GMP production of ISCOMs. A magnetic stirrer, dialysis tubing, and clean glass tubes will cover the basic needs. For analysis of starting materials and the final product (quantification and quality control) facilities for electron microscopy, ultracentrifugation, HPLC analysis of lipids and Quillaja saponins, and aminoacid analysis are required. The method for antigen quantification are also critical because methods based on antibody or dye-binding is often strongly influenced by the physical state of the antigen. Incorporation into ISCOMs may increase (or decrease) the surface area of the antigen compared with its exposure

in the native microorganism, or in monomeric solution or aggregated form. Also, chemical surface modification may alter the antigenicity and dye-binding properties of antigens.

3. Methods

3.1. Preparation of ISCOM-Matrix

1. Mix 10 mg of cholesterol and phospholipid (e.g., PC, PE, or mixtures of both) with 50 mg of Quil-A or 35 mg of Iscoprep.
2. Adjust the concentration of cholesterol to 1–2 mg/mL with, e.g., PBS and incubate for 1–2 h at 20–25°C.
3. Dialyze against 3–5 changes of buffer (>48 h), at 20–25°C.
4. Quantify, e.g., by HPLC or inclusion of a radioactive tracer, such as ^{3}H-cholesterol, and store at +4°C (or frozen at < –20°C) until use.

3.2. Preparation of ISCOMs (Hydrophobic Interactions)

3.2.1. Amphipathic Antigens (Native or Lipidated) in Detergent

1. Make a preparation of the antigen in detergent.
2. Mix antigen, lipids, and saponin according to **Table 4** and adjust the volume with PBS. Incubate for 1–2 h at room temperature prior to extensive dialysis against PBS.
3. Dialyze against 3–5 changes of buffer (24–48 h), the first 24 h at 20–25°C then at +4°C.

3.2.2. Antigen in 3–8 M urea (Gua-HCl, DMSO, EG, and so on)

1. If the antigen is solubilized in, e.g., urea, mix antigen, lipids, and saponin according to **Table 4** and adjust the volume with 3–8 *M* urea. Incubate for 1–2 h at room temperature prior to extensive dialysis against PBS. If the antigen is provided in another buffer and urea is used to increase the solubility, the incubation time may need extension to 18–24 h.
2. Dialyze against 3–5 changes of buffer (24–48 h), the first 24 h at 20–25°C, then at +4°C.

3.2.3. Low pH Procedure

1. Mix antigen, lipids, and saponin according to **Table 4** and add 1/10 of the final volume (e.g., 0.1 mL to 1 mL) of 1 *M* citrate pH 2.5. Mix thoroughly and incubate for 1–2 h at room temperature prior to extensive dialysis against PBS. Because of the low pH, a white precipitate forms. Dissolve the precipitate by resuspending the precipitate several times a day during dialysis until it is dissolved or diminished to minimum.
2. Dialyze against 3–5 changes of buffer (24–48 h), the first 24 h at 20–25°C, then at +4°C.

Table 4
Guideline for the Mixing of Antigens, Saponins, and Lipids for ISCOM Formation

	Detergent	Antigen	CHOL[1]	PL[2]	Quillaja saponin[3]
Weight Ratio		0.5–1	1	1	≤5 (Quil A, Spikoside) 3,5 (Iscoprep 703)
Final Concentration	1–2% (or more)	0.2–1 mg/mL			>1 mg/mL

The final concentration of detergent should preferably not exceed 2% (*see* **Notes 1** and **2**). A higher concentration may be used, but it is important to realize that the time of dialysis required to remove the detergent and complete ISCOM (or ISCOM-matrix) formation often becomes substantially longer. Under these circumstances, it may happen that other components in the mixture, particularly the phospholipid and Quillaja saponin component(s), may also be partly lost. The final concentration of CHOL and PL depends on the antigen concentration and must be balanced with Quillaja saponin, as indicated in this table.

[1]Cholesterol

[2]Phospholipid

[3]Other Quillaja saponin preparations may balance with cholesterol different ratios. If the supplier of the saponin is unable to give this information this has to be tested by mixing 1 mL volumes containing 1 mg of cholesterol (containing ^{3}H-cholesterol) with 1 mg of phospholipid (in 2% MEGA-10) with different amounts of the saponin preparation (e.g., 1, 3, and 10 mg). Proceed as described under **Subheading 3.1.** ***(1–3)***. Submit samples of the preparations for negative staining EM analysis (**Note 6**) and sucrose density gradient centrifugation (**Note 7**).

3.3. Preparation of ISCOMs (Conjugation to Preformed ISCOM-Matrix)

ISCOM-matrix can be activated for conjugation to thiol-containing (or modified) antigen using SPDP or MBS.

3.3.1. SPDP (Introduction of Protected Thiol Groups)

1. Add SPDP (maximum 12.5 mg/mL in anhydrous ethanol) to ISCOM-matrix in 0.1 *M* phosphate buffer pH 6.7 in a molar ratio of about five times the concentration of PE (PE conc. approx 0.5 mg/mL). Incubate for 1 h at room temperature.
2. Separate the ISCOM-matrix from SPDP by gel filtration, e.g., using prepacked desalting columns (PD-10 from Pharmacia and Upjohn, Kalamazoo, MI or Econo-Pac 10DG from Bio-Rad, Richmond, CA) equilibrated with N_2-saturated 0.1 *M* phosphate buffer containing 0.1 *M* ethylenediaminetetraacetic acid (EDTA), pH 6.7. Collect fractions of 5–6 drops in an enzyme-linked immunosorbent assay (ELISA) plate and pool the ISCOM-matrix containing fractions (e.g., detected through ^{3}H-cholesterol in the ISCOM-matrix).
3. Quantify/estimate the amount of modified ISCOM-matrix, e.g., by HPLC or inclusion of a radioactive tracer, such as ^{3}H-cholesterol and mix with antigen.

3.3.2. SPDP (Introduction of Thiol (-SH) Groups)

1. Add SPDP (maximum 12.5 mg/mL in anhydrous ethanol) to ISCOM-matrix in 0.1 *M* phosphate buffer pH 6.7 in a molar ratio of about five times the conc. of PE (PE conc. approx 0.5 mg/mL). Incubate for 1 h at room temperature.
2. Add diphtheria tetanus toxoid (DTT) to a final concentration of 10 m*M* and incubate for 30 min.
3. Separate the ISCOM-matrix from SPDP/DTT by gel filtration, e.g., using prepacked desalting columns (PD-10 from Pharmacia and Upjohn or Econo-Pac 10DG from Bio-Rad) equilibrated with N_2-saturated 0.1 *M* phosphate buffer containing 0.1 *M* (EDTA), pH 6.7. Collect fractions of 5–6 drops in an ELISA plate and pool the ISCOM-matrix containing fractions (e.g., detected through ^{3}H-cholesterol in the ISCOM-matrix).
4. Quantify/estimate the amount of modified ISCOM-matrix, e.g., by HPLC or inclusion of a radioactive tracer such as ^{3}H-cholesterol and mix with antigen.

3.3.3. MBS (Introduction of Thiol-Binding Maleimide Groups)

1. Add MBS (dissolved a small volume of DMSO) to ISCOM-matrix in 0.1 *M* phosphate buffer pH 6.7 in a molar ratio of about five times the conc. of PE (PE conc. approx 0.5 mg/mL). Incubate for 1 h at room temperature.
2. Separate the ISCOM-matrix from MBS by gel filtration, e.g., using prepacked desalting columns (PD-10 from Pharmacia and Upjohn or Econo-Pac 10DG from Bio-Rad) equilibrated with N_2-saturated 0.1 *M* phosphate buffer containing 0.1 *M* EDTA, pH 6.7. Collect fractions of 5–6 drops in an ELISA plate and pool the ISCOM-matrix containing fractions (e.g., detected through ^{3}H-cholesterol in the ISCOM-matrix).
3. Quantify/estimate the amount of modified ISCOM-matrix, e.g., by HPLC or inclusion of a radioactive tracer such as ^{3}H-cholesterol and mix with antigen.

If the antigens do not contain an accessible thiol group for conjugation to the activated ISCOM-matrix, the antigens need some chemical modification. Methods for the introduction of a protected thiol or a thiol-binding maleimide on the antigen at ε-amino groups (in principle, lysine side chains) and the introduction of a protected thiol or a thiol-binding maleimid on carbohydrate moieties are described. Both the protected thiol group and the thiol-binding maleimid will bind to an unprotected reduced thiol (-SH) on the ISCOM-matrix in a controled way.

3.3.4. Thiol-Containing Antigens

Antigens containing an accessible thiol can be used directly for conjugation to activated ISCOM-matrix after reduction.

1. Incubate the antigen in 10–100 m*M* DTT for 20–60 min in a buffer with a pH around 8.0.

2. Remove DTT by gel filtration or dialysis (e.g., 0.1 *M* phosphate, 10–100 m*M* EDTA, pH 6.7).
3. Quantify, e.g., using the method of Bradford *(58)* and store at +4°C under non-oxidizing conditions until use.

3.3.5. Amino-Group Modification—SPDP (Introduction of Protected Thiol Groups)

1. Transfer the antigen into 0.1 *M* phosphate buffer pH 8.0 (0.5–5 mg/mL, 0.5–1 mL volume) and add SPDP or MBS in a 2–50 times molar excess to the antigen. Incubate for 1 h at room temperature.
2. Separate the antigen from reaction products by dialysis or gel filtration, e.g., using prepacked desalting columns (PD-10 from Pharmacia and Upjohn or Econo-Pac 10DG from Bio-Rad) equilibrated with N_2-saturated 0.1 *M* phosphate buffer containing 0.1 *M* EDTA, pH 6.7. Collect fractions of 5–6 drops in an ELISA plate and pool the antigen-containing fractions (Micro-Bradford, *see* **Note 5**).
3. Quantify the amount of modified antigen, e.g., using the method of Bradford *(58)* and mix with activated ISCOM-matrix.

3.3.6. Amino-Group Modification—SPDP/DTT (Introduction Thiol Groups)

1. Transfer the antigen into 0.1 *M* phosphate buffer pH 8.0 (0.5–5 mg/mL, 0.5–1 mL volume) and add SPDP in a 2–50 times molar excess to the antigen. Incubate for 1 h at room temperature.
2. Add DTT to a final concentration of 10 m*M* and incubate for 30 min.
3. Separate the antigen from reaction products (SPDP/DTT) by dialysis or gel filtration, e.g., using prepacked desalting columns (PD-10 from Pharmacia and Upjohn or Econo-Pac 10DG from Bio-Rad) equilibrated with N_2-saturated 0.1 *M* phosphate buffer containing 0.1 *M* EDTA, pH 6.7. Collect fractions of 5–6 drops in an ELISA plate and pool the antigen-containing fractions (Micro-Bradford, *see* **Note 5**).
4. Quantify the amount of modified antigen, e.g., using the method of Bradford *(58)* and mix with activated ISCOM-matrix.

3.3.7. Amino-Group Modification—MBS (Introduction of Thiol-Binding Maleimide Groups)

1. Transfer the antigen into 0.1 *M* phosphate buffer pH 8.0 (0.5–5 mg/mL, 0.5–1 mL volume) and add MBS in a 2–50 times molar excess to the antigen. Incubate for 1 h at room temperature.
2. Separate the antigen from reaction products by dialysis or gel filtration, e.g., using prepacked desalting columns (PD-10 from Pharmacia and Upjohn or Econo-Pac 10DG from Bio-Rad) equilibrated with N_2-saturated 0.1 *M* phosphate buffer containing 0.1 *M* EDTA, pH 6.7. Collect fractions of 5–6 drops in an ELISA plate and pool the antigen-containing fractions (Micro-Bradford, *see* **Note 5**).

3. Quantify the amount of modified antigen, e.g., using the method of Bradford *(58)* and mix with activated ISCOM-matrix.

3.3.8. Carbohydrate Modification

1. Dissolve the glycoprotein in 0.1 *M* NaAc, pH 5.5 (antigen conc. 0.5–5 mg/mL).
2. Oxidize carbohydrates by addition of $NaIO_4$ from a fresh 100 m*M* solution of $NaIO_4$ in distilled water (keep out of light); sialic acid moieties, 1–10 m*M* $NaIO_4$, 0°C (on ice), 20 min; other carbohydrates, 1–10 m*M* $NaIO_4$, 0–20°C, 20 min.
3. Stop the reaction by addition of glycerol (approx 1.5 times molar excess to $NaIO_4$), incubate 5 min on ice (dark).
4. Remove reaction products by overnight dialysis or gel filtration, e.g., using prepacked desalting columns (PD-10 from Pharmacia and Upjohn or Econo-Pac 10DG from Bio-Rad) equilibrated with 0.1 *M* NaAc, pH 5.5. Try to keep the temperature used for the $NaIO_4$ oxidation during separation on the column (keep the main part of the column out of light). Collect fractions of 5–6 drops in an ELISA plate and pool the antigen containing fractions.
5. Make a 20 m*M* stock solution of PDPH or MPBH in DMSO and add to the oxidized protein at a final concentration 5 m*M*. Agitate slowly for 2 h, 20°C. Keep out of light.
6. Separate the antigen from reaction products by dialysis or gel filtration, e.g., using prepacked desalting columns (PD-10 from Pharmacia and Upjohn or Econo-Pac 10DG from Bio-Rad) equilibrated with N_2-saturated 0.1 *M* phosphate buffer containing 0.1 *M* EDTA, pH 6.7. Collect fractions of 5–6 drops in an ELISA plate and pool the antigen-containing fractions (Micro-Bradford, *see* **Note 5**).
7. Quantify the amount of modified antigen, e.g., using the method of Bradford *(58)* and mix with activated ISCOM-matrix.

3.4. Preparation of ISCOMs (Antigen Lipidation Techniques)

Hydrophilic antigens that need introduction of an hydrophobic moiety in order to incorporate into ISCOMs can be readily lipidated (attachment of a lipid tail) at ε-amino groups (in principle lysine side chains) using, e.g., hydroxysuccinimide esters of fatty acids or at carboxy groups (aspartic and glutamic acid residues) using carbodiimide and aminogroup containing lipids. Alternatively thiol-binding lipids can be attached to naturally occurring thiols (cystein) or at chemically introduced thiols. Reagent for antigen lipidation are listed in **Table 1**.

3.4.1. Amino-Group Lipidation

1. Dissolve or transfer the antigen in 0.1 *M* $NaCO_3$, pH 9.6 (1 mg/mL). Add sodium deoxycholate (from a 1–10% stock solution in 0.1 *M* $NaCO_3$, pH 9.6) to a final concentration of 0.1% and increase the temperature to 37°C.
2. Make a 10 mg/mL stock solution of N-hydroxypalmitic acid succinimide ester (NPS) or N-hydroxyoleic acid succinimide ester (NOS) in DMSO at 37°C.

3. Add NPS or NOS (from a fresh stock solution) in a 20–40 times molar excess to the antigen and mix thoroughly.
4. Incubate at 37°C overnight.
5. Add cholesterol, PC, and Quillaja saponin according to **Table 4**, and proceed with ISCOM formation as described under **Subheading 3.2.** To remove sodium deoxycholate, the dialysis should be initiated against a buffer with pH >8.0 (e.g., 0.1 *M* phosphate pH 8.5), then proceed to dialysis against PBS.

3.4.2. Carboxyl Acid Lipidation

1. Make a stock solution of the antigen (2–10 mg/mL) in distilled water or in MES (2-morpholinoethanesulphonic acid) pH 4.5–5.0.
2. Add 0.5 mg of solid S-NHS into a glass tube.
3. Add 1 mg of antigen and 1–2 mg of PE (both 37°C) to the solid S-NHS.
4. Adjust the volume to 1 mL with MES-buffer or water containing a final concentration of 15% (v/v) of DMF (or DMSO) and mix thoroughly.
5. Add 10 mg solid EDC into a small glass container fitted with a magnetic bar. Transfer the mixture of antigen, PE, and S-NHS to the solid EDC.
6. Mix and incubate for 2 h at 20–25°C on a magnetic stirrer.
7. Add cholesterol and Quillaja saponin according to **Table 4**, but NB omit the addition of phosphoplipid, and proceed with ISCOM formation as described in **Subheading 3.2.**

3.4.3. Thiol Group Lipidation

1. A thiolated antigen (*see* **Subheadings 3.3.1.** and **3.3.6.**) or a cystein containing antigen is dissolved in or transferred to 0.1 *M* phosphate buffer pH 8. Add DTT to a final concentration of 10 m*M* and incubate for 20–60 min at 4–20°C.
2. Remove reaction products by overnight (+4°C) dialysis against 10% PBS in distilled water or by gel filtration, e.g., using prepacked desalting columns (PD-10 from Pharmacia and Upjohn or Econo-Pac 10DG from Bio-Rad) equilibrated with 10% PBS in distilled water.
3. Concentrate, e.g., by lyophilization and redissolve in one-tenth of initial volume or use a "speed-vac" centrifuge to reduce the volume to one-tenth of the initial volume.
4. Dissolve a thiol-binding lipid (TBL) (PDP-DPPE, MBP-DPPE, and MB-DPPE, *see* **Table 1**) in a small volume of chloroform. "Dry" onto the bottom of a glass tube under a stream of N_2. Stop the process when the liquid becomes a gel-like semisolid and add 20% MEGA-10 to make a final concentration of 5–10 mg TBL per mL. Add 1 mg of TBL per mg of antigen and incubate overnight (or more) at 20°C.
5. Add cholesterol, PC, and Quillaja saponin according to **Table 4**, and proceed with ISCOM formation as described by **Subheading 3.2.**

3.5. Quality Control and Biochemical Characterization

Whichever method is used for ISCOM preparation, the goal is the same; to prepare a highly immunogenic particle of low toxicity, efficiently presenting an antigen with native conformation. To achieve such an ISCOM, the rate of antigen incorporation and the final composition of the ISCOM must be determined. It is not conclusive just to study he preparation by electron microscopy because this technique does not distinguish between ISCOMs and ISCOM-matrix.

Most of the problems concerning ISCOMs arise from when antigens that incorporate poorly (or not at all) are used and the resulting preparation is tested in animals without the required analyses of the final product. In the literature, we see several examples of poor or toxic ISCOMs, most likely resulting from problems with insufficient antigen incorporation, i.e., ISCOMs with a very high ratio (up to 100-fold) of Quillaja saponin to antigen. However, by analyzing the final ISCOMs to establish the antigen to Quil-A ratio, also suboptimal ISCOM preparations can be safely tested in laboratory animals. Special attention must be given to preparations for use in mice. Mice, in general, are sensitive to saponins but there is a great strain variation. Also, the mode of administration to mice plays a decisive role. Intravenous (iv) and intraperitoneal (ip) routes of administration should preferably be avoided, if used however, the dose of ISCOMs should be reduced to about 10% of that suitable for use sc or im, i.e., a maximum of 0.1–0.5 μg (antigen) or a dose of ISCOMs containing <1 μg of Quil-A. The increased toxicity of iv and ip administration is most likely related to the highly efficient and fast uptake of ISCOMs. In a dose response study of ISCOMs, about a 10-fold lower dose was required by the ip route compared to the sc route of administration to generate the same magnitude of response (Lövgren Bengtsson, unpublished).

4. Notes

1. For efficient removal of detergent (e.g., MEGA-10) the surface area vs the volume of dialysate should be as large as possible. In practice, we use a maximum volume of 3 mL in a 4–8-cm-long tube (9-mm wide). For larger volumes, divide the preparation into several tubings.
2. The preparation of detergent solubilized antigens is not within the scope of this chapter. It is however, of most importance to ensure that the antigens are soluble in the detergent used for solubilization. A common reason for failure to incorporate antigens into ISCOMs is that the antigens are not sufficiently solubilized as monomer, but rather in the form of small aggregates or protein micelles. Such preparations may very well be clear and free from opalescence.

   Preferably, the detergent is dialyzable and nonionic. It is possible to also use nondialyzable detergents for preparation of antigen if there is a substantial dilution factor of the detergent when the antigen is mixed with lipids and Quillaja saponins prior to dialysis. Nonionic detergents are usually less harmful to antigen conformation than ionic detergents.

   Also, nonionic detergent at concentrations exceeding 0.5–1% may be harmful for some antigens. Particularly conformational epitopes stabilized by hydrophobic interactions are vulnerable to small efficient detergents such MEGA-10, but often less sensitive to β-octyl-glucoside. We have found epitopes within the hemeagglutinin/neuraminidase antigen(s) on paramyxoviruses to be particularly sentisitive (unpublished observations), but also an antigen such as gp51 of bovine leukemia virus was sensitive to MEGA-10 ***(58)***.

Make sure that the detergent is removed, because ionic detergent may be irritant and toxic to laboratory animals.

3. For rapid detection and quantification of ISCOM-matrix, it is very helpful to include a small amount of radio-labeled cholesterol in the ISCOM-matrix. An alternative is to run a colorimetric assay for cholesterol, e.g., the "TC Cholesterol" assay from Boheringer Mannheim (Germany). A less sensitive, but rapid, method is to assay for the light-scattering effect of the ISCOM-matrix by reading the optical density at 310 nm.
4. The amount of antigen possible to conjugate preformed ISCOM-matrix varies from antigen to antigen depending on its size, degree of modification, and so on. A final composition of 1 mg of antigen bound per mg of cholesterol can serve as a goal and depending on several factors, a two- to three-fold excess of antigen may be required.
5. For detection of antigen in fractions eluted into a microtiter plate from, e.g., gel filtration, we take 5–10 μL from each fraction using a multichannel pipet into a new microtiter plate and add 50–200 μL of Bradford reagent ***(59)***. The protein-containing fractions are pooled after reading the optical density at 595 nm and the pool is further analyzed according to the method of Bradford ***(58)*** or any other suitable method for protein quantification.
6. Using, e.g., negative staining electron microscopy, the typical cage-like structure of ISCOMs and ISCOM-matrix can be verified. A sample of ISCOM or ISCOM-matrix is applied to carbon-coated grids and dialyzed against drops of 0.1 *M* phosphate buffer pH 7.2 or 0.1 *M* ammonium acetate, pH 6.8 prior to contrasting by 2% (w/v) ammonium molybdate ***(60)***.
7. For characterization of ISCOMs and ISCOM-matrix, a sample from each preparation is analyzed by analytical 10–50% (w/w) sucrose density gradient centrifugation (18 h at 200,000*g*, 10°C). The sucrose gradients are fractionated into 17 fractions, which are analyzed for protein (ISCOMs) content and for ^{3}H-cholesterol (if included) using a scintillator.

Acknowledgments

Many thanks to Jill Ekström, Katarina Ranlund, and Lena Sandberg for critical reading and expert technical suggestions. The main financial contributors to the work content of this chapter have been: The Swedish Board for Technical Development, Swedish Research Council for Engineering Sciences, The Swedish Council for Forestry and Agricultural Research, EEC, and Iscotec AB.

References

1. Morein, B., Lövgren Bengtsson, K., and Cox, J. (1996) Modern adjuvants. Functional aspects, in *Concepts in Vaccine Development* (Kaufmann, H. E., ed.), Walter de Gruyter, Berlin.

2. Morein, B., Sundquist, B., Höglund, S., Dalsgaard, K., and Osterhaus, A. (1984) ISCOM, a novel structure for antigenic presentation of membrane proteins from enveloped viruses. *Nature* **308,** 457–460.
3. Dalsgaard, K. (1978) A study on the isolation and characterisation of the saponin Quil A. Evaluation of its adjuvant activity with special reference to the application in foot-and-mouth disease. *Acta Vet. Scand.* (suppl), **69,** 1–40.
4. Lucy, J. A. and Glauert, A. M. (1964) Structure and assembly of macromolecular lipid complexes composed of globular micelles. *J. Mol. Biol.* **8,** 727–748.
5. Kersten, G. F. A., Spiekstra, A., Beuvery, E. C., and Crommelin, D. J. A. (1991) On the structure of immune-stimulating saponin-lipid complexes (ISCOMs). **BBA 1062,** 165–171.
6. Özel, M., Höglund, S., Gelderblom, H., and Morein, B. (1989) Quarternary structure of the immunostimulating complex (ISCOM). *J. Ultrastruct. Molec. Struct. Res.* **102,** 240–248.
7. Lövgren, K. and Morein, B. (1988) The requirement of lipids for the formation of immunostimulating complexes (ISCOMs). *Biotechnol. Appl. Biochem.* **10,** 161–172.
8. Lövgren, K., Lindmark, J., Pipkorn, R., and Morein, B. (1987) Antigenic presentation of small molecules and synthetic peptides conjugated to a preformed ISCOM as carrier. *J. Immunol. Meth.* **98,** 137–143.
9. Barr, I. G. and Mitchell, G. F. (1996) ISCOMs (immunostimulating complexes): the first decade. *Immunol. Cell. Biol.* **74,** 8–25.
10. Morein, B., Lövgren, K., Rönnberg, B., Sjölander, A., and Villacrés-Eriksson, M. (1995) Immunostimulating complexes. Clinical potential in vaccine development. *Clin. Immunother. Adis International Ltd.* **3,** 409–487.
11. Rimmelzwaan, G. F. and Osterhaus, A. D. (1995). A novel generation of viral vaccines based on the ISCOM matrix. *Pharm. Biotechnol.* **6,** 543–558.
12. Lövgren Bengtsson, K., and Sjölander, A. (1996) Adjuvant activities of ISCOMs and ISCOM matrix; two different formulations of Quillaja saponin and antigen. *Vaccine* **14,** 753–760.
13. Sjölander, A., Lövgren Bengtsson, K., and Morein, B. (1997) Kinetics, localization and cytokine profile of T cell responses to immune stimulating complexes (ISCOMs) containing human influenza virus envelope glycoproteins. *Vaccine* **15,** 1030–1038.
14. Bergström-Mollauglu, M., Lövgren, K., Åkerblom, L., Fossum, C., and Morein B. (1992) Antigen-specific increases in the number of spleenocytes expressing MHC Class II molecules following restimulation with antigen in various physical forms. *Scand J. Immunol.* **36,** 565–574.
15. Watson, D., Watson, N., Fossum, C., Lövgren, K., and Morein, B. (1992) Interactions between immune-stimulating complexes (ISCOMS) and peritoneal mononuclear Leucocytes. *Microbiol. Immunol.* **36,** 199–203.
16. Sjölander, A., van't Land, B., and Lövgren Bengtsson, K. (1997) ISCOMs containing purified Quillaja saponins upregulate both Th1-like and Th2-like immune responses. *Cell. Immunol.* **177,** 69–76.

17. Johansson, M. H. S. and Lövgren-Bengtsson, K. (1999) ISCOMs with different Quillaja saponin components differ in their immunomodulating activities. *Vaccine* **17,** 2894–2900.
18. Sundquist, B., Lövgren, K., and Morein, B. (1988) Influenza virus ISCOMs: antibody response in animals. *Vaccine* **6,** 49–52.
19. Lövgren, K. (1988) The serum antibody responses distributed in subclasses and isotypes following intranasal and subcutaneous immunization with influenza virus ISCOMs. *Scand. J. Immunol.* **27,** 241–245.
20. Mumford, J. A., Jesset, D., Dunleavy, U., Wood, J., Hannant, D., Sundquist, B., et al. (1994) Antigenicity and immunogenicity of experimental equine influenza ISCOM vaccines. *Vaccine* **12,** 857–863.
21. Mumford, J. A., Jesset, D., Rollinson, E. A., Hannant, D., and Draper, M. E. (1994) Duration of protective efficacy of equine influenza immunostimulating complex/tetanus vaccines. *Vet. Rec.*, **February 12,** 158–162.
22. Hannant, D., Jessett, D. M., O'Neill, T., Dolby, C. A., Cook, R. F., and Mumford, J. A. (1993) Responses of ponies to equine herpes virus-1 ISCOM vaccination and challenge with virus of the homologous strain. *Res. Vet. Sci.* **54,** 299–305.
23. Villacrés-Eriksson, M., Bergström-Mollauglu, M., Kåberg, H., and Morein, B. (1992) Involvement of interleukin-2 and interferon-gamma in the immune response induced by influenza virus ISCOMs. *Scand. J. Immunol.* **36,** 421–426.
24. Sjölander, A., Lövgren Bengtsson, K., Johansson, M., and Morein, B. (1996) Kinetics, localization and isotype profile of antibody responses to immune stimulating complexes (ISCOMs) containing human influenza virus envelope glycoproteins. *Scand. J. Immunol.* **43,** 164–172.
25. Villacrés-Eriksson, M., Bergström-Mollauglu, M., Kåberg, H., Lövgren, K., and Morein B. (1993) The induction of cell-associated and secreted interleukin-1 by ISCOMs, matrix or micelles in murine spleenic cells. *Clin. Exp. Immunol.* **93,** 120–125.
26. Villacres-Eriksson, M. (1995) Antigen presentation by naive macrophages, dendritic cells and B cells to primed T lymphocytes and their cytokine production following exposure to immunostimulating complexes. *Clin. Exp. Immunol.* **102,** 46–52.
27. Valensi, J. P., Carlsson, J. R., and Van Nest, G. A. (1994) Systemic cytokine profiles in BALB/c mice immunized with trivalent influenza vaccine containing MF59 oil emulsion and other adjuvants. *J. Immunol.* **153,** 4029–4039.
28. Behboudi, S., Morein, B., and Villacres-Eriksson, M. (1997) In vivo and in vitro induction of IL-6 by Quillaja saponaria molina triterpenoid formulations. *Cytokine* **9,** 682–687.
29. Villacres-Eriksson, M., Behboudi, S., Morgan, A. J., Trichieri, G., and Morein, B. (1997) Immunomodulation by Quillaja saponaria adjuvant formulations: In vivo stimulation of interleukin 12 and its effects on the antibody response. *Cytokine* **9,** 78–82.
30. Fossum, C., Bergström, M., Lövgren, K., Watson, D. L., and Morein, B. (1990) Effect of ISCOM and/or their adjuvant moiety (matrix) on the initial proliferative

and il-2 responses in vitro. Comparison of spleen cells from mice inoculated with ISCOMs and/or matrix. *Cell. Immunol.* **129,** 414–425.

31. Jones, P. D., Tha Hla, R., Morein B., Lövgren, K., and Ada, G. L. (1988) Cellular immune responses in the murine lung to local immunization with influenza A virus glycoproteins in micelles and immunostimulating complexes (ISCOMs). *Scand. J. Immunol.* **27,** 645–652.
32. Takahashi, H., Takeshita, T., Morein, B., Putney, S., Germain, R. N., and Berzofsky, J. (1990) Induction of CD8+ cytotoxic T cells by immunization with purified HIV-1 envelope proteins in ISCOMs. *Nature* **344,** 873–875.
33. Heeney, J. L., Teeuwsen, V. J., van Gils, M., Bogers, W. M., De Giuli Morghen, C., Radaelli, A., et al. (1998) beta-chemokines and neutralizing antibody titers correlate with sterilizing immunity generated in HIV-1 vaccinated macaques. *Proc. Natl. Acad. Sci.* **95,** 10,803–10,808.
34. Mowat, A. M., Donachie, A. M., Reid, G., and Jarret, O. (1991) Immune-stimulating complexes containing Quil A and protein antigen prime class 1 MHC-restricted T lymphocytes in vivo and are immunogenic by the oral route. *Immunology* **72,** 317–322.
35. Hu, K. F., Elvander, M., Merza, M., Akerblom, L., Brandenburg, A., and Morein, B. (1998) The immunostimulating complex (ISCOM) is an efficient mucosal delivery system for respiratory syncytial virus (RSV) envelope antigens inducing high local and systemic antibody responses. *Clin. Exp. Immunol.* **113,** 235–243.
36. Ekström, L., Hu, K.-F., Lövgren-Bengtsson, K., and Morein, B. (1999) ISCOM and ISCOM-matrix enhance by intranasal route the IgA responses to OVA and rCTB in local and remote mucosal secretions. *Vaccine* **17,** 2690–2701.
37. Dalsgaard, K., Hilgers, L., and Trouvé, G. (1990) Classical and new approaches to adjuvant use in domestic animals, in *Immunomodulation in Domestic Food Animals. Adv. Vet. Sci. Comp. Med.,* vol. 35 (Blecha, F. and Charley, B., eds.), Academic, San Diego, CA, pp. 121–160.
38. Cox, J., Coulter, A., Macfarlane, R., Beezum, L., Bates, J., Wong, T-Y., and Drane, D. (1997) Development of an influenza-ISCOM™ vaccine, in *Vaccine Design: The Role of Cytokine Networks* (Gregoriadis et al., eds.), Plenum, New York.
39. Rönnberg, B., Fekadu, M., and Morein, B. (1995) Adjuvant activity of non-toxic *Quillaja Saponaria Molina* components for use in ISCOM-matrix. *Vaccine* **13,** 1375–1382.
40. Cox, J. and Coulter, A. (1997) Adjuvants—a classification and review of their mode of action. *Vaccine* **15,** 248–256.
41. Lundén, A., Parmely, S. F., Lövgren Bengtsson, K., and Araujo, F. G. (1997) Use of recombinant antigen (SAG2) expressed as a glutathione-S-transferase fusion protein to immunize mice against Toxoplasma gondii. *Parasitol. Res.* **83,** 6–9.
42. Sjölander, S., Hansen, J.-E., Lövgren Bengtsson, K., Åkerblom, L., and Morein, B. (1996) Induction of homologous virus neutralizing antibodies in guinea-pigs immunized with two human immunodeficiency virus type 1 glycoprotein gp120-ISCOM preparations. A comparison with other adjuvant systems. *Vaccine* **14,** 344–352.

43. Bomford, R. (1980a) The comparative selectivity of adjuvants for humoral and cell mediated immunity. I. Effect on the antibody response to bovine serum albumin and sheep red blood cells of Freund's incomplete and complete adjuvants, allhydrogel, *Corynebacterium parvum, Bordetella pertussis,* muramyldipeptide and saponin. *Clin. Exp. Immunol.* **39,** 426–434.
44. Bomford, R. (1980b) The comparative selectivity of adjuvants for humoral and cell mediated immunity. II. Effect on delayed-type hypersensitivity in the mouse and guinea pigs, and cell-mediated immunity to tumour antigens in the mouse of Freund's incomplete and complete adjuvants, allhydrogel, Corynebacterium parvum. Bordetella pertussis, muramyldipeptide and saponin. *Clin. Exp. Immunol.* **39,** 435–441.
45. Bomford, R. (1984) Relative adjuvant efficacy of Al(OH)3 and Saponin is related to the immunogenicity of the antigen. *Int. Archs. Allergy Appl. Immun.* **75,** 280–281.
46. Jones, G. E., Jones, K. A., Machell, J., Brebner, J., Anderson, I. E., and How, S. (1995) Efficacy trials with tissue-culture grown, inactivated vaccines against chlamydial abortion in sheep. *Vaccine* **13,** 715–723.
47. Snodgrass, D. R., Campbell, I., Mwenda, J. M., Chege, G., Seleman, M.A-, Morein, B., and Hart, C. A. (1995) Stimulation of rotavirus IgA, IgG and neutralising antibodies in baboon milk by parenteral vaccination. *Vaccine* **13,** 408–413.
48. Lövgren, K. and Sundquist, B. (1994) Comparison of four different adjuvant formulations with two types of antigens; influenza virus protein micelles and ovalbumin. IBC Conf. on Novel Vaccine Strategies, Washington, Feb. 23–25.
49. Browning, M., Reid, G. R., Osborne, R., and Jarret, O. (1992) Incorporation of soluble antigens into ISCOMs: HIV gp120 ISCOMs induce virus neutralizing antibodies. *Vaccine* **10,** 585–590.
50. Reid, G. (1992) Soluble proteins incorporate into ISCOMs after covalent attachment of fatty acid. *Vaccine* **10,** 597–602.
51. Scheepers, K. and Becht, H. (1994) Protection of mice against an influenza virus infection by oral vaccination with viral nucleoprotein incorporated into immunostimulating complexes. *Med. Microbiol. Immunol.* **183,** 265–278.
52. Wilson A. D., Lövgren-Bengtsson K., Villacres-Ericsson M., Morein B, and Morgan A. J. (1999) The major Epstein-Barr virus (EBV) envelope glycoprotein gp340 when incorporated into ISCOMs primes cytotoxic T-cell responses directed against EBV lymphoblastoid cell lines. *Vaccine* **17,** 1282–1290.
53. Morein, B., Ekström, J., and Lövgren, K. (1990) Increased immunogenicity of a non-amphipathic protein (BSA) after inclusion into ISCOMs. *J. Immunol. Meth.* **128,** 177–181.
54. Bomford, R., Stapleton, M., Winsor, S., Beesley, J. E., Jessup, E. A., Price, K. R., and Fenwick, G. R. (1992) Adjuvanticity and ISCOM formation by structurally diverse saponins. *Vaccine* **10,** 572–577.
55. Phillips, N. C., Gagné, L., Ivanoff, N., and Riveau, G. (1996) Influence of phospholipid composition on antibody response to liposome encapsulated protein and peptide. *Vaccine* **14,** 898–904.

56. Calder, P. C. (1993) The effects of fatty acids on lymphocyte functions. *Braz. J. Biol. Res.* **26,** 901–917.
57. Calder, P. C. (1998) Fat chance of immunomodulation. *Immunol. Today* **19,** 244–247.
58. Merza, M., Linné, T., Höglund, S., Portetelle, D., Burny, A., and Morein, B. (1989) Bovine leukemia virus ISCOMs: biochemical characterization. *Vaccine* **7,** 22–28.
59. Bradford, M. M. (1976) A rapid and sensitive method for the quantitation of microgram quantities of protein utilising the principle of protein-dye-binding. *Anal. Biochem.* **72,** 248.
60. Sundquist, B., Lövgren, K., Höglund, S., and Morein, B. (1988) Influenza virus ISCOMs: biochemical characterization. *Vaccine* **6,** 44–58.

15

QS-21 Adjuvant

Charlotte Read Kensil

1. Introduction

1.1. Source

QS-21 is an immunological adjuvant derived from a natural source: the bark of the South American tree *Quillaja saponaria* Molina. Crude extracts of *Quillaja saponaria* bark were found to have adjuvant activity in foot-and-mouth disease vaccines in cattle *(1)*. These extracts consisted of a complex mixture of tannins, polyphenolics, and triterpene glycoside "saponins." The adjuvant activity was determined to be in the saponin fraction *(2)*. This was later fractionated by high-performance liquid chromatography (HPLC) into at least 23 different triterpene glycoside saponins with a varying range of biological activity for adjuvanticity, surfactant properties, and toxicity *(3)*. QS-21 was identified as a saponin with potent adjuvant activity and low toxicity *(3)*. It can be purified to near homogenity via preparative HPLC. The high level of purity and standardization of the QS-21 saponin adjuvant has enabled evaluation of this compound in clinical trials of experimental vaccines.

1.2. General Adjuvant Properties

QS-21 stimulates strong antibody- and cell-mediated responses in animals. QS-21 has been shown to stimulate strong antibody responses to T-dependent protein antigens in mice *(3–5)*, guinea pigs *(6)*, rhesus monkeys *(7)*, and baboons *(8)*. Antibody responses induced by QS-21-adjuvanted vaccines were shown to be higher than antibody responses with aluminum hydroxide-adjuvanted vaccines and were similar to those obtained with Freund's complete-adjuvanted (FCA) vaccines *(3,6)*. QS-21 is also a strong adjuvant for

From: *Methods in Molecular Medicine, Vol. 42:*
Vaccine Adjuvants: Preparation Methods and Research Protocols
Edited by: D. T. O'Hagan © Humana Press, Inc., Totowa, NJ

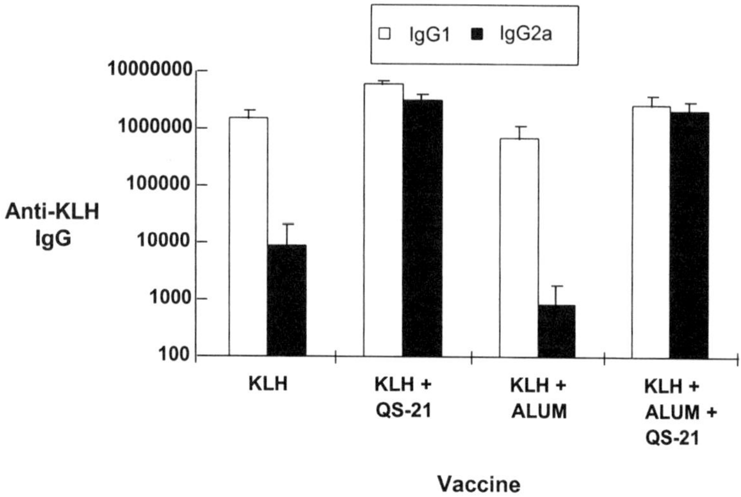

Fig. 1. Influence of QS-21 on mouse IgG subclasses. Balb/c mice (five per group) were immunized with KLH (2.5 μg) without adjuvant, with 20 μg QS-21, 2.5 μg aluminum hydroxide or the combination of QS-21/aluminum hydroxide. Vaccines were given by sc route on days 0, 14, and 28. Sera was collected at day 42 for analysis of anti-KLH IgG_1 or IgG_2a by EIA.

murine antibody responses to T-independent polysaccharide antigens, such as *Escherichia coli* polysaccharide ***(9)***. More recently, a QS-21 adjuvant effect on serum immunoglobulin G (IgG) responses was shown with an HIV (*env*) DNA vaccine administered by intramuscular (im) or intranasal (in) route ***(10)***.

QS-21 has been shown to influence murine IgG subclass response by enhancing levels of IgG_2a ***(3–5,9)*** to protein and polysaccharide antigens. **Figure 1** shows an example of the adjuvant effect of QS-21 on IgG_1 and IgG_2a antibodies with a protein antigen vaccine. Keyhole limpet hemocyanin (KLH) vaccines in three adjuvant formulations (QS-21/PBS, aluminum hydroxide, and QS-21/aluminum hydroxide) or in saline were given by subcutaneous (sc) route to Balb/c mice three times at 2-wk intervals, followed by measurement of KLH-specific IgG subclasses in serum. IgG_1 titers induced by the vaccines were generally similar between formulations, however, IgG_2a titers were significantly enhanced by the addition of QS-21, both in the presence and absence of aluminum hydroxide (which induced the lowest IgG_2a titers when used alone).

QS-21 also enables the induction of murine antigen-specific $CD8^+$ cytotoxic T lymphocytes (CTL) to exogenous antigens, such as ovalbumin ***(11)*** and respiratory syncytial virus fusion protein ***(5)***. This response is higher than that evoked by FCA and is associated with enhanced production of interleukin 2 (IL-2) and interferon-γ (IFN-γ) by antigen-stimulated splenocytes ***(12)***. A sys-

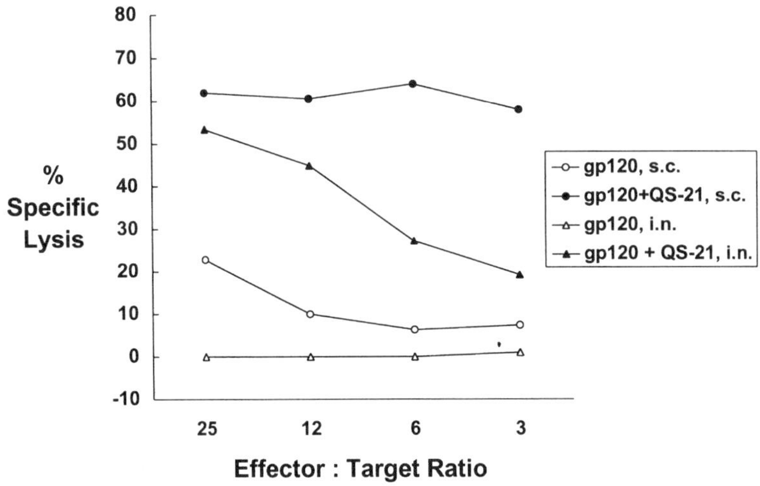

Fig. 2. QS-21 enhancement of CTL response to a subunit vaccine. Balb/c mice were immunized with purified recombinant HIV-1_{IIIB} gp120 *(23)* with and without 10 μg QS-21 by either sc or in routes on days 0, 14, and 28. Splenocytes were collected at day 42 and were stimulated by incubation with peptide 18 *(24)* in RPMI-1640 medium for 6 d prior to assay on ^{51}Cr-loaded p18-coated P815 target cells. The data shown were background-subtracted for lysis of P815 cells.

temic CTL response to QS-21-containing vaccines can be induced by both parenteral and mucosal immunization routes. **Figure 2** shows the CTL response to r-gp120 [from human immunodeficiency virus type 1 (HIV-1) IIIB strain, produced in insect cells] administered sc and in using antigen restimulated splenocytes from immunized animals. QS-21 induced a substantial increase in CTL by both routes.

The safety and adjuvant effect of QS-21 has been evaluated in completed and ongoing human clinical trials of various antigens. A dose of 100 μg of QS-21 was used without significant toxicity and was shown to significantly improve the responder rate and median IgG titer to the tumor antigen GM2 in response to a GM2-KLH vaccine *(13)* in comparison to nonadjuvanted vaccine or vaccine adjuvanted with Detox adjuvant (**Fig. 3**). Immune responses to QS-21 itself were measured by EIA and were not observed in this trial *(14)*. QS-21 was also used together with maximum permissable level (MPL) and an oil-in-water (o/w) emulsion in an adjuvant system known as SBAS2 in a Phase I trial of a malaria vaccine that consisted of a recombinant circumsporozoite antigen. This antigen in SBAS2 was shown to protect six out of seven individuals against challenge whereas o/w and MPL/aluminum hydroxide were not protective *(15)*. At present, more than 1600 volunteers have received QS-21 in completed or ongoing trials of 29 different vaccines.

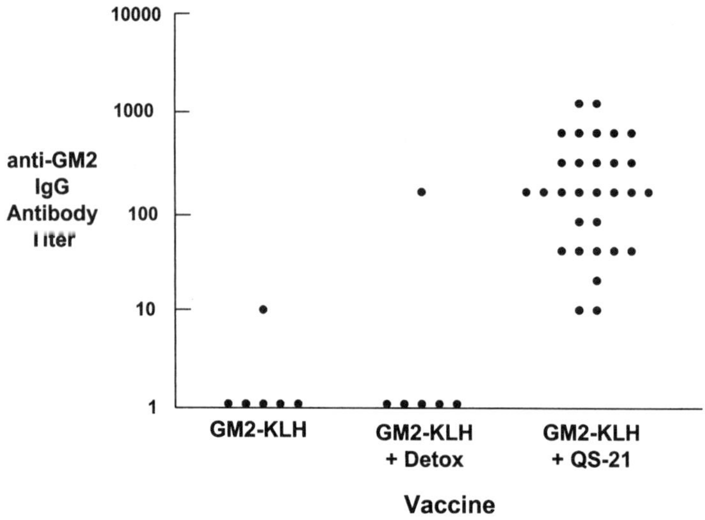

Fig. 3. Serological response to GM2-KLH/QS-21 in melanoma patients. Melanoma patients (AJCC Stage III or IV, disease-free after surgery) were immunized with GM2-KLH without adjuvant, with Detox adjuvant, and with QS-21 (100 µg). Anti-GM2-IgG titers shown are the peak titers postimmunization. Data is from Table 1 of **ref. *13***.

1.3. General Structure and Physicochemical Properties

QS-21 was shown by ^{1}H and ^{13}C-NMR and fast-atom bombardment-mass spectrometry to be an acylated 3,28-o-bisdesmodic triterpene saponin of molecular weight 1990 ***(16)***. The structure of QS-21 is shown in **Fig. 4**.

QS-21 is anionic at neutral pH, because of the carboxyl group on glucuronic acid. It is insoluble in aqueous solution in the protonated form, but soluble in the sodium salt form where QS-21 forms micelles in solution. The critical micellar concentration of QS-21 was estimated to be 26 µ*M* in phosphate-buffered saline (PBS) at pH 7.0 ***(17)***. However, micelle formation is not required for adjuvant activity as significant adjuvant effect has been observed at QS-21 concentrations below the critical micellar concentration ***(17)***. Although QS-21 may associate with hydrophobic antigens or hydrophobic sites of amphipathic antigens, this association is not required for adjuvant effect. QS-21 induces strong antibody and CTL responses to undenatured OVA despite lack of association. In addition, strong adjuvant effect is still observed if QS-21 is given up to 24 hours in advance of the antigen at the same injection site (Aquila Biopharmaceuticals, Inc., Framingham, MA, unpublished data). QS-21 is typically utilized in aqueous antigen formulations as a simple mixture of buffered antigen and QS-21. Emulsification is not required for QS-21 adjuvanted

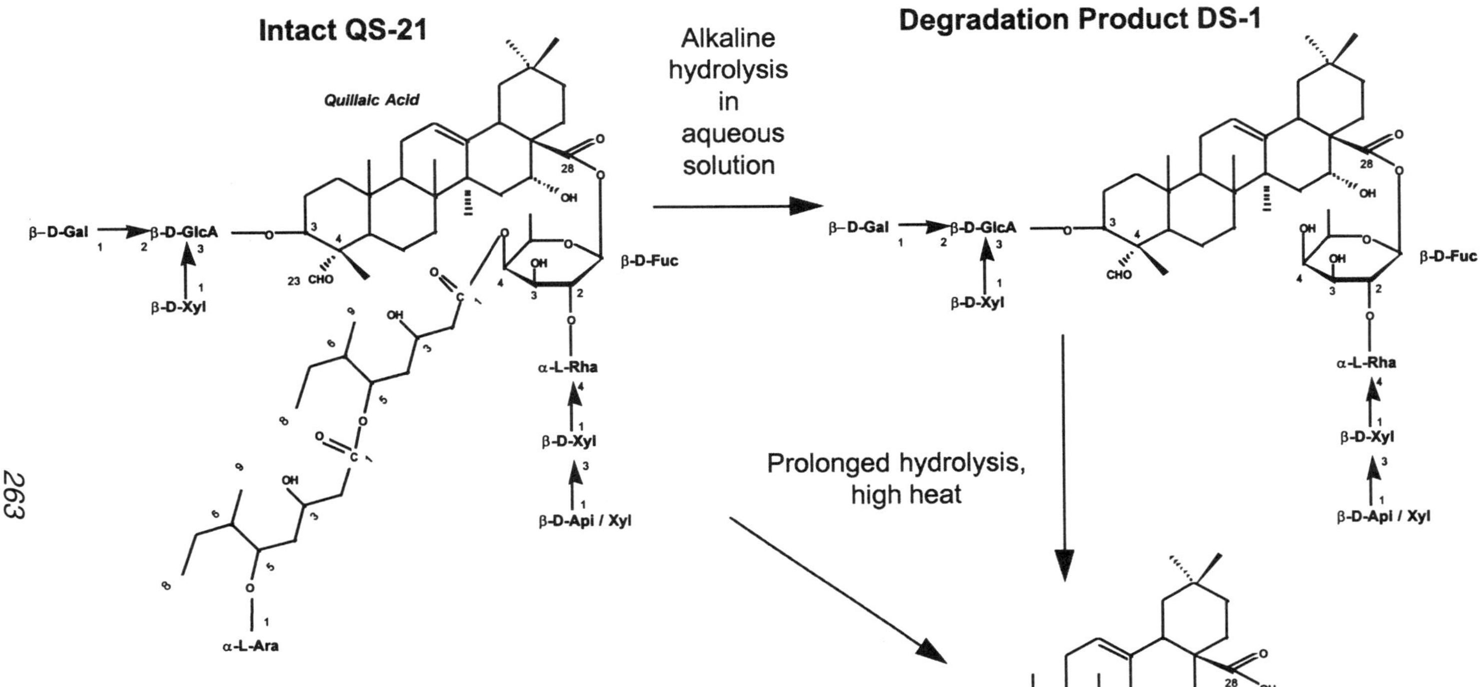

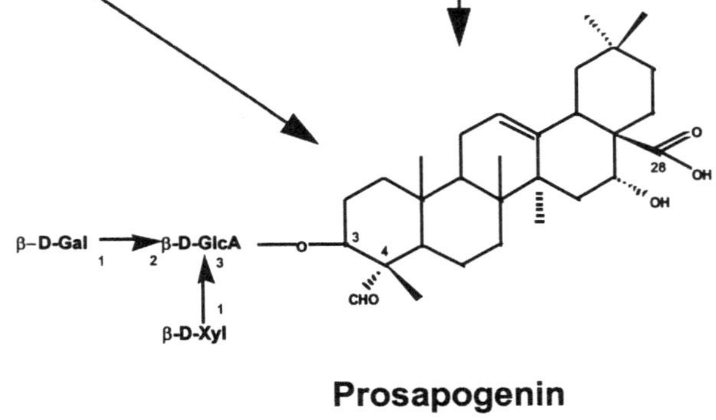

Fig. 4. QS-21 and aqueous degradation products. QS-21 consists of two equilibrium isomers formed by a reversible acyl shift from a predominant isomer QS-21a (acylated at the 4-hydroxyl on fucose) and a minor isomer QS-21b (acylated at the 3-hydroxyl on fucose). DS-1 is the primary degradation product occuring in aqueous solution during storage under refrigeration (2–8°C). The prosapogenin of QS-21 is observed only upon extended incubation at high heat.

vaccines although QS-21 has also been shown to be useful in emulsion-type formulations ***(15)***. Although QS-21 is typically used as the sole adjuvant in most experimental vaccines, QS-21 has also been shown to be useful in combination with aluminum hydroxide ***(17)***, combination with PLGA-encapsulated antigens ***(6)***, and with MPL/o/w ***(15)***.

2. Materials

2.1. QS-21

2.1.1. Pharmaceutical Properties and Storage

QS-21 is manufactured by Aquila Biopharmaceuticals, Inc., and is supplied as a lyophilized, odorless, white powder, which is stored at ≤–20°C until formulation (up to 3 yr postmanufacture). It is ≥98% pure by RP-HPLC, has ≤10 endotoxin units/mg QS-21, ≤10 colony-forming units (CFU)/mg QS-21, and ≤5% residual moisture.

2.1.2. Spectroscopic Identification

Positive ion fast-atom bombardment mass spectrometry can be employed for spectroscopic identification. The most frequently observed pseudomolecular ion peaks are 2012 $[M + Na]^+$, 2028 $[M + K]^+$, and 2034 $[M - H + 2Na]^+$ for a QS-21 sample dissolved in 5% acetic acid and analyzed in a matrix of metanitrobenzoic acid.

Natural abundance ^{13}C-NMR on QS-21 in deuterated dimethyl sulfoxide (DMSO) relative to tetramethylsilane may be utilized to confirm specific functional group carbons. These include the aldehyde carbon C-23 (209.6 ppm), the C-28 ester-bond carbon (175.1 ppm), the fatty-acid ester carbons (170.8, 170.9 ppm), the triterpene double-bond carbons C-13 (143.1 ppm), and C-12 (121.3 ppm), as well as carbons at the C-1 position in specific sugars that distinguish QS-21 from other saponins.

2.2. Formulation Reagents

1. Dulbecco's phosphate-buffered saline, without calcium or magnesium.
2. Saline for injection.
3. 0.1 *N* NaOH.
4. 0.2 µm Gelman Acrodisk filter.

2.3. Analytical Reagents for Quantitation

2.3.1. Quantitation of QS-21

1. QS-21 standard: 2 mg/mL in 30% acetonitrile/ 70% water v/v.
2. Water (HPLC grade).
3. Acetonitrile (HPLC grade).

4. Trifluoroacetic acid (TFA, HPLC grade).
5. Vydac C4 column (4.6 mm × 25 cm, 300 Å pore size, 5 μm).

2.3.2. Quantitation of Protein Antigen

1. BSA protein standard (Pierce Chemical, Rockford, IL).
2. Micro-BCA reagent (Pierce Chemical).

3. Methods

3.1. Preparation of QS-21 Stock Solution for Further Vaccine Formulation

3.1.1. Preparation of 1 mg/mL QS-21 Stock Solution in Buffered Saline

1. Accurately weigh QS-21. It may be necessary to use a static gun to aid in sample handling. Transfer quantitatively into a pyrogen-free container.
2. Add Dulbecco's phosphate-buffered saline, without calcium or magnesium, pH 7.2–7.5, to a final QS-21 concentration of 1 mg/mL.
3. Mix via magnetic stirrer until solution clarifies. Solution may be initially opaque, but should clarify.

3.1.2. Preparation of 1 mg/mL QS-21 Stock Solution in Unbuffered Saline

1. Accurately weigh QS-21. Transfer quantitatively into a pyrogen-free glass container.
2. Add saline (0.9% NaCl) to a final QS-21 concentration of 1 mg/mL to resuspend the QS-21. QS-21 will be insoluble because it is in the acid form.
3. Titrate with 0.1 *N* NaOH, added in increments. Use 5 μL of 0.1 *N* NaOH for each mg of QS-21. Monitor the pH to confirm that the pH does not exceed 7.4 to avoid alkaline hydrolysis (*see* **Note 3**). The purpose of this step is to solubilize the QS-21 by conversion into the sodium salt form.

3.1.3. Sterilization of QS-21 Stock Solution

1. Filter sterilize through a 0.2-μ membrane (Gelman acrodisk or equivalent). Although recoveries from a 1-mg/mL solution are expected to exceed 95%, it is recommended that the QS-21 concentration of the sterilized solution be quantitated by HPLC.
2. QS-21 solutions should not be autoclaved (*see* **Note 3**).

3.1.4. HPLC Quantitation of QS-21

1. Prepare a standard QS-21 stock solution for development of a standard curve on the HPLC. Dissolve QS-21 at 2 mg/mL (w/v) in 30% acetonitrile/70% water (v/v). This solution may be aliquotted into autosampler vials and stored at –40°C for 18 mo. It should be thoroughly thawed, mixed, and warmed to room temperature before use.

2. Obtain a Vydac C4 column, 5-μ particle size, 300 Å pore size (4.6 mm diameter × 25 cm length). Equilibrate the column in 30% acetonitrile/70% water/0.15% trifluoroacetic acid (v/v/v) on an HPLC system at a flow rate of 1.0 mL/min with ultraviolet (UV) monitoring at 214 nm.
3. Set up an HPLC autosampler to sample volumes equivalent to 0, 10, 30, 50, 70, 90, and 110 μg QS-21 from the 2 mg/mL stock solution. Each QS-21 amount should be assayed in triplicate.
4. Set up the HPLC to assay samples using a linear gradient of 30% acetonitrile/ 70%water/0.15% TFA to 45% acetonitrile/55% water/0.15% TFA over a 30-min period at a 1.0 mL/min flow rate.
5. There should be one main peak corresponding to QS-21a (see legend and structure in **Fig. 4**). Integrate the peak area and plot on the y-axis vs QS-21 amount in μg on the x-axis. Do a linear curve fit and determine the correlation value r for the curve because it should exceed 0.975.
6. Assay test sample in triplicate. Determine amount of QS-21 from the standard curve. In aqueous solution, QS-21 will consist of both QS-21a and QS-21b peaks (see legend and structure in **Fig. 4**). The total quantity of QS-21 is determined from the sum of QS-21a and QS-21b peaks (*see* **Note 1**).
7. Upon subsequent analyses, the QS-21 standard curve does not need to be repeated if an assay of 100 μg of the working standard yields the expected result (±10%). The standard curve should be redetermined at three-month intervals or upon failure of the working standard sample to meet specifications, whichever is earlier. The standard curve should also be redetermined after HPLC maintenance (such as lamp replacement) or replacement of the column.

3.2. Vaccine Formulation

3.2.1. Formulation with Antigen

3.2.1.1. Soluble Antigens

1. Mix the sterile stock solution of QS-21 with a sterile stock of soluble antigen with the dose of each adjusted to the optimum for the animal to be immunized. A typical effective QS-21 dose is 10–20 μg for mice, 25–50 μg for guinea pigs or rats, and 50–100 μg for rabbits, rhesus monkeys, and baboons. The volume of the vaccine is then adjusted to the final formulation volume (0.2 mL for mice, 0.5–1.0 mL for larger animals) with sterile saline or sterile-buffered saline. Although QS-21 is a relatively mild surfactant that is not expected to denature proteins, extensive studies on the effect of QS-21 on conformation-dependent epitopes have not been carried out. Therefore, assays for such epitopes should be considered.
2. The formulated vaccine should be visually inspected for clarity. Although the stock solution of QS-21 (at 1 mg/mL) may have an opalescent appearance upon prolonged storage, it should clarify upon dilution to the concentration typically used in vaccine formulations (50–200 μg/mL).

3. After the combination of QS-21 with a soluble antigen, the vaccine formulation may be sterilized by filtration. An HPLC confirmation of the QS-21 concentration in the filter-sterilized formulation is recommended.

3.2.1.2. Alum-Adsorbed Antigens

QS-21 may also be added to aluminum hydroxide-precipitated antigens. QS-21 is added to the aluminum-hydroxide precipitated antigen as a simple admixture.

1. Formulate the antigen/aluminum hydroxide according to a standard adsorption procedure. Use sterile technique and sterile components. Confirm the binding of antigen to the aluminum hydroxide through a protein assay on the supernatant.
2. Add sterile QS-21 to the aluminum hydroxide in the desired dose, using sterile technique. The same doses of QS-21 are recommended for soluble antigen vaccines and for alum-adsorbed vaccines.
3. Assay for protein binding. QS-21 will bind weakly to aluminum hydroxide under certain conditions (if present at greater than critical micellar concentrations) and may displace a weakly bound antigen from the alum, particularly if a minimum ratio of alum to protein is used (*see* **Note 5**).

3.2.2. Quantitation of Antigen, Adjuvant

3.2.2.1. Quantitation of Protein Antigen

The micro-BCA assay (Pierce Chemical) may be used according to product insert. QS-21, at concentrations up to 1 mg/mL, does not interfere in this assay.

3.2.2.2. Quantitation of QS-21 (HPLC Analysis)

This method is suitable for determination of QS-21 concentration in vaccines containing ≥100 μg/mL QS-21 in an aqueous buffer formulation at physiological pH. It can be used if antigen or buffer components do not coelute with QS-21 on the HPLC column.

1. Add 200 μL sample to 87 μL acetonitrile and 2.9 μL of 1 *N* acetic acid (final concentration: 30% acetonitrile, v/v and 10 m*M* acetic acid). Transfer to an autosampler vial.
2. Assay 150 μL via HPLC according to the assay described in **Subheading 3.1.4.**
3. Assay antigen and buffer controls.
4. The quantity of QS-21 can be determined from the standard curve. The total quantity of QS-21 is determined from the sum of QS-21a and QS-21b peaks (*see* **Note 1**).

4. Notes

1. Equilibrium Isomers: **Figure 4** shows the active solution forms and inactive degradation products of QS-21 occuring in aqueous solution. The two active

Table 1
Shelf-Life of QS-21 at 4°C

	Shelf-life (time to 10% degradation) at 4°C	
pH	50 µg/mL QS-21	500 µg/mL QS-21
6.0	680 d (23 mo)	3700 d (120 mo)[a]
7.0	90 d (3 mo)	750 d (25 mo)

[a]Estimate from 18-mo stabiity data.

isomeric solution forms of QS-21 in aqueous solution result from a reversible hydroxide-catalyzed acyl shift of the fatty acid from the four-position of fucose (predominant isomer QS-21a) to the three-position of fucose (minor isomer QS-21b). These equilibrium isomers can be distinguished by nuclear magnetic resonance (NMR) ***(13)*** and by RP-HPLC ***(15)***. Both isomers are active as adjuvants in animals ***(18)***. The powder form of QS-21 is entirely QS-21a. QS-21b appears after formulation into aqueous solution. It can be detected as an HPLC peak with a relative retention time (rrt) to QS-21a of 0.90–0.91 (where rrt = k' QS-21b/k' QS-21a) when analyzed by the HPLC method described in **Subheading 3.1.4.** For determination of total QS-21 amount in aqueous solution, the HPLC peaks corresponding to QS-21a and QS-21b are summed.

2. Degradation Products: QS-21 contains three ester bonds. The ester bond between the fatty-acid domain and the 4-hydroxyl of fucose is the most labile bond in the molecule and is the critical factor that determines stability in aqueous solution. The primary degradation products that are generated by hydrolysis of this ester are a deacylated triterpene glycoside (designated DS-1, rrt of 0.25–0.26) and a fatty-acid domain consisting of two short chain fatty acids (3,5-dihydroxy-6-methyl-octanoic acid) connected through an ester linkage from the C-1 position of the terminal fatty acid to the 5-hydroxyl of the fatty acid linked to fucose; the terminal fatty acid is glycosylated with arabinose at the 5-hydroxyl. The ester between the two fatty acids degrades only after hydrolysis of the fatty-acid domain from DS-1. These degradation products were shown to be inactive as adjuvants for antibody and CTL induction ***(19)***. Upon prolonged degradation at high temperature (60°C), the ester between the quillaic acid C-28 and fucose is hydrolyzed, yielding the prosapogenin of QS-21 (relative retention time of 0.34–0.36).
3. Dependence of Stability on pH, QS-21 Concentration: The stability of QS-21 in solution is mainly pH- and QS-21 concentration-dependent ***(18)***. QS-21 is susceptible to deacylation at alkaline pH. Hence, lower pH (down to pH 5.5) can be used to stabilize QS-21. Lower pH's are not recommended because QS-21 is poorly soluble in the acid form. The micelle form of QS-21 is more stable than the monomer form. **Table 1** shows the expected shelf-life in aqueous solution at various pH and QS-21 concentrations. QS-21 stability should be tested with each new antigen because antigen pH may affect stability. QS-21 stability may also be affected if it is formulated into an emulsion-based or liposome-based formulation.

4. Lyophilized Formulations: In contrast to aluminum hydroxide and most emulsion-based formulations, QS-21 can be lyophilized without loss of activity. Hence, QS-21 could potentially be utilized in lyophilized vaccine formulations. As an example, recombinant OspA antigen from *Borrelia burgorferi* was colyophilized with QS-21 and was then rehydrated with a saline diluent. The immunogenicity of this formulation for inducing antibody to *B. burgdorferi* lysate in C3H/Hej mice was equivalent to that of a liquid formulation that was not subjected to lyophilization (Aquila Biopharmaceuticals, unpublished data). However, the use of QS-21 in lyophilized formulations is dependent upon the stability of individual antigens to the freeze-drying process. In addition, excipients and bulking agents might be required for production of stable single-dose lyophilized vaccines.
5. Combination with Aluminum Hydroxide-Adsorbed Antigens: QS-21 is used frequently in combination with aluminum hydroxide-adsorbed antigens. Generally, the antibody responses to the QS-21/aluminum hydroxide combination are equal or slightly higher than those obtained by QS-21 alone ***(17,20)***. QS-21/aluminum hydroxide combinations have also been used successfully to induce CTL to subunit antigens ***(11)***. QS-21 will bind to aluminum hydroxide if present in micellar form (>50 μg/mL) and in a cationic buffer such as Tris-HCl. QS-21 binds more weakly in a dianionic buffer such as phosphate that competes for positively charged sites on the aluminum. It is likely that any adsorbed QS-21 is rapidly desorbed from the alum in vivo. This is supported by the observation that QS-21 dose response curves in Tris-buffered saline/alum and phosphate-buffered saline/alum for adjuvanting antibody response to ovalbumin in mice are similar (Aquila Biopharmaceuticals, unpublished data).
6. Combination with Slow Release Antigen Delivery Systems: QS-21 has also been combined with slow-release antigen delivery systems. Cleland et al. ***(21)*** compared soluble QS-21 and QS-21 coencapsulated with antigen as coadjuvants for poly(lactic-coglycolic) acid (PLGA)-encapsulated gp120. Both encapsulated and soluble QS-21 were adjuvants for the PLGA-encapsulated antigen. The addition of soluble QS-21 to PLGA-encapsulated antigen increased guinea pig serum antibody titers by fivefold compared to PLGA-antigen alone (measured at 10 wk after sc immunizations at 0 and 8 wk). Another fivefold increase was observed in the group receiving coencapsulated antigen/adjuvant. However, a single-shot vaccine formulation consisting of a mixture of separate formulations of encapsulated *gp120* and encapsulated QS-21 was recommended over coencapsulation in order to assure reproducible ratios of antigen to adjuvant ***(22)***. Methods for encapsulation of QS-21 are described by Cleland et al. ***(22)***.

References

1. Espinet, R. G. (1951) Nouveau vaccin antiaphteux a complexe glucoviral. *Gac. Vet.* **13,** 268.
2. Dalsgaard, K. (1974) Saponin adjuvants. III. Isolation of a substance from *Quillaja saponaria* Molina with adjuvant activity in foot-and-mouth disease vaccines. *Arch. Gesamte Virusforsch.* **44,** 243–254.

3. Kensil, C. R., Patel, U., Lennick, M., and Marciani, D. (1991) Separation and characterization of saponins with adjuvant activity from *Quillaja saponaria* Molina cortex. *J. Immunol.* **146,** 431–437.
4. Ma, J., Bulger, P. A., Davis, D. R., Perilli-Palmer, B., Bedore, D. A., Kensil, C. R., et al. (1994) Impact of the saponin adjuvant QS-21 and aluminium hydroxide on the immunogenicity of recombinant OspA and OspB of Borrelia burgdorferi. *Vaccine* **12,** 925–932.
5. Hancock, G. E., Speelman, D. J., Frenchick, P. J., Mineo-Kuhn, M. M., Baggs, R. B., and Hahn, D. J. (1995) Formulation of the purified fusion protein of respiratory syncytial virus with the saponin QS-21 induces protective immune responses in Balb/c mice that are similar to those generated by experimental infection. *Vaccine* **13,** 391–400.
6. Cleland, J. L., Barron, L., Daugherty, A., Eastman, D., Kensil, C., Lim, A., et al. (1996) Development of a single-shot subunit vaccine for HIV-1. 3. Effect of adjuvant and immunization schedule on the duration of the humoral immune response to recombinant MN gp120. *J. Pharm. Sci.* **85,** 1350–1357.
7. Newman, M. J., Wu, J. Y., Coughlin, R. T., Murphy, C. I., Seals, J. R., Wyand, M. S., et al. (1992) Immunogenicity and toxicity testing of an experimental HIV-1 vaccine in nonhuman primates. *AIDS Res. Hum. Retroviruses* **8,** 1413–1418.
8. Powell, M. F., Cleland, J. L., Eastman, D. J., Lim, A., Murthy, K., Newman, M. J., et al. (1994) Immunogenicity and HIV-1 virus neutralization of MN recombinant glycoprotein 120/HIV-1 QS21 vaccine in baboons. *AIDS Res. Hum. Retroviruses* **10 (Suppl. 2),** S105–S108.
9. Coughlin, R. T., Fattom, A., Chu, C., White, A. C., and Winston, S. (1995) Adjuvant activity of QS-21 for experimental E. coli 018 polysaccharide vaccines. *Vaccine* **13,** 17–21.
10. Sasaki, S., Sumino, K., Hamajima, K., Fukushima, J., Ishii, N., Kawamoto, S., et al. (1998) Induction of systemic and mucosal immune responses to human immunodeficiency virus type 1 by a DNA vaccine formulated with QS-21 saponin adjuvant via intramuscular and intranasal routes. *J. Virol.* **72,** 4931–4939.
11. Newman, M. J., Wu, J. Y., Gardner, B. H., Munroe, K. J., Leombruno, D., Recchia, J., et al. (1992) Saponin adjuvant induction of ovalbumin-specific CD8+ cytotoxic T lymphocyte responses. *J. Immunol.* **148,** 2357–2362.
12. Kensil, C. R., Wu, J. Y., and Soltysik, S. (1995) Structural and immunological characterization of the vaccine adjuvant QS-21. *Pharm. Biotechnol.* **6,** 525–541.
13. Helling, F., Zhang, S., Shang, A., Adluri, S., Calves, M., Koganty, R., et al. (1995) GM2-KLH conjugate vaccine: increased immunogenicity in melanoma patients after administration with immunological adjuvant QS-21. *Cancer Res.* **55,** 2783–2788.
14. Livingston, P. O., Adluri, S., Helling, F., Yao, T. J., Kensil, C. R., Newman, M. J., et al. (1994) Phase 1 trial of immunological adjuvant QS-21 with a GM2 ganglioside-keyhole limpet haemocyanin conjugate vaccine in patients with malignant melanoma. *Vaccine* **12,** 1275–1280.

15. Stoute, J. A., Slaoui, M., Heppner, D. G., Momin, P., Kester, K. E., Desmons, P., et al. (1997) A preliminary evaluation of a recombinant circumsporozoite protein vaccine against *Plasmodium falciparum* malaria. *The N. Eng. J. Med.* **9,** 86–91.
16. Jacobsen, N. E., Fairbrother, W. J., Kensil, C. R., Lim, A., Wheeler, D. A., and Powell, M. F. (1996) Structure of the saponin adjuvant QS-21 and its base-catalyzed isomerization product by ^{1}H and natural abundance ^{13}C NMR spectroscopy. *Carbohydr. Res.* **280,** 1–14.
17. Kensil, C. R., Newman, M. J., Coughlin, R. T., Soltysik, S., Bedore, D., Recchia, J., et al. (1993) The use of Stimulon adjuvant to boost vaccine response. *Vaccine Res.* **2,** 273–281.
18. Cleland, J. L., Kensil, C. R., Lim, A., Jacobsen, N. E., Basa, L., Spellman, M., et al. (1996) Isomerization and formulation stability of the vaccine adjuvant QS-21. *J. Pharm. Sci.* **85,** 22–28.
19. Kensil, C. R., Soltysik, S., Wheeler, D. A., and Wu, J. Y. (1996) Structure/function studies on QS-21, a unique immunological adjuvant from *Quillaja saponaria. Adv. Exp. Med. Biol.* **404,** 165–172.
20. Powell, M. F., Eastman, D. J., Lim, A., Lucas, C., Peterson, M., Vennari, J., et al. (1995) Effect of adjuvants on immunogenicity of MN recombinant glycoprotein 120 in guinea pigs. *AIDS Res. Hum. Retroviruses* **11**, 203–209.
21. Cleland, J. L., Powell, M. F., Lim, A., Barron, L., Berman, P. W., Eastman, D. J., et al. (1994) Development of a single-shot subunit vaccine for HIV-1. *AIDS Res. Hum. Retroviruses* **10 (Suppl. 2),** S21–S26.
22. Cleland, J. L., Lim, A., Barron, L., Duenas, E. T., and Powell, M. F. (1997) Development of a single-shot subunit vaccine for HIV-1: Part 4. Optimizing microencapsulation and pulsatile release of MN rgp120 from biodegradable microspheres. *J. Controlled Release* **47,** 135–150.
23. Murphy, C. I., McIntire, J. R., V.R.Davis, D., Hodgon, H., Seals, J. R., and Young, E. (1993) Enhanced expression, secretion, and large-scale purification of recombinant HIV-1 gp120 in insect cells using the baculovirus egt and p67 signal peptides. *Protein Express. Purif.* **4,** 349.
24. Takahashi, H., Cohen, J., Hosmalin, A., Cease, K. B., Houghten, R., Cornette, J., et al. (1988) An immunodominant epitope of the HIV gp160 envelope glycoprotein recognized by class I MHC molecule-restricted cytotoxic T lymphocytes. *Proc. Natl. Acad. Sci. USA* **85,** 3105.

16

MPL® Immunostimulant: *Adjuvant Formulations*

J. Terry Ulrich

1. Introduction

Interest in new methods of potentiating the immune response against vaccine antigens has increased considerably over the past decade. In part, this interest is in response to vaccine initiatives that have established aggressive goals for improving existing vaccines and for developing much-needed new vaccines. Many of the candidate vaccine antigens being developed as part of this effort are synthetic or recombinant subunit structures that are often poorly immunogenic and as such, are unable to elicit protective immune responses in the absence of an adjuvant. Fortunately, our understanding of disease pathogenesis and the immunological mechanisms of protection have increased considerably over the past few years, thus providing an improved rational basis for the development of new adjuvants.

A promising candidate adjuvant in this setting is MPL® immunostimulant, a monophosphoryl lipid A preparation derived from the lipopolysaccharide (LPS) of *Salmonella minnesota*, R595 ***(1,2)***. The manufacturing process, chemistry, and quality control of MPL has been recently reviewed ***(3)***. An important characteristic of the adjuvant activity of MPL is its ability to enhance the generation of specific immunity without being directly associated with an antigen. This property, which is shared by the LPS from which MPL is derived ***(4,5)***, is partially a reflection of the ability of MPL to induce the synthesis and release of cytokines that promote the generation of specific immune responses ***(6)***. These cytokines can be induced in the absence of antigen, and can stimulate cells that are distal to the site of induction. This is in contrast to the action of depot-type adjuvants, such as alum or oil-in-water (o/w) emulsions, which

From: *Methods in Molecular Medicine, Vol. 42:*
Vaccine Adjuvants: Preparation Methods and Research Protocols
Edited by: D. T. O'Hagan © Humana Press, Inc., Totowa, NJ

function by creating an antigen reservoir at the injection site, and therefore must be intimately associated with antigen to be effective. Because of its mode of action, MPL can be used either alone or in combination with these depot-type adjuvants. The choice of an MPL adjuvant formulation will depend on several factors such as (1) the nature of the antigen; (2) the characteristics of the desired immune response; and (3) the level of local reactogenicity that is tolerable.

An aqueous dispersion of MPL provides the simplest adjuvant formulation. MPL in this type of formulation exists in an aggregated form. This is because MPL is composed of a series of closely related monophosphoryl lipid A species that all possess well-defined hydrophobic and hydrophilic domains *(3)*. As with all lipids, these highly amphiphilic structures do not dissolve in water to yield a solution of fully solvated molecules, but instead form particulate structures in which the hydrophobic regions are excluded from the aqueous phase whereas the hydrophillic domains remain solvated. The concentration of single (unaggregated) molecules in an aqueous solution of MPL has not been measured. However, the solubility of a closely related compound, the Re LPS from *Escherichia coli* D31m4, was found to be 30 n*M* by equilibrium dialysis *(7)*. Because MPL possesses essentially the same hydrophobic domain (i.e., fatty acyl groups), but an attenuated hydrophilic region as compared to Re LPS, it is likely that the solubility of MPL is in the low nanomolar range. The nature of the aggregates formed by MPL in aqueous solution is not known, although it was found by electron microscopy that MPL forms liposome-like structures when dispersed in dilute aqueous triethylamine (TEA) by sonication *(8)*.

Aqueous dispersions of MPL in isotonic buffers can provide a strong adjuvant effect when admixed with soluble protein antigens ***(9,10)***. The contribution of MPL to the induced immune response is often more apparent in these simple formulations than in those cases where the antigen is incorporated into a depot-type adjuvant, such as an o/w emulsion. An advantage of these vaccine preparations, comprising only MPL plus antigen, is that they tend to be well tolerated and induce little or no local tissue reaction at the injection site.

A substantial amount of experimental work has demonstrated that o/w emulsions are an effective way of using MPL as an adjuvant (reviewed in **ref. *3***). The effectiveness of such formulations can be rationalized in terms of the expected behavior of MPL in an emulsion environment. In general, a key attribute of emulsions is that they contain an oil–water interface phase with which soluble antigens with some degree of amphiphilic character can associate. By associating with the oil phase, the antigen becomes more particulate, and therefore more efficiently taken up by antigen-presenting cells (APCs). In addition, the oil phase can also serve as a depot for antigen at the injection site. MPL can be readily dissolved in the oil component of an emulsion prior to dispersal in the aqueous phase (*see* **Subheading 3.2.**), and it is likely that essentially all of the MPL remains associated with the oil phase following combination with the aqueous phase. This localization of both antigen and MPL in the same particulate structure allows for more efficient delivery of antigenic and immunostimulatory signals to the same cells.

In the past, the emulsions used with MPL have been of the o/w type, consisting of 1–2% oil and a surfactant such as Tween-80 at a concentration of 0.2–0.5%. Commonly used oils in these emulsions have included mineral oil, squalane, and squalene (a biodegradable precursor of cholesterol biosynthesis). The type of oil used in these emulsions is important, because it can influence both the immunogenicity and tissue reactogenicity of the vaccine formulation. Several methods for preparing o/w emulsions have been described, including homogenization ***(11–13)***, sonication ***(14–16)***, and microfluidization ***(17–19)***. Several of these methods have described the incorporation of MPL, as well as other immunostimulants for enhancing adjuvant activity.

It is the purpose of this chapter to outline the methodology for suitably dispersing MPL into an aqueous formulation, as well as to describe the preparation of a simple o/w emulsion containing MPL. With these stock formulations in hand, the investigator needs only to make appropriate mixtures with antigen for initiating vaccine studies.

2. Materials

2.1. Preparation of MPL-TEoA Aqueous Dispersion

1. MPL from *S. minnesota*, R595. Purchased from Ribi ImmunoChem Research, Inc., Hamilton, MT as a TEA salt. Product codes: R350–2.0 mg; R351–10.0 mg.
2. Triethanolamine (TEoA) [2,2′,2″-nitrilotriethanol].
3. Sterile water-for-injection (WFI), USP, nonpyrogenic.
4. Ultrasonic bath with heater (Lab-Line Instruments, Model 9303. Melrose Park, IL).
5. Miscellaneous glassware, sterile/depyrogenated.
6. Serum vial ring seals, 20 mm.
7. Crimper for 20-mm ring seals.

2.2. Preparation of MPL Oil-in-Water Emulsion

1. MPL. *See* **Subheading 2.1., item 1**. Method scaled to 10.0 mg of MPL lyophilized TEA salt.
2. Squalene (2,6,10,15,19,23-hexamethyl-2,6,10,14,18,22-tetracosahexene). Acros Organics, Fisher Chemical Co., Santa Monica, CA. Product code: 20747.
3. Polyoxyethylenesorbitan monooleate (Tween-80).
4. Lecithin, granular from Soybean (Acros Organics, Fisher Chemical Co.), Product code: 41310-2500.

5. Dulbecco's phosphate-buffered saline (DPBS), Ca^{++}/Mg^{++} free (Sigma Chemical Co., St. Louis, MO). Product code: D8537.
6. Ultrasonic bath with heater (*see* **Subheading 2.1., item 4**).

3. Methods

3.1. Preparation of Stock MPL/TEoA Aqueous Dispersion Formulation

1. Prepare 20–30 mL of a fresh solution of 0.5% v/v TEoA in WFI. Filter sterilize using 0.2-µm filter.
2. Remove ring seal from 2.0 or 10.0 mg vial of MPL-lyophilized TEA salt, remove stopper, and aseptically add 0.98 mL of 0.5% v/v TEoA/WFI for each 1.0 mg of MPL salt to be treated (*see* **Note 1**).
3. Replace stopper and crimp new 20-mm ring seal in place and vortex vial briefly (15–30 s) to disperse the MPL salt.
4. Suspend vial in preheated (65°C) ultrasonic bath and sonicate for 30 min using maximum power (*see* **Note 2**).
5. After sonication, remove vial from ultrasonic bath (*Caution*: ring seal will be very hot), visually examine solution for any evidence of particulates.
6. Repeat **step 4** for an additional 5–10 min, if necessary, to produce a slightly translucent solution.
7. Allow vial and contents to cool to room temperature, remove ring seal, and aseptically add 20 µL of 1 N HCl for each 0.98 mL of 0.5% w/v TEoA/WFI added initially. Mix by vortexing (*see* **Note 3**).

3.2. Preparation of Stock MPL Oil-in-Water Emulsion Formulation

1. Prepare 25 mL of squalene/lecithin as follows: Into a suitable, glass, depyrogenated vessel, add 25 mL of squalene. Weigh 3.0 g of granular lecithin and add to the squalene. Place in preheated (65°C) water bath for 10–15 min to completely dissolve the lecithin in the squalene. Sonication will aid in dissolving the lecithin. The squalene/lecithin solution will have a light-yellow color. Pass the squalene/lecithin solution through a 0.2-µm sterile filter. Unused squalene/lecithin can be stored at 4–7°C for up to 6 mo.
2. Remove ring seal from 10.0-mg vial of MPL-lyophilized TEA salt, remove stopper, and aseptically add 1.0 mL of sterile squalene/lecithin. Replace stopper and vortex vial to dissolve MPL. Heat to 65°C for 1–2 min to aid in dissolving the MPL.
3. Remove stopper and add 9.0 mL of sterile 0.5% v/v Tween-80 in Ca^{+}/Mg^{++}-free DPBS directly to vial. Replace stopper and reseal vial using a 20-mm ring seal and crimper.
4. Suspend vial in preheated (65°C) ultrasonic bath and sonicate for 20 min at maximum power (*see* **Note 2**, also **Note 5**).
5. After sonication, cool vial to room temperature, remove ring seal, and add 0.01% w/v thimerosal. Mix well, reseal, and store at 4–7°C. DO NOT FREEZE (*see* **Note 4**).

3.3. Use of MPL Adjuvant Formulations

The formulations prepared as aforementioned are considered stock preparations of MPL at 1.0 mg/mL and as such, require dilution for use with antigens. It is the intent of the following to provide general guidelines for the use of these preparations as adjuvants for vaccine antigens in experimental animal models.

1. An effective adjuvant dose of either MPL formulation with a vaccine antigen must be determined experimentally by the investigator. Using mice in our laboratory, we have found that MPL doses that range between 5–50 μg have been useful with soluble protein or peptide antigens, as well as with polysaccharide-protein conjugates.
2. To use the MPL-TEoA (1.0 mg/mL) stock formulation, dissolve the antigen in DPBS and combine with MPL-TEoA to achieve the desired MPL and antigen concentration per dose. It is advisable to prepare fresh mixtures of antigen and MPL from the 1.0 mg/mL stock for each required set of booster injections. Antigen mixed with appropriately diluted 0.5% v/v TEoA-WFI, without MPL, should be used as an experimental control.
3. The 1.0 mg/mL stock MPL-TEoA formulation is compatible with alum-adsorbed antigens. We have found it helpful to prepare the antigen/alum adsorbate at two times final concentration and add a equal volume of appropriately diluted MPL-TEoA stock with mixing. It has been our experience that after 10–15 min of mixing, essentially 100% of the MPL is bound to the alum (*see* **Note 6**).
4. To use the MPL o/w emulsion (1.0 mg/mL MPL–10% oil) stock formulation, add the antigen as a solution in DPBS, such that the stock o/w emulsion is diluted either 1 : 10 or 1 : 5, which yields a final oil concentration of 1% and 2%, respectively. The concentration of MPL will be either 100 or 200 μg/mL. For mouse studies, we inject 0.05–0.25-mL volumes of the above dilutions to achieve MPL doses that range between 5–50 μg. Because 1–2% o/w emulsions without MPL are adjuvant active, it is important to prepare a vehicle (10% o/w emulsion), which can be diluted appropriately with antigen to serve as a control vaccine formulation.
5. In our laboratory, we use either intramuscular (im) or subcutaneous (sc) injections of the final vaccine formulation. Our preferred site for sc injections is in the inguinal region. We adhere to an immunization schedule of a primary immunization, followed by boosts at 21-d intervals as needed. Bleeds are taken at 14-d intervals, serum stored at –20°C until antibody determinations are made. Spleens and lymph nodes are removed from selected mice in experimental groups at various time-points and used for in vitro measurements of cellular immunity (*see* **Note 7**).
6. The MPL formulations discussed in this chapter each utilize buffered aqueous solutions at neutral pH. MPL is stable under such conditions for at least 6 mo when stored at 4–7°C. The chemical and physical stability of individual antigens

in the formulations described in this chapter must be assessed on a case-by-case basis.

4. Notes

1. MPL-lyophilized TEA salt is supplied as a research product in 2.0 or 10.0-mg vials. The dry weight is based on the actual weight of MPL in the salt. It is impractical to attempt to weigh the lyophilized salt because of its electrostatic nature. Therefore, it is recommended that the entire contents of the vial be used for formulation and that the excipients be added directly to the vial.
2. It is advisable to suspend the vial in the ultrasonic bath by a string, with one end attached around the neck of the vial and the other end attached to a clamp on a ring stand placed over the bath. Submerge the vial up to the neck in the bath.
3. After addition of 1 N HCl, pH will be 7.2 ± 0.2. Store stock 1.0 mg/mL MPL-TEoA solution at 4–7°C. DO NOT FREEZE. For long-term storage, add 0.01% w/v thimerosal as a preservative. MPL-TEoA stock is biologically and chemically stable for at least 6 mo when stored at 4–7°C and at pH 7.2 ± 0.2.
4. The 1.0 mg/mL MPL-10% o/w emulsion is biologically and chemically stable for at least 6 mo, however, there may be some physical separation of the emulsion during long-term storage at 4–7°C. If this occurs, warm the emulsion to room temperature and vortex briefly (10–30 s) before removing an aliquot for vaccine formulation.
5. Homogenization is an alternative method for preparation of the o/w emulsion to that described in **Subheading 3.2., step 4.** The equipment used in our laboratory for homogenization is a T-25 ULTRA-TURRAX homogenizer fitted with S25N-8G dispersing element (VWR Scientific Products, S. Plainfield, NJ). This method requires that the homogenizer dispersing element be immersed into the oil/T80-PBS mixture and the mixture homogenized for 30 min at 25,000 rpm to form the o/w emulsion. Some foaming may occur during homogenization, however, this can be minimized by immersing the dispersing element to a depth of approximately 2.0 cm.
6. An experimental vaccine formulation for use in mice was prepared as an alum (Alhydrogel®, 2%, Superfos Biosector w/s, Vedback, Denmark) adsorbate of a recombinant hepatitis B surface antigen (rHBsAg, Rhein Biotech GmbH, Dusseldorf, Germany). Briefly, the procedure was as follows: While mixing (magnetic bar stirrer), 0.5 mL (10 mg) of Alhydrogel was added dropwise, over a period of 2–3 min, to 9.5 mL of DPBS containing 100 μg of rHBsAg. After the addition of alum, the suspension was allowed to mix for an additional 30 min. This stock alum adsorbate of rHBsAg contained 1.0 mg/mL alum and 10 μg/ml rHBsAg. For vaccine formulations, an equal volume of alum adsorbate was mixed with an equal volume of DPBS or DPBS containing 250 μg/mL of the stock MPL-TEoA formulation described in **Subheading 3.1.** Mice were injected subcutaneously (inguinal region) with 0.2-mL volumes of the vaccines on day 0

Table 1
The Effect of MPL on the Antibody Response to a rHBsAg/Alum Adsorbate Vaccine

Vaccine	Anti-HBsAg titer^{-1}	
	IgG1-specific	IgG2a-specific
HBsAg/Alum	128K	64K
HBsAg/Alum + MPL®	256K	1024K

See **Note 7** for experimental details. Titer end point is the reciprocal of the serum dilution having an OD ≥ 0.100. K = 10^3.

and day 21. A mouse dose contained 1.0 µg rHBsAg, 100 µg alum, ± 25 µg MPL. A typical antibody response on day 35 of the experiment measuring IgG1-specific and IgG2a-specific anti-rHBsAg antibody titers is shown in **Table 1**. The adjuvant effect of MPL in this system is observed as promoting a strong IgG2a response. Recently, a clinical study has shown that the addition of MPL to a commercially available hepatitis B vaccine, Engerix-B®, promoted 100% seroprotection (antibody levels ≥ 10 mIUmL^{-1}) of the subjects by 60 days following the 1-mo booster injection, as compared to a 58% seroprotection rate, at the same time-point, for the group given the vaccine without MPL ***(20)***.

7. The following is an example of the experimental use of the stock MPL-TEoA and MPL o/w emulsion adjuvant formulations. We have used each formulation in combination with the rHBsAg, discussed in **Note 6**, to evaluate the MPL adjuvant effect in mice on both the antibody response and cytotoxic T-lymphocyte (CTL) response. In these experiments, a standard dose of 1.0 µg rHBsAg diluted in DPBS was combined with either stock MPL adjuvant formulation by simple mixing. The mice were injected on day 0 and boosted on day 21. CTL assays using spleen cells from 2–3 mice per group were done on day 35 and the remaining mice bled for serum antibody titers on day 48. Details of the CTL assay and a description of the target cell have been reported ***(21)***. Serum antibody titers were determined by a conventional enzyme-linked immunosorbent assay (ELISA) methodology in 96 well plates using the rHBsAg as a plate coating antigen. As shown in **Table 2**, the MPL o/w emulsion was an effective adjuvant over a broad MPL dose range for the induction of CTLs to the rHBsAg class I, L^d restricted, CTL epitope S_{28-39} (IPQSLDSWWTSL). In addition, the o/w emulsion containing MPL induced a strong IgG2a antibody response when compared to the vehicle o/w emulsion control. Finally, the simple addition of the MPL-TEoA formulation to rHBsAg provides a modest enhancement of the CTL response, but a strong enhancement of the IgG2a specific antibody response when compared to the antigen in DPBS only.

Table 2
Adjuvant Activity of the MPL-TEoA and MPL O/W Emulsion Formulations on the Antibody Response and CTL Response to rHBsAg

		% Cytotoxicity		Anti - HBsAg titer^{-1}	
	MPL	E/T			
Adjuvant	dose (µg)	50:1	25:1	IgG1-specific	IgG2a-specific
MPL® O/W	50	89	65	256K	1024K
	25	80	64	512K	1024K
	5	64	45	256K	512K
	1	44	30	256K	256K
Vehicle O/W	0	28	18	128K	64K
MPL-TEoA	15	45	22	32K	512K
DPBS	0	17	12	32K	16K

See **Note 7** for experimental details. E/T = effector/target ratio. Titer end point is the reciprocal of the serum dilution serum having an OD ≥ 0.100. K = 10^3.

References

1. Qureshi, N., Mascagni, P., Ribi, E., and Takayama, K. (1985) Monophosphoryl lipid A obtained from lipopolysaccharides of *Salmonella minnesota* R595: Purification of the dimethyl derivative by high performance liquid chromatography and complete structural determination. *J. Biol. Chem.* **260,** 5271–5278.
2. Myers, K. R., Truchot, A. T., Ward, J., Hudson, Y., and Ulrich, J. T. (1990) A critical determinant of lipid A endotoxic activity, in *Cellular and Molecular Aspects of Endotoxin Reactions* (Nowotny, A., Spitzer, J. J., and Ziegler, E. J., eds.), Elsevier Science, Amsterdam, pp. 145–156.
3. Ulrich, J. T. and Myers, K. R. (1995) Monophosphoryl lipid A as an adjuvant. Past experiences and new directions, in *Vaccine Design: The Subunit and Adjuvant Approach* (Powell, M. F. and Newman, M. J. eds.), Plenum, New York, pp. 495–524.
4. Johnson, A. G. (1964) Adjuvant action of bacterial endotoxins on the primary antibody response, in *Bacterial Endotoxins* (Landy, M. and Braun, W., eds.), Rutgers University Press, New Brunswick, NJ, pp. 252–262.
5. Munoz, J. (1964) Effects of vacteria and bacteria products on antibody response, in *Advances in Immunology* (Dixon, F. J. and Kunkel, H. G., eds.), Academic, New York, pp. 397–440.
6. Gustafson, G. L. and Rhodes, M. J. (1992) Bacterial cell wall products as adjuvants: early interferon gamma as a marker for adjuvants that enhance protective immunity. *Res. Immunol.* **143,** 483–488.
7. Takayama, K., Din, Z. Z., Mukerjee, P., Cooke, P. H., and Kirkland, T. N. (1990) Physicochemical properties of the lipopolysaccharide unit that activates B lymphocytes. *J. Biol. Chem.* **265,** 14,023–14,029.

8. Ribi, E., Cantrell, J. L., Takayama, K., Ribi, H. O., Myers, K. R., and Qureshi, N. (1986) Modulation of humoral and cell-mediated immune responses by a structurally established nontoxic lipid A, in *Immunobiology and Immunopharmacololgy of Bacterial Endotoxins* (Szentivanyi, A. and Friedman, H., eds.), Plenum, New York, pp. 407–419.
9. Schneerson, R., Fattom, A., Szu, S. C., Bryla, D., Ulrich, J. T., Rudbach, J. A., et al. (1991) Evaluation of monophosphoryl lipid A (MPL) as an adjuvant: Enhancement of the serum antibody response in mice to polysaccharide-protein conjugates by concurrent injection with MPL. *J. Immunol.* **147,** 2136–2140.
10. Devi, S. J. N., Schneerson, R., Egan, W., Ulrich, T., Bryla, D., Robbins, J. B., and Bennett, J. E. (1991) *Cryptococcus neoformans* Serotype A glucuronoxylomannan-protein conjugate vaccines: Synthesis, characterization, and immunogenicity. *Infect. Immun.* **59,** 3700–3707.
11. Meyer, T. J., Ribi, E. E., Azuma, I., and Zbar, B. (1974) Biologically active components from mycobacterial cell walls. II. Suppression and regression of strain-2 guinea pig hepatoma. *J. Natl. Cancer Inst.* **52,** 103–111.
12. Granger, D. L., Yamamoto, K. I., and Ribi, E. E. (1976) Delayed hypersensitivity and granulomatous response after immunization with protein antigens associated with a mycobacterial glycolipid and oil droplets. *J. Immunol.* **116,** 482–488.
13. Vosika, G. J., Schmidtke, J. R., Goldman, A., Parker, R., Ribi, E. E., and Gray, G. R. (1980) Phase 1 study of intradermal immunotherapy with oil-attached *Mycobacterium smegmatis* cell wall skeleton and trehalose dimycolate. *Cancer Immunol. Immunother.* **7,** 221–224.
14. Bekierkunst, A., Levij, I. S., Yarkoni, E., Vilkas, E., Adam, A., and Lederer, E. (1969) Granuloma formation induced in mice by chemically defined mycobacterial fractions. *J. Bacteriol.* **100,** 95–102.
15. Yarkoni, E., Rapp, H. J., and Zbar, B. (1977) Immunotherapy of a guinea pig hepatoma with ultrasonically prepared mycobacterial vaccines. *Cancer Immunol. Immunother.* **2,** 143–146.
16. Bomford, R., Stapleton, M., Winsor, S., McKnight, A., and Andronova, T. (1992) The control of the antibody isotype response to recombinant human immunodeficiency virus gp120 antigen by adjuvants. *AIDS Res. Hum. Retroviruses* **8,** 1765–1771.
17. Lidgate, D. M., Fu, R. C., Byars, N. E., Foster, L. C., and Fleitman, J. S. (1989) Formulation of vaccine adjuvant muramyldipeptides. 3. Processing optimization, characterization, and bioactivity of an emulsion vehicle. *Pharm. Res.* **6,** 748–752.
18. Ott, G., Barchfeld, G. L., and Van Nest, G. (1995) Enhancement of humoral response against human influenza vaccine with the simple submicron oil/water emulsion adjuvant MF59. *Vaccine* **13,** 1557–1562.
19. Traquina, P., Morandi, M., Contorni, M., and Van Nest, G. (1996) MF59 adjuvant enhances the antibody response to recombinant hepatitis B surface antigen vaccine in primates. *J. Infect. Dis.* **174,** 1168–1175.

20. Thoelen, S., Van Damme, P., Mathei, C., Leroux-Roels, G., Desombere, I., Safary, A., et al. (1998) Safety and immunogenicity of a hepatitis B vaccine formulated with a novel adjuvant system. *Vaccine* **16,** 708–714.
21. Schirmbeck, R., Deml, L., Melber, K., Wolf, H., Wagner, R., and Reimann, J. (1995) Priming of class I-restricted cytotoxic T lymphocytes by vaccination with recombinant protein antigens. *Vaccine* **13,** 857–865.

17

Cytokines As Vaccine Adjuvants: *The Use of Interleukin-2*

Martin A. Giedlin

1. Introduction

Live attenuated virus and bacterial vaccines are generally more potent than subunit or nucleic acid vaccines because of the host's vigorous inflammatory response to them. The challenge to building effective subunit or nucleic acid vaccines is incorporating those factors in the regimen that mimic an infection, resulting in a robust and protective immune response. Numerous cytokines have been shown to significantly modulate the inflammatory process, including interleukin-12 (IL-12), granulocyte-macrophage colony stimulating factor (GM-CSF), and interleukin-2 (IL-2), (*reviewed* in ***1*** and ***2***). The addition of recombinant or nucleic acid-derived cytokine(s) to a vaccine regimen can therefore enhance the endogenous immune response to the vaccine antigen.

Cytokines are a group of secreted low-molecular weight proteins that have a major role in cell-to-cell communication. Similarly to hormones, cytokines serve as messengers of the immune system. However, in contrast to the wide-ranging effects of hormones in the body, cytokines are most effective in local microenvironments. Cytokines are secreted in response to a number of stimuli, and bind to specific receptors that trigger signal-transduction pathways that can effect the gene expression and function of the target cells. The receptors exhibit very high affinity for the cytokine ligand (10^{-10}–$10^{-12}M$), and because of this high affinity, local picomolar amounts of cytokine can mediate biological effects. The end result of this process can be the enhancement or suppression of the immune response to a particular antigen, depending on the spectrum of cytokines elicited during the immune response.

From: *Methods in Molecular Medicine, Vol. 42: Vaccine Adjuvants: Preparation Methods and Research Protocols*
Edited by: D. T. O'Hagan © Humana Press, Inc., Totowa, NJ

In broad terms, CD4+ T-helper (T_H) cells are activated following recognition of an antigen-class II major histocompatibility complex (MHC) on an antigen-presenting cell (APC), such as tissue macrophages, dendritic cells, and B lymphocytes. Once activated, the T_H cells divide and expand into antigen-specific clones of effector cells. During this expansion period, the T_H cells can secrete various cytokines that can affect the activation and response of B cells, cytotoxic T cells, and other cells that mediate the immune response. Different patterns of cytokine secretion can influence the type of immune response that develops. A T_H1 response, characterized by the secretion of IL-2, interferon γ (IFNγ), IL-12, and GM-CSF, preferentially activates T-cytotoxic cells and macrophages (cell-mediated immune response or CMI), whereas, a T_H2 cytokine profile (IL-4, IL-10, IL-5) activates mainly B lymphocytes (humoral immune response). Therefore, in designing an antigen-cytokine/adjuvant immunization regimen, knowledge of the type of immune response desired (CMI or humoral) will influence the choice of cytokine.

A number of cytokines have been studied as vaccine adjuvants. Exogenous IL-1, IL-2, IFNγ, GM-CSF, and IL-12 have all shown some enhancement of the immune response to protein antigen when given systemically ***(3)***. IL-12, GM-CSF, and IL-2 have been studied the most extensively as vaccine adjuvants in both infectious diseases and cancer. The dose and schedule of cytokine administration is very important in maximizing response to vaccine while limiting toxicities. High bolus doses of IL-2 can result in hypotension, exacerbation of underlying autoimmune disease, and induce vascular leak syndrome. IFNγ can be immunosuppressive at high doses, and certain regimens of IL-12 can result in mortality. Therefore, the doses and regimens that minimize systemic toxicity are required for vaccines treating nonlife-threatening diseases, whereas more-aggressive cytokine regimens can be employed in those therapeutic vaccines treating cancer.

1.1. Interleukin-12 (IL-12)

IL-12 or natural-killer cell stimulatory factor (NKSF) was identified and cloned on the basis of its ability to induce IFNγ from T cells and natural-killer (NK) cells and enhance their activity (***4***; available from Genetic Institute, Boston, MA). The cytokine is composed of two unrelated glycoproteins of approximately 40,000 Dalton mol wt (*p*40) and 35,000 Dalton mol wt (*p*35). The cytokine is primarily secreted by activated monocytes, dendritic cells, and some Epstein-Barr Virus (EBV)-transformed B-cell lines. The active heterodimer is 70,000 Dalton mol wt with a single disulfide bond. The receptor is expressed on activated T cells and NK cells and has an affinity for the ligand in the 100–600 pmol range.

Because IL-12 is secreted by activated professional APCs, the cytokine can influence T-cell development during antigen priming. This influence has been shown to be preferential toward the development of T_H1 cells ***(5)***. Therefore, if vaccines are intended to drive the immune response toward a T_H1 profile, the addition of IL-12 to the immunization regimen would be beneficial. This has been shown to be true in a model of experimental murine *Leishmania* ***(6)***. Susceptible Balb/c mice were injected on days 0 and 10 with soluble Leishmanial antigen (SLA) plus IL-12 protein. The mice were then challenged 14 d later with *Leishmania major*. The combined immunization regimen conferred protection and was mediated by IFNγ. Antigen or IL-12 alone had no protective effect. Therefore, IL-12 can shift T-helper cell phenotype from susceptible T_H2 to the resistant T_H1 path. Similar results have been shown in a murine model of experimental toxoplasmosis ***(7)***. Gene therapy of IL-12 coadministered with a DNA immunogen has been shown to be effective in generating a enhanced cellular immune response over DNA antigen alone ***(8)***.

Recombinant mouse IL-12 has also been shown to have an adjuvant effect with tumor vaccines in murine syngeneic tumor models when administered 10 times intraperitoneally following immunization with irradiated tumor cells ***(9)***. It is important to note that IL-12 is species specific, so that murine IL-12 has to be used in murine tumor models. Interleukin-12 gene therapy has been shown to be effective in murine tumor models, where the IL-12 genes were delivered in transfected, cytokine-secreting tumor cells ***(10,11)***. The avoidance of IL-12 toxicities, seen with some systemic recombinant protein regimens, may be avoided with the local low concentrations of the cytokine provided by gene therapy. Clearly, both the systemic and local administration of IL-12 during the immunization process can enhance the host's immune response to antigen.

1.2. Granulocyte-Macrophage Colony Stimulating Factor (GM-CSF)

GM-CSF was originally identified as a survival and growth factor for hematopoietic progenitor cells and a differentiation and activating factor for granulocyte and monocyte cells ***(12)***. Recently, it has been shown to enhance the maturation of dendritic cell precursors ***(13)***. It is a glycoprotein of approximately 16,000 Dalton mol wt (127 amino acids [aa] in the human) containing two disulfide bonds ***(14)***. It is secreted by activated T cells, macrophages, fibroblasts, and endothelial cells. The high-affinity receptor is a complex of low-affinity α-chain (CD116) and the affinity converting β-chain (KH97 in the human, AIC2B in the mouse). The β-chain is shared with IL-3 and IL-5 α-chains.

Because GM-CSF acts on APC populations, it, too, can influence the early T-cell priming events. Whereas studies with recombinant GM-CSF (Immunex,

Seattle, WA) have been reported with both protein and peptide-based vaccines ***(15)***, this cytokine has been extensively studied as a gene therapy approach with either DNA vaccines or as cytokine-secreting transduced tumor cells ***(16,17)***. These studies demonstrated that local administration of GM-CSF in combination with an antigen source, particularly in poorly immunogenic murine syngeneic tumor models, can stimulate potent, specific, and long-lasting antitumor immunity.

1.3. Biology and Molecular Characterization of IL-2

IL-2 is a pluripotent globular glycoprotein of 15,000 mol wt. It was first described as a T-cell growth factor (TCGF) ***(18,19)***. It is now known to stimulate growth and differentiation in not only T cells, but also B cells, NK cells, lymphokine-activated killer (LAK) cells, monocyte/macrophages, and neutrophils (*reviewed* in ***20–22***). The biological activity of IL-2 is mediated through the IL-2 receptor (IL-2R) complex, comprising three distinct polypeptide chains: α-chain (TAC, p55, CD25), β-chain (p75, CD122), and γ-chain (p64, γ_c) ***(23)***. The IL-2R β-chain is also part of the IL-15 receptor complex ***(24)***. The IL-2R γ_c-chain has been shown to be part of the IL-4R, IL-7R, IL-9R, IL-13R, and the IL-15R receptor complexes ***(25)***. The intermediate affinity (*kd* 10^{-9} *M*) dimeric IL-2R complex is comprised of β/γ_c chains and are primarily found on resting T, B, and NK cells, monocyte/macrophages, and neutrophils ***(26)***. The high affinity (*kd* 10^{-11} *M*) IL-2R trimeric complex is comprised of $\alpha/\beta/\gamma_c$ chains and is primarily expressed on antigen-activated T and B cells, activated monocytes, and a subpopulation of NK cells ***(23,25–27)***. The differential expression of the intermediate and high-affinity IL-2R complexes on different leukocyte subsets, in combination with IL-2 plasma concentrations, influences the biological activity of IL-2.

1.4. Vaccine Adjuvant

The local administration of IL-2 alone induces the migration of immune cells to the site of injection, increases local expression of major histocompatibility (MHC) class II antigens, and enhances skin antigen reactivity ***(28)***. Activation of monocytes and dendritic cells is also improved ***(29–31)***. Additional studies in animal models and in vitro human systems suggest that exogenous IL-2 could be a valuable adjunct in the treatment of specific opportunistic infections in immunosuppressed individuals infected with human immunodeficiency virus (HIV) ***(32–38)***.

Systemic IL-2 administration of HIV-infected individuals leads to T-cell proliferation as evidenced by the increase in spontaneous blast transformation ex vivo. This IL-2 induced T-cell proliferation results in a prominent and sustained polyclonal increases in circulating CD4+ T cells, with preferential expansion of the naïve T cell subset *(39)*. Some data also suggest that IL-2 decreases the frequency of apoptotic peripheral blood mononuclear cells (PMBCs) obtained from HIV-infected patients, which may contribute to the increase in circulating CD4+ T cells *(40)*. HIV-specific T-cell proliferation is augmented by IL-2 in vitro *(41)*. In vitro exposure to IL-2 of CD8+ T cells from some patients with advanced disease improved the capacity of these cells to suppress HIV replication *(42)*. Exogenous IL-2 partially reverses the deficit in NK-cell activity seen in AIDS patients *(43)*. IL-2 also induces B-cell activation and antibody synthesis in vitro. Therefore, IL-2's pleotropic effect on the immune response can potentially enhance vaccine efficacy in individuals with virally impaired immune systems.

Table 1 (**refs.** ***44–50***) provides a summary of published articles describing the use of IL-2 as a vaccine adjuvant in infectious disease animal models. Viral *(44,46,49,50)*, bacterial *(45)*, and parasitic *(48)* vaccine model systems have benefited from the incorporation of systemic recombinant IL-2 into the immunization regimen. The doses of recombinant IL-2 have ranged from 1 µg/kg to 1 mg/kg, with the lower doses being administered over 3–5 d following antigen. The recombinant IL-2 has been delivered separately or incorporated into the antigen/adjuvant mixture *(45,47,48)*. At relatively high IL-2 doses, genetic unresponsiveness, as measured by serum antibody, can be overcome to certain antigens by expanding the number of antigen-specific $_{TH}$ cells, pushing the number of responding cells above detectable levels *(47,48)*. IL-2 administration is probably expanding the number of vaccine-generated antigen-specific effector cells that are expressing the high-affinity IL-2R, although careful frequency analysis by limiting dilution-type methods have not been reported. The doses of recombinant IL-2 are well below what has been reported as the maximally tolerated dose (MTD) (approximately 10–12 mg/kg QD for 5–7 days iv in mice) *(51)*.

There is a dose–response relationship associated with systemic administration of recombinant IL-2 *(46)*. Nunberg and colleagues demonstrated in the murine rabies vaccine challenge model that the adjuvant effect of IL-2 was lost at doses above or below 0.1 µg/g (100 µg/kg). This relationship has been noted before *(2)* and illustrates the fine line between overcoming nonresponsiveness at relatively high IL-2 doses and inducing suppression *(52,53)*. Therefore, the dose, timing, and schedule of recombinant IL-2 administration should be optimized for each vaccine system. The route of administration should also be determined, although intraperitoneal (ip) or subcutaneous (sc) administration seems preferable to intravenous (iv) (because of longer systemic exposure), particularly when dosing twice a day over five days.

Modified forms of recombinant IL-2, for example, polyethylene glycol-modified recombinant IL-2, have been reported to enhance the efficacy of vaccines *(46)*. This modification increased the residence time of the IL-2,

Table 1
Uses of IL-2 as a Vaccine Adjuvant for Infectious Diseases and Genetic Unresponsiveness

Animal vaccine	Adjuvant route	IL-2 dose/regimen	Results	Ref.
HSV (rgD; 50 μg) Day 1, 14 Day 1,14,38 guinea pigs	alum sc[5]	rIL-21 ; 66 μg/kg sc qd -Days 0–17 with double vaccination -Days 15–26 with triple vaccination -challenge intravaginally 1 wk after last IL-2 dose	-increased cytoxicity -decreased virus shedding -unchanged antibody titers	*44*
H. pleuropneumoniae swine	oil	3.3–33 μg/kg multiple following each immunization	-enhanced protection	*45*
Rabies (Dura-Rab-3) 0.5 mL/mouse Day 0 and 7 mice	none	30–100 μg/kg -QDx5 following each vaccination -Challenge intracerebrally with CVS-11 strain on D21	-enhanced efficacy 25-fold -increased cellular response -no change in antibody titers	*46*
Whale sperm myoglobin component IV 100 μg, single mice	CFA[2]	75 μg/kg,single -incorporated with antigen/adjuvant -bled on Days 10–46	-overcame *Ir* gene low responsiveness -increase antibody titer 10-50-fold	*47*
Malarial peptide R32tet$_{32}$ 50 μg/injection, single sc, base of tail mice	CFA, IFA[3]	1 mg/kg (17 μg/mouse) -formulated with antigen/adjuvant -draining lympho nodes harvested on Days 8–10; sera on Day 28	-overcame genetic unresponsiveness in H-2^k mice	*48*
Rabies (inactivated vaccine) 25 μg ip on Day 0 and 7 mice	none	1.6 μg/mouse (180,000 IU) ip[6] on Day 0, 4, and 7 intracerebral challenge on Day 14 with 30 μL of CVS-26 (30 LD$_{50}$)	-increased protection 50-fold	*49*
Pseudorabies swine	IFA	10^5 CU[4]/kg	-enhanced serum antibody -unchanged CMI response -unchanged weight gain -unchanged virus shedding	*50*

[1]Chiron/Cetus Proleukin® recombinant human IL-2. [2]Complete Freund's Adjuvant. [3]Incomplete Freund's Adjuvant. [4]1 Cetus Unit (CU) = 6 International Units (IU) of IL-2 activity; [5]subcutaenous, intraperitoneal.

therefore, reducing the number of administrations from once every day for five days to once a week *(51)*. The immunogenicity of Proleukin recombinant IL-2 was also reduced (*54*; *see* **Notes**). Polyethylene glycol-modified recombinant IL-2 has been shown to increase the protective properties of a *Mycobacterium* subunit vaccine in a guinea pig aerosol challenge model *(55)*. Similar enhancements have been reported in a guinea pig model of recurrent herpes simplex virus (HSV) using liposomal-formulated recombinant IL-2 *(56)*. The encapsulation of polyethylene glycol-modified IL-2 can extend the systemic exposure to IL-2 out to more than 20 d *(57)*. Modifications of Proleukin have can also reduce the specific activity of recombinant IL-2, so care must be taken in deciding what properties, long-half-life or high activity, is needed (*see* **Note 2**). Therefore, controled release of low local IL-2 concentrations over time may be attractive in the vaccine setting.

Systemic IL-2 has also been shown to have a role in enhancing the antitumor response of a variety of putative cancer vaccines (**Table 2**; **refs.** *58–61*). Single-agent IL-2 has been shown to be efficacious in a variety of murine syngeneic tumor models *(51)*. However, optimal response, as measured by survival, reduction of tumor growth, or number of metastatic lesions, is near the MTD. Incorporation of systemic IL-2 into a cancer vaccine regimen can significantly reduce the amount of recombinant IL-2 needed to achieve higher response rates as compared to high dose IL-2 alone. The range of tumor antigen sources that have shown increased efficacy with recombinant IL-2 have included irradiated whole tumor cells *(61–63)*, vaccinia tumor oncolysates *(58)*, recombinant virus *(59,60)*, and tumor-lysate pulsed dendritic cells *(64)*. The mechanism of the IL-2 enhanced antitumor activity is primarily mediated by CD8+ T cells, although CD4+ T cells play a significant role *(63)*.

1.5. Summary

Systemic IL-2 can be a powerful vaccine adjuvant in both infectious disease and oncology indications. In humans, IL-2 can increase the frequency of elderly responders to flu and tetanus vaccination *(65,66)*. Numerous human clinical trials utilizing systemic IL-2 with tumor antigen (peptides, lysate, irradiated cells, and so on) are currently ongoing. Although any one cytokine may augment the immune response to a given vaccine, a combination of cytokines in the immunization process might be needed to mimic the inflammatory response needed to generate an optimal immune response. The administration of GM-CSF and IL-12 with the antigen, to enhance T-cell priming, followed by 3–5 d of systemic IL-2 to preferentially expand the antigen-activated high-affinity IL-2R-expressing T cells, might be a regimen applicable to most vaccines. This would be especially true if one or more of the cytokines and/or antigens can be delivered as nucleic acid. Finally, because successful vaccines

Table 2
Uses of IL-2 As Vaccine Adjuvant in Cancer Models

Vaccine animal	Model adjuvant route	IL-2 dose/regimen	Results	Ref.
CC-36 colorectal carcinoma carcinoma established liver mets Balb/c mice	Vaccinia Oncolysate Intrasplenic Day 0; (10^5) 0.2 ml (10^6 cells) sc, flanks Day 4, Day 10	Roche rIL-2 (10^6) U/ml)[1] ip 25,000 U bid Days 11–13	-40% improved survival -lower liver weight -with IFNα, total protection	***58***
CT26 pulmonary mets +/– β-galactosidase (β-gal) expression Balb/c mice	iv, 10^5 rVV or rFPV[2] with β-gal 5×10^6–10^7 PFU Day 3 or Day 6	Chiron rIL-2 300,000 IU bid ip for 3 days 12 hrs post immunization or 90,000 IU bid ip for 6 days 12 hrs post immunization	-increased anti-β-gal CTL -increased survival -tumor recurred that was β-gal negative	***59***
MC-38 colon carcinoma expressing CEA C57BI/6 mice	3×10^5 sc Day 0 rV-CEA 10^7 PFU/10 μL tail scarification Day 7 or Day 10	Chiron rIL-2 -with 1% mouse serum -73 hr post rV-CEA daily for 5 days -0.1–5.0 μg/mouse ip bid	-complete tumor regression in 60–70% tumor-bearing mice (vs 30% with rV-CEA only) -protective against rechallenge -protective against rechallenge -increased CTL	***60***
MC-12 fibrosarcoma (C57BL/6 × Balb/c) F1	irradiated MC-12 100 μg Day 0, D35 Challenge on D56 sc	natural IL-2 20,000 IU/0.5 mL ip bid × 5 Days Days 3–8, Days 38–42	-controls = 25/26 tumor + -Vaccine = 15/25 tumor + -Vaccine + IL-2 = 4/25	***61***

[1]1 Roche IL-2 U = 3 IU; [2] rVV= vaccinia virus, rFPV = fowlpox virus.

are antigen and disease dependent, more experimental work needs to be done to elucidate the proper mix of antigen and cytokine for safe and effective vaccines.

2. Materials

Proleukin® (aldesleukin) recombinant human IL-2 is manufactured by Chiron Corporation (Emeryville, CA). Proleukin® is a 15 kD protein manufactured by recombinant technology and is similar to the natural IL-2 found in humans. It differs from the native molecule by being nonglycosylated (*Escherichia coli* derived), lacking an alanine at the N-terminal, and having a serine substituted for a cysteine at amino acid position 125. Proleukin® is supplied as a lyophilized cake in vials containing 1.3 mg of protein (22 mIU).

Studies of bioactivity after dilution of reconstituted Proleukin® in diluents of 5% Dextrose Injection, USP (D5W), containing varying percentages of Human Serum Albumin, USP (HSA), have been performed. A final concentration of 0.1% HSA in D5W has been found to be optimal for maximum recovery of Proleukin® IL-2 biological activity at concentrations below 100 μg/mL. Some loss of bioactivity has been observed with increasing percentages of HSA. Other protein sources can be used for preclinical animal experiments, e.g., mouse serum (1%), bovine serum albumin (0.1%). Reconstituted and diluted Proleukin® contains no bacteriostatic agents. Aseptic technique should be carefully observed during preparation and administration; however, reconstituted Proleukin® should not be filtered. Following reconstitution, samples of Proleukin® kept at 4°C (39°F) for up to 14 d have been subsequently cultured for 48 h and found to be free of microbial contamination. Alternatively, dilutions can be frozen for up to 1 yr at –80°C and retain activity, as long as exogenous carrier protein is in the diluent.

3. Methods

Each vial of Proleukin® should be reconstituted with 1.2 mL of Sterile Water for Injection, USP. Reconstitution or dilution with Bacteriostatic Water for Injection, USP, or 0.9% Sodium Chloride Injection, USP, should be avoided because of the potential for precipitation. Vials should be entered once only for reconstitution and once only to remove an aliquot for further dilution, in order to minimize the chance of contamination. The resulting solution should be a clear, colorless liquid. When reconstituted as directed, each mL contains 18 MIU of Proleukin.

For sc, iv, or ip administration, Proleukin® must be further diluted with medium along with 0.1% HSA or other protein source to maintain its stability for 14 d at 2°–8°C. Always dilute the reconstituted stock of Proleukin® into the protein containing diluent.

4. Notes

1. Immunogenicity: Proleukin has been shown to be immunogenic in rodents and rabbits when administered intravenously or subcutaneously (***39*** and data on file). Peak antibody titers can be seen on day 7 during a daily iv administration of 1 mg/kg for 14 d. No relationship has been formally established between onset of anti-Proleukin antibody and efficacy.
2. Storage and Bioactivity: Proleukin, when properly reconstituted and diluted into protein containing medium, can maintain its biological activity for up to 1 yr at –80°C (unpublished results). However, it is recommended that each investigator routinely monitor the biological activity of Proleukin by bioassay using murine HT-2 (ATCC # CRL-1841) cells and the National Biological Standards Board (NBSB, National Institute for Biological Standards and Control, Hertfordshire, U.K.) IL-2 standard. Briefly, IL-2 samples and standards are serially diluted in triplicate and then added to the murine HT-2 cells in a microtiter plate. The HT-2 cell line is completely dependent on IL-2 for growth and proliferates in a dose-dependent manner in response to exogenous IL-2. The amount of cell proliferation is measured by the incorporation of the tetrazolium salt 3-(4,5 dimethylthiazol-2-y1)-2,5-diphenyltetrazolium bromide (MTT) into the cells after 18–24 h of culture. The MTT salt crystals are solubilized with acid and the wells read at 570 nm.

References

1. Heath, W. W. and Playfair, J. H. L. (1992) Cytokines as immunological adjuvants. *Vaccine* **10,** 427–434.
2. Hughes, H. P. A. and Babiuk, L. A. (1992) The adjuvant potential of cytokines. *Biotechnol. Therapeut.* **3,** 101–117.
3. Heath, A. W. (1995) Cytokines as adjuvants, in *Vaccine Design: The Subunit and Adjuvant Approach* (Pavell, M. F. and Neuman, M. J., eds.), Plenum, New York.
4. Wolf, S. F., Sieburth, D., and Sypek, J. (1994) Interleukin 12: a key modulator of immune function. *Stem Cells* **12,** 154–168.
5. Germann, T., Gately, M. K., Schoenhaut, D. S., Lohoff, M., Mattner, F., Fischer, S., et al. (1993) Interleukin-12/T cell stimulating factor: a cytokine with multiple effects on T helper type 1 (TH1) but not on TH2 cells. *Europ. J. Immunol.* **23,** 1762–1770.
6. Afonso, L. C., Scharton, T. M., Vieira, L. Q., Wysocka, T., Trinchieri, G., and Scott, P. (1994) IL-12 functions as an effective adjuvant in a vaccine against *Leishmania major* by directing the development of leishmanial specific CD4+ T h1 cells. *Science* **263,** 235–237.
7. Letscher-Bru, V., Villard, O., Risse, B., Sauke, M., Klein, J.-P., and Kien, T. T. (1998) Protective effect of vaccination with a combination of recombinant surface antigen 1 and interleukin-12 against Toxoplasmosis in mice. *Infec. Immun.* **66,** 4503–4506.

8. Kim, J. J., Ayyavoo, B., Bagarazzi, M. L., Chattergoon, M. A., Dang, K., Wang, B., et al. (1997) In vivo engineering of a cellular immune response by coadministration of IL-12 expression vector with a DNA immunogen. *J. Immunol.* **158,** 816–826.
9. Kursawa, H., Wysocka, M., Aruga, E., Chang, A. E., Trinchieri, G., and Lee, W. M. F. (1998) Recombinant interleukin-12 enhances cellular immune response to vaccination only after a period of suppression. *Cancer Res.* **58,** 491–499.
10. Rodolfo, M., Silocchi, C., Melani, C., Cappetti, B., Arioli, I., Parmiani, G., and Colombo, M. P. (1996) Immunotherapy of experimental metastases by vaccination with interleukin-12 gene-transduced adenocarcinoma cells sharing tumor-associated antigens. *J. Immunol.* **157,** 5536–5542.
11. Tahara, H., Zitvogel, L., Storkus, W. J., Zeh, H. J., McKinney, T. G., Schreiber, R. D., et al. (1995) Effective eradication of established murine tumors with IL-12 gene therapy using a polycistronic retroviral vector. *J. Immunol.* **154,** 6466–6474.
12. Metcalf, D. (1985) The granulocyte-macrophage colony-stimulating factors. *Science* **229,** 16–22.
13. Tarr, P. E., Lin, R., Mueller, E. A., Kovarik, M., Guillaume, M., and Jones, T. C. (1996) Evaluation of tolerability and antibody response after recombinant human granulocyte-macrophage colony-stimulating factor (rhGM-CSF) and a single dose of recombinant hepatitis B vaccine. *Vaccine* **14,** 1199–1204.
14. Callard, R. and Gearing, A. eds. (1994) GM-CSF, in *Cytokine Facts Book.* Academic, New York, pp. 139–143.
15. Disis, M. L., Bernhard, H., Shiota, F. M., Hand, S. L., Gralow, J. R., Huseby, E. S., et al. (1996) Granulocyte-macrophage colony-stimulating factor: an effective adjuvant for protein and peptide-based vaccines. *Blood* **88,** 202–210.
16. Weiss, W. R., Ishii, K. J., Hedstrom, R. C., Sedegah, M., Ichino, M., Barnhart, K., et al. (1998) A plasmid encoding murine granulocyte-macrophage colony-stimulating factor increases protection conferred by a malaria DNA vaccine. *J. Immunol.* **161,** 2325–2332.
17. Dranoff, G., Jaffee, E., Lazenby, A., Golumbek, P., Levitsky, H., Brose, K., et al. (1993) Vaccination with irradiated tumor cells engineered to secrete murine granulocyte-macrophage colony-stimulating factor stimulates potent, specific, and long-lasting anti-tumor immunity. *Proc. Natl. Acad. Sci. USA* **90,** 3539–3543.
18. Morgan, D. A., Ruscetti, F. W., and Gallo, R. (1976) Selective in vitro growth of T lymphocytes from normal human bone marrows. *Science* **193,** 1007–1008.
19. Mier, J. W. and Gall, R. C. (1985) The purification and properties of human T cell growth factor. *J. Immunol.* **128,** 1122–1127.
20. Atkins, M. B. and Mier, J. W., eds. (1993) *Therapeutic Applications of Interleukin-2.* Marcel Dekker, New York.
21. Schumann, R. R., Nakaral, T., Gruss, H. J., Brach, M. A., Vanm Arnim, U., Kirschning, C., et al. (1996) Transcript synthesis and surface expression of the

interleukin-2 receptor (alpha-, beta-, and gamma chain) by normal and malignant myeloid cells. *Blood* **87,** 2419–2427.

22. Bartlett, Y. (1998) Potential monitoring value of functional interleukin-2 receptors on human neutrophils. *Clinic. Diagnos. Lab. Immunol.* **5,** 270.
23. Taniguchi, T. and Minami, Y. (1993) The IL-2/IL-2 receptor system: a current overview. *Cell* **73,** 5–8.
24. de Jong, J. L., Farner, N. L., Widmer, M. B., Giri, J. G., and Sondel, P. M. (1996) Interaction of IL-15 with the shared IL-2 receptor beta and gamma c subunits: the IL-15/beta/gamma c receptor-ligand complex is less stable than the IL-2/beta/gamma c receptor-ligand complex. *J. Immunol.* **156,** 1339–1248.
25. Callard, R. and Gearing, A., eds. (1994) IL-2 and IL-2R, in *The Cytokine Facts Book*. Academic, London and New York, pp. 39–45.
26. Caligiuri, M. A. (1993) Low-dose recombinant interleukin-2 therapy: rationale and potential clinical applications. *Seminars in Oncol.* **20,** suppl. 9, 3–10.
27. David, D., Bani, L., Moreau, J-L., Demaison, C., Sun, K., Salvucci, O., et al. (1998) Further analysis of interleukin-2 receptor subunit expression on the different human peripheral blood mononuclear cell subsets. *Blood* **91,** 165–172.
28. McElrath, M. J., Kaplan, G., Burkhardt, R. A., and Cohn, Z. A. (1990) Cutaneous responses to recombinant interleukin-2 in human immunodeficiency virus-1 seropositive individuals. *Proc. Natl. Acad. Sci. USA* **87,** 5783–5787.
29. Murray, H. W., DePamphilis, J., Schooley, R. T., and Hirsch, M. S. (1988) Circulating Interferon gamma in AIDS patients treated with interleukin-2. *N. Engl. J. Med.* **318,** 1538–1539.
30. Murray, H. W., Welte, K., Jacobs, J. L., Rubin, B. Y., Mertelsmann, R., and Roberts, R. B. (1985) Production of and in vitro response to interleukin 2 in the acquired immunodeficiency syndrome. *J. Clinic. Investig.* **76,** 1959–1964.
31. Bykovskaja, S. N., Buffo, S. J., Bunker, M., Shang, H., Majors, A., Herbert, M., et al. (1998) Interleukin-2 induces development of dendritic cells from cord blood CD34+ cells. *J. Leukocyte Biology* **63,** 620–630.
32. Benedetto, N., Auriault C., Darcy F., Lando D., Watier H., and Capron, A. (1991) Effect of rIFNγ and IL-2 treatments in mouse and nude rat infections with *Toxoplasma gondii. Europ. Cytokine Net.* **2,** 107–114.
33. Jeevan, A. and Asherson, G. L. (1988) Recombinant interleukin-2 limits the replication of *Mycobacterium lepraemurium* and *Mycobacterium bovis* BCG in mice. *Lymphokine Res.* **7,** 129–140.
34. Reddehase, M. J., Mutter, W., and Koszinowski, U. H. (1987) In vivo application of recombinant interleukin 2 in the immunotherapy of established cytomegalovirus infection. *J. Exp. Med.* **165,** 650–656.
35. Bonavida, B., Katz, J., and Gottlieb, M. (1986) Mechanism of defective NK cell activity in patients with acquired immunodeficiency syndrome (AIDS) and AIDS-related complex. *J. Immunol.* **137,** 1157–1163.
36. Toosi, Z., Kleinhenz, M. E., Ellner, J. J. (1986) Defective interleukin-2 production and responsiveness in human pulmonary tuberculosis. *J. Exp. Med.* **163,** 1162–1172.

37. Sheridan, J. F., Aurelian, L., Sonnenberg, A. D., and Quinn, T. C. (1984) Cell-mediated immunity to cytomegalovirus (CMV) and herpes simplex virus (HSV) antigens in the acquired immunodeficiency syndrome: interleukin-1 and interleukin-2 modify in vitro responses. *J. Clinic. Immunol.* **4,** 304–311.
38. Dix, R. D., Giedlin, M., and Cousins, S. W. (1997) Systemic cytokine immunotherapy for experimental cytomegalovirus retinitis in mice with retrovirus-induced immunodeficiency. *Investigat. Opthalmol. Visual Sci.* **38,** 1411–1417.
39. Connors, M., Kovacs, J. A., Kreva, S., Gea-Banacloche, J. C., Sneller, M. C., Flanigan, M., et al. (1997) HIV infection induces changes in CD4+ T-cell phenotype and depletions within the CD4+ T-cell repertoire that are not immediately restored by antiviral or immune-based therapies. *Nature Med.* **3,** 533–540.
40. Fei, P. C., Solmone, M., Viora, M., Vanacore, P., Pugliese, O., Giglio, A., et al. (1994) Apoptosis in HIV infection: protective role of IL-2. *J. Biolog. Regulators Homerostatic Agents* **8,** 60–64.
41. Bell, S. J. D., Cooper, D. A., Kemp, B. E., Doherty, R. R., and Penny, R. (1992) Heterogenous effects of exogenous IL-2 on HIV-specific cell-mediated immunity (CMI). *Clinic. Exp. Immunol.* **90,** 6–12.
42. Barker, E., Mackewicz, C. E., and Levy, J. A. (1995) Effects of TH1 and TH2 cytokines on CD8+ T-cell response against human immunodeficiency virus: implications for long-term survival. *Proc. Natl. Acad. Sci. USA* **92,** 11,135–11,139.
43. Zerhouni, B., Sanhadji, K., Kehrli, L., Livrozet, J. M., and Touraine, J. L. (1997) Interleukin (IL)-2 deficiency aggravates the defect of natural killer cell activity in AIDS patients. *Thymus.* **24,** 147–156.
44. Weinberg, A. and Merigan, T. C. (1988) Recombinant interleukin 2 as an adjuvant for vaccine-induced protection. *J. Immunol.* **140,** 294–299.
45. Nunberg, J. H., Doyle, M. V., and Newell, A. D. (1988) Interleukin-2 as an adjuvant to vaccination, in *Technological Advances in Vaccine Development* (Lasky, L., ed.), Alan R Liss, New York.
46. Nunberg, J. H., Doyle, M. V., York, S. M., and York, C. J. (1989) Interleukin 2 acts as an adjuvant to enhance the potency of inactivated rabies virus vaccine. *Proc. Natl. Acad. Sci. USA* **86,** 4240–4243.
47. Kawamura, H., Rosenberg, S. A., and Berzofsky, J. A. (1985) Immunization with antigen and interleukin 2 in vivo overcomes *Ir* gene low responsiveness. *J. Exp. Med.* **162,** 381–386.
48. Good, M. F., Pombo, D., Lunde, M. N., Maloy, W. L., Halenbeck, R., Koths, K., et al. (1988) Recombinant IL-2 overcomes genetic nonresponsiveness to malaria sporozoite peptides: correlation of effect with biological activity of IL-2. *J. Immunol.* **141,** 972–977.
49. Schijns, V. E. C. J., Claasen, I. J. T. M., Vermeulem, A. A., Horsinek, M. C., and Osterhaus, A. D. M. E. (1994) Modulation of antiviral immune responses by exogenous cytokines: Effects of tumor necrosis factor-α, interleukin-1α, interleukin-2, and interferon-γ on the immunogenicity of an inactivated rabies vaccine. *J. General Virol.* **75,** 55–63.

50. Kawashima, K. and Platt, K. B. (1989) The effect of human recombinant interleukin-2 on the porcine immune response to a pseudorabies virus subunit vaccine. *Veterin. Immunol. Immunopathol.* **22,** 345–353.
51. Zimmerman, R. J., Aukerman, S. L., Katre, N. V., Winkelhake, J. L., and Young, J. D. (1989) Schedule dependency of the antitumor activity and toxicity of polyethylene glycol-modified interleukin 2 in murine tumor models. *Cancer Res.* **49,** 6521–6528.
52. Schmidt, W., Schweighoffer, T., Herbst, E., Maass, G., Berger, M., Schilcher, F., et al. (1995). Cancer vaccines: the interleukin 2 dosage effect. *Proc. Natl. Acad. Sci. USA* **92,** 4711–4714.
53. Delaney, B. and Kaminsky, N. E. (1993) High concentrations of interleukin-2 selectively suppress T-cell dependent humoral immune responses. *Immunopharmacology* **26,** 119–127.
54. Katre, N. V. (1990) Immunogenicity of recombinant IL-2 modified by covalent attachment of polyethylene glycol. *J. Immunol.* **144,** 209–213.
55. Baldwin, S. L., D'Souza, C., Roberts, A. D., Kelly, B. P., Frank, A. A., Lui, M.A., et al. (1998) Evaluation of new vaccines in the mouse and guinea pig model of tuberculosis. *Infec. Immun.* **66,** 2951–2959.
56. Ho, R. J. Y., Burke, R. L., and Merigan, T. C. (1992) Liposome-formulated interleukin-2 as an adjuvant of recombinant HSV glycoprotein gD for the treatment of recurrent genital HSV-2 in guinea pigs. *Vaccine* **10,** 209–213.
57. Hora, M. S., Rana, R. K., Numberg, J. H., Tice, T. R., Gilley, R. M., and Hudsen, M. E. (1990) Controlled release of interleukin-2 from biodegradable microspheres. *Biotechnology* **8,** 755–758.
58. Arroyo, P. J., Bash, J. A., and Wallack, M. K. (1990) Active immunotherapy with vaccinia colon oncolysate enhances the immunomodulatory and antitumor effects of interleukin-2 and interferon-α in a murine hepatic metastasis model. *Cancer Immunol. Immunother.* **31,** 305–311.
59. Bronte, V., Tsung, K., Rao, J. B., Chen, P. W., Wang, M., Rosenberg, S. A., and Restifo, N. P. (1995) IL-2 enhances the function of recombinant poxvirus-based vaccines in the treatment of established pulmonary metastases. *J. Immunol.* **154,** 5282–5292.
60. McLaughlin, J. P., Schlom, J., Kantor, J. S., and Greiner, J. W. (1996) Improved immunotherapy of a recombinant carcinoembryonic antigen vaccinia vaccine when given with interleukin-2. *Cancer Res.* **56,** 2361–2367.
61. Vondrys, P., Simova, J., Takacova, S. Jandlove, T., and Bubenik, J. (1997) Recombinant interleukin-2 acts as an adjuvant and helps to increase the efficacy of tumor vaccines. *Folia Biologica (Praha)* **43,** 39,40.
62. Everse, L. A., Bernsen, M. R., Dullens, H. F. J., and Otter, W. D. (1997) Priming of the antitumor response promotes efficacy of interleukin-2 therapy. *Cancer Immunol. Immunother.* **44,** 221–229.
63. Harada, M., Matsuzaki, G., Shinomiya, Y., Kurosawa, S., Ito, O., Okamoto, T., et al. (1994) Generation of tumor-specific cytotoxic T lymphocytes in vivo by

combined treatment with inactivated tumor cells and recombinant interleukin-2. *Cancer Immunol. Immunother.* **38,** 332–338.

64. Shimiza, K., Fields, R. C., Giedlin, M., Mulé, J. J. (1999) Systemic administration of interleukin-2 enhances the therapeutic efficacy of dendritic cell-based tumor vaccines. *PNAS(USA)* **96,** 2268–2273.
65. Provinciali, M., Di Sefano, G., Colombo, M., Della Croce, F., Gandolfi, M. C., Daghetta, L., et al. (1994) Adjuvant effect of low-dose interleukin-2 on antibody response to influenza virus vaccination in healthy elderly subjects. *Mechan. Aging Develop.* **77,** 75–82.
66. Fagiolo, U., Bordin, M. C., Biselli, R., D'Amelio, R., Zamarchi, R., and Amadori, A. (1997) Effect of rIL-2 treatment on anti-tetanus toxoid response in the elderly. *Mechan. Aging Develop.* **93,** 205–214.

18

DNA As an Adjuvant

David C. Neujahr and David S. Pisetsky

1. Introduction

DNA is a complex macromolecule with immunological properties that depend on base sequence. Although mammalian DNA is immunologically inert, DNA from bacteria has potent immunostimulatory properties that result from short sequence motifs called CpG motifs or immunostimulatory sequences (ISS). These motifs, which have the general structure of two 5′ purines, an unmethylated CpG motif, and two 3′ pyrimidines, occur much more commonly in bacterial DNA than mammalian DNA because of two main factors: CpG suppression and the frequent methylation of cytosine in this position in mammalian DNA *(1)*. As a result, bacterial DNA displays (in code-like fashion) sequences emblematic of foreignness. This code allows DNA to function as a danger signal in the induction of innate immunity *(2)*.

Although the role of bacterial DNA in stimulating normal host defense is uncertain, the immunological properties of this molecule are nevertheless highly relevant to emerging vaccine technologies. Thus, bacterial DNA has adjuvant properties. These properties, which have been most clearly demonstrated in the murine system, include the induction of cytokines [interferon gamma, alpha, beta; tumor necrosis factor alpha; interleukin 6, 12, and 18 (IFN-γ, IFN-α/β, TNF-α, IL-6, IL-12, IL-18)] as well as the direct stimulation of murine B cells *(3–6)*. The basis of DNA stimulation has been assessed using three major sources of DNA: natural DNA, synthetic phosphodiester oligonucleotides (Po oligos), and phosphorothioate oligonucleotides (Ps oligos). Ps compounds are DNA derivatives in which one of the nonbridging oxygens in the phosphodiester backbone is replaced by a sulfur atom. This substitution leads to nuclease resistance, as well as changes in other physical properties of DNA such as melting temperature *(7)*.

From: *Methods in Molecular Medicine, Vol. 42:*
Vaccine Adjuvants: Preparation Methods and Research Protocols
Edited by: D. T. O'Hagan © Humana Press, Inc., Totowa, NJ

In general, Ps oligos are much more potent than Po oligos, leading to their use as adjuvants and immunomodulators. The spectrum of activities of Ps and Po oligos, however, may differ. For example, Ps oligos can effectively stimulate human B cells in vitro whereas Po oligos as well as natural DNA are inactive. Furthermore, immune stimulation by Ps oligos may show different structure–function relationships than Po oligos *(8)*. Among Ps oligos, immune stimulation is not as much dependent on the number and sequence of CpG motifs as Po oligos. Furthermore, immune stimulation by Ps oligos appears to be a feature of the modified backbone, as well as sequence *(9)*, indicating caution in extrapolating from results with Ps oligos to Po oligos and natural DNA. The marked differences in responsiveness of human and murine cells to Po oligos should also be a caveat in interpreting studies on immune activities of DNA.

At present, there are two major settings in which adjuvant properties of bacterial DNA, as illustrated in **Fig. 1**, are relevant. The first setting is DNA vaccination where the vector itself contains ISS. This approach involves the administration of plasmid DNA encoding a protein targeted for a therapeutic or protective response. This vector is taken up into cells where it can be expressed and can induce immune responses. The encoded protein to be targeted can be a foreign protein from a virus, bacteria, or protozoa, for example, as well as an endogenous protein such as a tumor-specific antigen.

DNA vaccines have theoretic advantages over conventional vaccines because they lead to both CD4 and CD8 responses, provide for a long-term source of protein for immunization, and allow antigen presentation within the context of self-MHC molecules *(10)*. Whereas the plasmid vector may be administered by various routes (i.e., intramuscular, intradermal, gene gun), ultimately, bone marrow-derived antigen-presenting cells (APC) are key to the response *(11)*.

The plasmid vectors used for these vaccinations are propagated in bacteria and, as such, bear bacterial sequences needed for replication and other functions such as antibiotic resistance. Furthermore, because of their growth in bacteria, these vectors show a bacterial pattern of base methylation and have unmethylated cytosines. The combination of bacterial sequence and methylation status ensures the presence of ISS centering on unmethylated CpG motifs. The number of ISS in these vectors will vary depending on the base sequence of various encoded genetic elements. Because of these structural features, these vectors have built-in adjuvants.

Vector ISS can enhance vaccine responses as well skew the response to a Th1 pattern because of the stimulation of IL-12, IFN-γ, as well as IFN-α/β. The potential importance of such sequences is highlighted by several lines of experimental evidence in animal models. Thus, most responses induced by DNA vaccines are Th1-like in mice and show a predominance of IgG_2a. Sec-

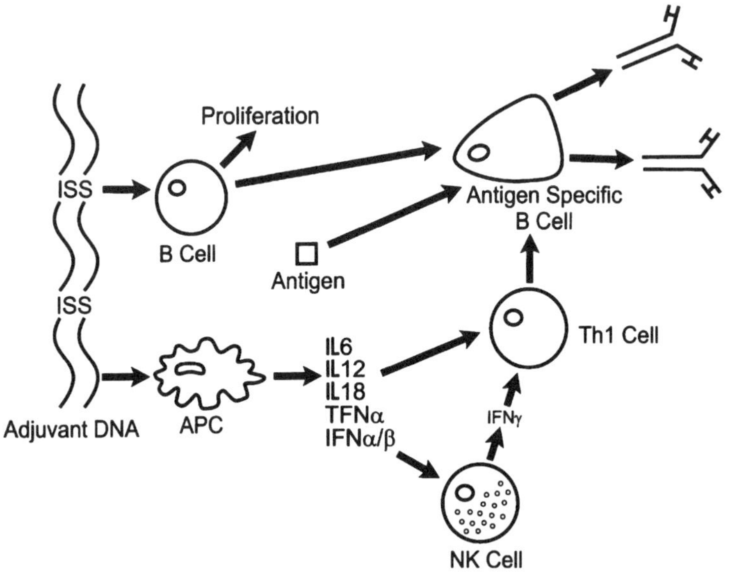

Fig. 1. Mechanisms for the adjuvant effect of DNA. In this schematic, adjuvant DNA represents either plasmid DNA or an oligonucleotide containing an ISS.

ond, methylation of a vector can eliminate the vaccine response. Third, the magnitude of the vaccine response may vary with the number of ISS in encoded genetic elements. And, fourth, the presence of CpG motifs in the vector may influence the development of Th1 vs Th2 responses, with this balance shifted by coadministration of a noncoding vector with a CpG motif *(12,13)*.

Whereas vector ISS can induce cytokines leading to a Th1 response, the in vivo response may depend on other factors. The nature of the protein encoded by the vector may also influence the pattern of responsiveness as shown by induction of a Th2 response by a vector encoding a soluble malaria protein *(14)*. In addition, the method for DNA delivery may alter the Th1/Th2 balance. When delivered by gene gun techniques, plasmids that contain CpG motifs can elicit a Th2 response, despite their capacity to stimulate IL-12 and the interferons *(15)*. The adjuvant properties of DNA vectors may also vary depending on the setting because the genetic background of experimental animals can influence the pattern of immune responsiveness. For example, BI0.D2 mice generate a much stronger Th1 response than Balb/c mice to Leishmania *(16)*.

Although the responsiveness of animals to DNA vaccines has been impressive, studies on humans are still in their initial phases. The responses of humans to DNA adjuvants has had limited investigation, although certain differences between mouse and human are already apparent. Thus, human B cells

Table 1
Clinical Settings for DNA Adjuvants

Use of DNA adjuvants	Goal(s)	Examples
Viral Infection	Induction of CD4 and CD8 responses	DNA vaccines for Hep B, HSV, and influenza ***(18,34,35)***.
Bacterial Infection	Induction of CD4 and CD8 responses	DNA vaccines for tuberculosis ***(36)***.
Parasitic Infection	Cellular and humoral immunity toward organism	Oligos and DNA vaccines for malaria and leishmania ***(24,37,38)***.
Cancer	Increase interferon, induce antitumor responses	Antitumor effect of bacterial DNA ***(3)***. CpG oligo enhancement of anti-Id responses ***(25)***.
Allergy	Decrease IgE responses	DNA vaccines for dust mite and latex allergens ***(19,39)***.
Autoimmunity	Anti-TCR	DNA based thearpy for EAE ***(20)***.

do not respond to natural DNA or Po oligos under conditions in which these compounds are potent mitogens for murine B cells ***(8)***. In addition, induction of cytokine responses in human cells appears to be more sporadic than murine cells ***(17)***. Whether these differences will affect vaccine responses is unknown, although the absence of B-cell mitogenicity may make the plasmid vectors less effective in humans than other species.

The second setting in which DNA can serve as an adjuvant involves coadministration of DNA or an oligo with a conventional vaccine such as a protein or subunit. In this situation, the effect of the adjuvant is likely to be local and involve cytokine stimulation as well as enhancement of APC function by inducing the expression of Class II or costimulatory molecules. Perhaps as a consequence of these activities, Ps oligos containing ISS can also promote CTL responses when used as adjuvants ***(18)***.

Table 1 provides examples of the settings in which the immunomodulatory effects of DNA are important in the induction of protective responses, either as integral components of DNA vaccines or as synthetic oligonucleotide adjuvants. In the case of allergic disease, protection results from a redirection of the response from IgE ***(19)***. Although not extensively investigated so far, DNA adjuvants can also be used in the treatment and prevention of autoimmune disease by inducing, for example, an anticlonotypic T-cell response or a response to an MHC antigen ***(20)***.

Both Ps and Po compounds can be used for these adjuvant purposes, although Ps compounds may be preferable because of their resistance to nuclease digestion, as well as their long in vivo half-life ***(7)***. These compounds can be less than 30 bases in length and can be modified to contain sequences to enhance cell uptake. Thus, the presence of extended sequences of dG residues can dramatically increase macrophage cytokine production by an ISS ***(21)***. This effect results from the binding of dG sequences to the Type A macrophage scavenger receptor (MSR). This receptor has broad specificity for polyanions, including dG-rich DNA ***(22)***.

In assessing adjuvant properties of bacterial DNA, as well as synthetic oligos, we have focused on in vitro assays of cytokine production, as well as B-cell mitogenesis using murine spleen culture. Available evidence indicates that in vitro and in vivo assays provide similar information concerning the relative immunostimulatory activity of DNAs, although a recent study noted discrepancies among Ps oligos ***(9)***. Furthermore, although DNA sequences for B cell and macrophage stimulation are similar, some compounds may differ in the stimulation of IL-12 compared to TNF-α ***(23)***.

Similar to other adjuvants, DNA and synthetic oligos likely have both systemic and local effects. For example, in a murine model of Leishmaniasis, CpG containing oligos injected 20 d after infection were able to redirect the immune system toward a curative Th1 response ***(24)***. These findings point to generalized effects that do not require direct contact with antigen. On the other hand, in a murine lymphoma model, administration of Ps oligos on the same flank as an idiotype (Id) protein led to higher anti-Id titers, as well as tumor resistance, than observed when the oligo was injected in the opposite flank ***(25)***. Whereas studies on the use of ISS containing oligos together with conventional adjuvants are limited, findings by Sun et al. indicate that Ps oligos in Freund's incomplete adjuvant (FIA) are more potent than Ps oligos delivered in saline. Similarly, insect DNA was inactive as an adjuvant in saline, but had significant effect when delivered in FIA ***(26)***.

Given the potent effects of ISS DNA, concerns about safety inevitably arise. To the extent that ISS DNA can shift the balance of the immune system, treatment with a DNA adjuvant could lead to adverse reactions by modifying the host response to an infection or, alternatively, inducing or potentiating autoimmune reactions. Although treatment of mice with ISS DNA does not in itself induce anti-DNA autoantibodies, immunization with complexes of bacterial DNA with a protein carrier in Freund's complete adjuvant leads to a significant anti-DNA response that, in certain strains of mice, is associated with nephritis

(27,28). It is possible that the safety of DNA adjuvants will be affected by the vaccine formulation with adverse immune reactions increased depending on the nature of the immunizing antigen as well as the vehicle (e.g., FIA). In this regard, safety of Ps and Po compounds may differ in man because of the B-cell stimulatory activity of Ps compounds, as well as their enhanced potency and longer half-life in vivo.

Ultimately, the test of an adjuvant will be the in vivo setting and involve both a specific protein (or vector), as well as a specific animal species. In optimizing this approach, it will therefore be important to assess the influence of vaccine formulation, as well as any physical association between antigen and DNA adjuvant. As a prelude to in vivo studies, in vitro assays allow high through-put screening and assessment of issues such as the basis of DNA binding and uptake. The approach outlined below can be readily adapted to the study of human cells as these technologies enter greater trials in patients.

2. Materials

1. Mice. Mice 6–8 wk old BALB/c females maintained in a pathogen-free facility receiving food and water.
2. Control nucleic acids. The following Po oligos can serve as positive and negative controls, respectively: 5′TCCATGACGTTCCTGATGCT-3′ and 5′-CTTCAA GAATTCTCATGTTTG-3′ (Midland Certified Reagents, Midland, TX). Store nucleic acids at 4°C where they are stable for up to 6 mo.
3. LPS from *Escherichia coli* 0111:B4 (Sigma, St. Louis, MO). Dilute to 1 mg/mL final concentration in RPMI-1640. Store at 4°C with stability up to 6 mo.
4. RPMI-1640 (Life Technologies, Gaithersberg, MD) fortified with 1.5 m*M* L-glutamine, 5% FCS (Hyclone, Logan, UT), 50 μ*M* 2-ME, and gentamicin (0.5 mL/100 mL media).
5. Limulus Amebocyte Lysate Assay kit (BioWhittaker, Walkersville, MD).
6. LAL stop solution. 10% SDS (Bio-Rad, Hercules, CA) in ddH_2O.
7. Titertek Microplate Reader (Flow Laboratories, McLean,VA).
8. Enzyme-linked immunosorbent assays (ELISA) reagents: All antibodies are from PharMingen, San Diego, CA. Antibodies are rat antimouse IFN-γ (cat.#18181D), biotinylated rat antimouse IFN-γ (cat.#18112D), rat antimouse IL-12 p40/p70 (cat#18491D), and biotinylated rat antimouse IL-12 p40/p70 (cat #18482D).
9. IFN-γ and IL-12 standards (PharMingen): IFN-γ standards are reconstituted in sterile ddH_2O and stored as 25-μL aliquots of 5×10^4 U/mL. IL-12 standards are reconstituted in ddH_2O and stored as 10-μL aliquots of 10-μg/mL. All standards are stored at –70°C with stability up to 1 yr.
10. HRP-Avidin (Zymed, San Francisco, CA). Store at 4°C.
11. RBC lysis solution: Add 90 mL of sterile 0.16 *M* NH_4Cl to 10 mL of sterile 0.17 *M* Tris- HCl pH 7.6. Store at 4°C.

12. DNase reagents: DNase I (Sigma), reconstitute to 1 mg/mL in ddH_2O and store in 10-µL aliquots at –20°C with stability up to 1 yr. 0.1 *M* $MgCl_2$, 0.5 *M* Tris-HCl pH 7.5, stable at room temperature.
13. 3H-thymidine (NEN, Boston, MA) prepared by adding 200 µL of stock 3H-thymidine (1 mCi/mL) to 10 mL serum-free RPMI. Store diluted 3H-thymidine at 4°C.
14. A Packard Instrument Tri-carb 4530 Beta scintillation counter or equivalent.
15. Cytoscint liquid scintillation cocktail (ICN, Costa Mesa, CA).
16. Plasticware: 96-well tissue-culture plates (Costar, Cambridge, MA), 96-well polypropylene plates (Sigma, 96-well Immulon 2 ELISA plates (Dynex, Chantilly, VA).
17. TMB/citrate buffer. Prepare citrate buffer as 0.1 *M* citric acid pH 4.0 and store at 4°C. Prepare TMB(3,3′,5,5′-tetramethylbenzidine dihydrochloride, Sigma) as 0.75% solution in 0.5-mL aliquots. Degas solution before placing in aliquots. Store TMB at –20°C. Make TMB/Citrate/H_2O_2 detection solution immediately before use.

3. Methods

3.1. Principles of Assays for Immunostimulatory DNA

Although bacterial DNA induces multiple activities (*see* **Note 1**), assay of IL-12, IFN-γ, and 3H-thymidine incorporation represents an efficient and cost-effective means of comparing activities of DNA. In addition, these assays allow comparisons of effects on different cell types. IL-12 is produced by macrophages *(29)*. IFN-γ is produced by NK cells in response to bacterial DNA and IL-12 *(30)*. 3H-thymidine incorporation reflects B cell activation. The general methods outlined below utilize primary cell cultures, but can be modified for cell lines as well.

An important issue in assessing adjuvant properties of a DNA concerns the presence of endotoxin. All DNA samples are assessed for endotoxin contamination by the Limulus Amebocyte Lysis assay. As an additional control, the activity of DNA digested by DNase 1 treatment is tested. In these experiments, splenocytes are obtained by primary cell culture and are incubated along with plasmid DNA for assessment of cytokine by ELISA and proliferation by 3H-thymidine incorporation. As controls, we recommend the use of active and inactive oligonucleotides, as well as LPS.

3.2. Manipulation of Nucleic Acids Prior to Culture

A variety of methods exist for the purification of endotoxin-free nucleic acids and the choice of these depends on the intended application *(31)* (**Note 2**). Methods described below pertain to plasmid DNA.

1. Dilute purified plasmid DNA in endotoxin-free ddH_2O to a final concentration of 1.0 mg/mL in a sterile 1.5-ml Eppendorf tube. This represents the stock from which subsequent dilutions will be made. Dilute control oligonucleotides to a final concentration of 1 mg/mL.
2. In a 96-well microtiter plate, pipet 100 µL of LPS at a concentration of 0.1 µg/mL in ddH_2O. Perform serial 1:2 dilutions with the LPS solution to provide standards ranging from 0.1 µg/mL to 12 pg/mg. The final volume in each well should be 50 µL. In a separate set of wells, add 5 µL of stock DNA to 95 µL of ddH_2O and perform serial 1:2 dilutions to provide concentrations ranging from 50 µg/mL to 0.8 µg/mL.
3. Incubate the microtiter plate at 37°C for 5 min. Following incubation, add 50 µL of the Limulus Amebocye Lysate solution, which is provided in the LAL kit. Mix the plate gently by tapping it several times, then incubate at 37°C for 10 min.
4. Following incubation, add 100 µL of LAL chromogenic substrate provided by the kit to each well. Mix plate gently and incubate at 37°C for 6 min. Standards should begin to turn yellow immediately.
5. Add 100 µL of 10% SDS solution to each well to stop the colorometric reaction (*see* **Note 3**).
6. Measure the absorbance at 405–410 nm of the samples with a microtiter plate reader.
7. Under these conditions, the absorbance at 405–410 nm is linear between 390 pg/mL and 24 pg/mL LPS. From these values, the concentration of endotoxin present in the DNA can be calculated from each dilution. The endotoxin concentration should be less than 5 ng/mg DNA.
8. Prior to cell culture experiments, make plasmid DNA single stranded by incubation in a boiling water bath for 15 min, followed by rapid cooling on ice (*see* **Note 4**).

3.3. DNase Digestion of DNA

The following technique provides enough digested DNA to perform one in vitro assay.

1. In a 600-µL sterile Eppendorf tube, combine 40 µL stock DNA, 5 µL of sterile O.1 *M* $MgCl_2$, 5 µL of sterile 0.5 *M* Tris-HCl pH 7.5, and 2.5 µL of Bovine Pancreas DNase 1 (1 mg/mL).
2. Incubate the tube in a 37°C water bath 1 h (*see* **Note 5**).
3. Following incubation, place the tube in a boiling water bath for 15 min, followed by rapid cooling in ice water.
4. Save 2 µL of digested DNA. Use this sample to assess for complete digestion by gel electrophoresis.

3.4. Preparation of Primary Splenocyte Cultures

1. For assays of IL-12, 5×10^5 cells/well are used. For assays of IFN-γ, 1×10^6 cells/well are used. Balb/c mice at 6–8 wk of age will generally yield 1×10^8 splenocytes.
2. Sacrifice mice by cervical dislocation.

3. Sterilize the abdomen with 70% ethanol and open the peritoneum with sterile forceps and scissors. Remove the spleen from the surrounding connective tissue being careful not to perforate the bowel.
4. Wash spleen gently two times in tissue-culture plates with RPMI containing gentamicin.
5. Under a sterile hood, gently tease apart the spleen using the coarse surfaces of sterile glass slides.
6. Pipet the homogenized spleen into a sterile 15-mL conical tube and allow debris to settle. Carefully transfer the cells to a new conical tube.
7. Centrifuge the cells for 5 min at 450*g* using a table top centrifuge.
8. Decant media from cells and disrupt pellet by gently flicking the tube. Resuspend cells in 5 mL of RBC lysis solution and allow debris to settle for 2 min. Pellet cells by centrifugation as before.
9. Wash cells two more times with 5 mL of RPMI media.
10. Resuspend cells in 10 mL RPMI/10% FCS/50 μ*M* 2-ME. Remove a small aliquot to use for cell count.

3.5. Stimulation of Splenocytes by DNA

1. In a sterile 96-well polypropylene plate, dilute DNA source. Plasmids should be diluted in triplicate wells to a concentration of 100 μg/mL in 110 μL of RPMI/5% FCS 50 μ*M* 2-ME with gentamicin. Perform serial 1:10 dilutions so that the concentration of the DNA ranges from 100 μg/mL to 0.1 μg/mL. The final volume in each well will be 100 μL.
2. In a separate set of wells, dilute LPS to a concentration of 10 μg/mL followed by serial 1:10 dilutions.
3. Add 100 μL of mouse splenocytes obtained in **Subheading 3.4.** to wells in a Costar 96-well tissue-culture plate. Transfer 100 μL of diluted plasmid DNA from the polypropylene plate to the tissue-culture plate to provide a final volume of 200 μL. The highest concentration of plasmid will be 50 μg/mL.
4. Place the 96-well tissue-culture plate in an incubator at 37°C with 5% CO_2.

5a. For cytokine experiments, remove supernatants for assay of IL-12 after 18–24 h and for assay of IFN-γ after 48 h. Plates should be centrifuged briefly prior to removal of supernatants. Carefully remove 100 μL from each well avoiding transfer of cells. Transfer the supernatants to 96-well polypropylene plates. If storage of supernatants is required, seal the plate with parafilm and store at –20°C. Cytokines stored this way are generally stable for 2–3 wk.

5b. For thymidine incorporation, add 25 μL of RPMI containing 3H-thymidine to each well. Incubate for an additional 7 h. Following labeling, absorb cell lysates to glass filters using a microharvester. For each well, wash 20 volumes of ddH_2O through the filter.

3.6. General ELISA Protocol

1. Dilute coating monoclonal antibodies to a final concentration of 1 μg/mL in PBS pH 8.5.

2. Add 100 µL of diluted coating antibody to each well of a 96-well Immulon 2 ELISA plate. Seal the plate with parafilm to prevent evaporation. Allow antibody to coat for 12–18 h at 4°C (*see* **Note 6**).
3. Wash plate four times with PBS/0.1%Tween-20. An automated plate washer is useful in this and subsequent wash steps. Slap the plate against a pile of paper towels to remove residual fluid.
4. Block the wells by adding 200 µL of PBS/1%BSA pH 7.4. Store at room temperature for 30 min.
5. While blocking, prepare samples and standards to be tested. Prepare all samples in a 96-well polypropylene plate prior to use in ELISA to a volume of 100 µL/well. For dilution of samples, add 10 µL of sample to 90 µL of PBS/0.5% BSA/0.05% Tween-20. Dilute stock standards in PBS/0.5% BSA/0.05% Tween-20 to a final concentration of 250 U/mL for IFN-γ and 25 µg/mL for IL-12. Perform 10 serial 1:2 dilutions on the standards.
6. Wash the plate four times, as in **step 3**. Transfer the diluted standards and samples to the ELISA plate. Allow binding to occur at room temperature for 3 h. For increased sensitivity, this step can be extended to an overnight incubation at 4°C.
7. Dilute the biotinylated detection antibody in PBS/0.5% BSA/0.05% Tween-20 to a final concentration of 0.5–1.0 µg/mL.
8. Wash the ELISA plate four times, as in **step 3**. Add 100 µL of dilute detection antibody to each well of the ELISA. Incubate at room temperature for 1 h.
9. Dilute Avidin/HRP 1:5000 in PBS/BSA/Tween. Wash the ELISA plate six times as in **step 3** and apply 100 µL to each well. Incubate room temperature for 30 min.
10. Wash plate at least eight times, as in **step 3**. Between washes prepare developing solution by adding 1 mL of 0.75% TMB and 17 µL of 30% H_2O_2 to 50 mL of citrate buffer. To each well, add 200 µL of developing solution. Place plate in dark while developing. Allow plate to develop for 20–30 min before measuring absorbance.
11. Measure the absorbance at 380 nm using a microplate reader. At this wavelength, values for the highest concentration of standard should range from 2.0 to 1.5 OD. If OD values are low, continue incubation and measure absorbance after 10 additional min.
12. The concentration of cytokines in a sample can be calculated from a standard curve using a program such as Cricket Graph or Microsoft Excel. The linefit function of these programs can be used to generate an exponential relationship between OD and cytokine concentration.

3.7. Calculating Thymidine Incorporation

1. After harvesting cells on glass filters, transfer filters into a scintillation vial and add 5 mL of scintillation fluid.
2. Record cpm from vial in a liquid scintillation counter calibrated for 3H energy.
3. Data from thymidine incorporation experiments can be recorded in cycles per minute (cpm). Alternatively, data can be displayed as Δcpm by subtracting the cpm obtained from cells stimulated with media alone (*see* **Notes 7** and **8**).

4. Notes

1. Because of the interest in adjuvant properties of DNA and induction of Th1 responses, we have described methods for measuring IL-12, IFN-γ, and B-cell mitogenesis. There are many other assays of immunostimulation, with the choice dependent on the intended application for the DNA. Similar methods can be used to measure Th2 cytokines, IL-4, and IL-10, as well as TNF-α. In this regard, TNF-α can be induced by plasmids or oligonucleotides. Although TNF-α is a mediator of septic shock induced by bacterial DNA ***(32)***, it is doubtful that this activity poses any significant safety issues under conditions in which DNA vaccines or oligos would be utilized.
2. A wide variety of protocols exist for the purification of plasmid DNA. It is critical that DNA be free of contaminating endotoxin because the presence of this material can confound interpretation of the activity of DNA vaccines or oligos. A number of commercially available kits exist for the removal of endotoxin from DNA. We have utilized the Qiagen endotoxin removal kit to obtain plasmid DNA which is free of detectable levels of LPS. There are other approaches to address the issues of endotoxin contamination. Cell-culture experiments can be performed in the presence of polymyxin B, using a concentration shown to inhibit the mitogenic effects of LPS. We have found that polymyxin B at concentrations as low as 2 μg/mL can abrogate the effects of LPS in vitro with little effect on the immunostimulatory effects of DNA. Investigators may consider the use of endotoxin-resistant C3H/HeJ mice. Our experiments have shown that splenocytes from C3H/HeJ mice respond to DNA similar to other strains.
3. For increased sensitivity with the LAL assay, the incubation step with the chromogenic substrate can be extended to 30 min or more.
4. Although any preparation of purified DNA can be used for stimulation, we commonly use single-strand DNA (ssDNA), which has been subjected to heat denaturation. We have found that ssDNA recapitulates the activity of native DNA and eliminates uncertainty in relative content of single- vs double-stranded regions. Oligonucleotides used in these experiments are synthesized as single-stranded species and do not require heat denaturation. At present there is little information on the relative safety and efficacy of single- vs double-stranded DNA, although their in vivo clearance may differ.
5. Nucleic acids that have been digested by DNase I can have apparent inhibitory effects on proliferation assays because unlabeled nucleotides dilute the labeled thymidine. As a result, the recorded Δcpm can be negative and prevent detection of contaminants. To address this issue, we recommend performing a phenol/chloroform extraction of the digest, followed by precipitation in ethanol. This step will efficiently remove nucleotides and DNase, but will preserve any undigested DNA as well as contaminants which copurify with the DNA.
6. IL-12 exists in vivo as a 70 kDa dimer composed of 40 and 35 kDa subunits. The *p35* subunit is constitutively produced by many cells, whereas the *p40* subunit is expressed by macrophages upon stimulation ***(29)***. The reagents for the IL-12 ELISA presented here detect the *p40* subunit. Commercially available reagents

for the detection of *p70* can be purchased. In our hands we have found a correlation between *p40* and *p70* levels, although *p40* levels are generally 5- to 10-fold higher than those of *p70*.

7. The 3H-thymidine incorporation assay allows comparison of the mitogenicity of plasmid DNAs. A potential complication arises when attempting to measure the mitogenic ability of oligonucleotides. Mitogenicity of oligos with a high thymidine content can be underestimated because thymidine resulting from breakdown dilutes the radioactive thymidine pool ***(33)***. As an alternative approach to assess mitogenesis we have used 3H-uridine (NEN, Boston, MA) as the radioactive label. In this way, we have found activity in oligos which appeared inactive by thymidine incorporation.
8. The use of control oligonucleotides allows comparison with a DNA known to have prominent immunostimulatory properties. Using the culture conditions in the methods section, the positive control oligo elicits response in the range of 100 U/mL IFN-γ, 5 ng/mL IL-12 (*p40*), or a Δcpm of 20,000 when the concentration of DNA is 50 μg/mL. We have observed significant increases in these values when conditions such as culture time and cell concentration are increased, but these manipulations also lead to increased background readings to the assays.

References

1. Pisetsky, D. S. (1996) Immune activation by bacterial DNA: a new genetic code. *Immunity* **5,** 303–310.
2. Matzinger, P. (1994) Tolerance, danger, and the extended family. *Ann. Rev. Immunol.* **12,** 991–1045.
3. Yamamoto, S., Yamamoto, T., Shimada, S., Kuramoto, E., Yano, O., Katoka, T., et al. (1992) DNA from bacteria, but not from vertebrates, induces interferons, activates natural killer cells and inhibits tumor growth. *Microbiol. Immunol.* **36,** 983–997.
4. Klinman, D. M., Yi, A-K., Beaucage, S. L., Conover, J., and Krieg, A. M. (1996) CpG motifs present in bacterial DNA rapidly induce lymphocytes to secrete interleukin 6, interleukin 12, and interferon γ. *Proc. Natl. Acad. Sci. USA* **93,** 2879–2883.
5. Sparwasser, T., Miethke, T., Lipford, G., Erdmann, A., Hacker, H., Heeg, K., et al. (1997) Macrophages sense pathogens via DNA motifs: induction of tumor necrosis factor-α-mediated shock. *Eur. J. Immunol.* **27,** 1671–1679.
6. Krieg, A. M., Yi, A., Matson, S., Waldschmidt, T. J., Bishop, G. A., Teasdale, R., et al. (1995) CpG motifs in bacterial DNA trigger direct B-cell activation. *Nature* **374,** 345–349.
7. Stein, C. A., Subasinghe, C., Shinozuka, K., and Cohen, J. S. (1988) Physiochemical properties of phosphorothioate oligodeoxynucleotides. *Nucl. Acids Res.* **16,** 3209–3221.
8. Liang, H., Nishioka, Y., Reich, C. F., Pisetsky, D. S., and Lipsky, P. E. (1996) Activation of human B cells by phosphorothioate oligodeoxynucleotides. *J. Clin. Invest.* **98,** 1119–1129.

9. Montieth, D. K., Henry, S. P., Howard, R. B., Flournoy, S., Levin, A. A., Bennett, C. F., et al. (1997) Immune stimulation—a class effect of phosphorothioate oligodeoxynucleotides in rodents. *Anti-Cancer Drug Design* **12,** 421–432.
10. Vogel, F. R. and Sarver, N. (1995) Nucleic acid vaccines. *Clin. Microbiol. Rev.* **8,** 406–410.
11. Corr, M., Lee, D. J., Carson, D. A., and Tighe, H. (1996) Gene vaccination with naked plasmid DNA: mechanism of CTL priming. *J. Exp. Med.* **184,** 1555–1560.
12. Leclerc, C., Deriaud, E., Rojas, M., and Whalen, R. G. (1997) The preferential induction of a Th1 immune response by DNA-based immunization is mediated by the immunostimulatory effect of plasmid DNA. *Cell. Immunol.* **179,** 97–106.
13. Sato, Y., Roman, M., Tighe, H., Lee, D., Corr, M., Nguyen, M-D., et al. (1996) Immunostimulatory DNA sequences necessary for effective intradermal gene immunization. *Science* **273,** 352–354.
14. Mor, G., Klinman, D. M., Shapiro, S., Hagiwara, E., Sedegah, M., Norman, J. A., et al. (1995) Complexity of the cytokine and antibody response elicited by immunizing mice with Plasodium yoelii circumsporozoite protein plasmid DNA. *J. Immunol.* **155,** 2039–2046.
15. Feltquate, D. M., Heaney, S., Webster, R. G., and Robinson H. L. (1997) Different T helper cell types and antibody isotypes generated by saline and gene gun DNA immunization. *J. Immunol.* **158,** 2278–2284.
16. Hsieh, C. S., Macatonia, S. E., O'Garra, A., and Murphy, K. M. (1995) T cell genetic background determines default T helper phenotype development in vitro. *J. Exp. Med.* **181,** 713–721.
17. Mashiba, H., Matsunaga, K., Tomoda, H., Furusawa, M., Jimi, S., and Tokunaga, T. (1988) In vitro augmentation of natural killer activity of peripheral blood cells from cancer patients by a DNA fraction from *Mycobacterium bovis* BCG. *Japan. J. Med. Sci. Biol.* **41,** 197–202.
18. Davis, H. L., Weeranta, R., Waldschmidt, T. J., Tygrett, L., Schorr, J., and Kreig, A. M. (1998) CpG DNA is a potent enhancer of specific immunity in mice immunized with recombinant hepatitis B surface antigen. *J. Immunol.* **160,** 870–876.
19. Hsu, C-H., Chua, K-Y., Tao, M-H., Lai, Y-L., Wu, H-D., Huang S-K., et al. (1996) Immunoprophylaxis of allergen-induced immunoglobulin E synthesis and airway hyperresponsiveness in vivo by genetic immunization. *Nat. Med.* **2,** 540–544.
20. Waisman, A., Ruiz, P. J., Hirschberg, D. L., Gelman, A., Oksenberg, J. R., Brocke, S., et al. (1996) Suppressive vaccination with DNA encoding a variable region gene of the T-cell receptor prevents autoimmune encephalomyelitis and activates Th2 immunity. *Nat. Med.* **2,** 899–905.
21. Kimura, Y., Sonehara, K., Kuramoto, E., Makino, T., Yamamoto, S., Yamamoto, T., et al. (1994) Binding of oligoguanylate to scavenger receptors is required for oligonucleotides to augment NK cell activity and induce IFN. *J. Biochem.* **116,** 991–994.
22. Pearson, A. M., Rich, A., and Krieger, M. (1993) Polynucleotide binding to macrophage scavenger receptors depends on the formation of base-quartet-stabilized four-stranded helices. *J. Biol. Chem.* **268,** 3546–3554.

23. Lipford, G. B., Sparwasser, T., Bauer, M., Zimmermann, S., Koch, E-S., Heeg, K., et al. (1997) Immunostimulatory DNA: sequence-dependent production of potentially harmful or useful cytokines. *Eur. J. Immunol.* **27,** 3420–3426.
24. Zimmermann, S., Egeter, O., Hausmann, S., Lipford, G. B., Rocken, M., Wagner, H., et al. (1998) CpG oligonucleotides trigger protective and curative Th1 responses in lethal murine leishmaniasis. *J. Immunol.* **160,** 3627–3630.
25. Weiner, G. J., Liu, H-M., Wooldridge, J. E., Dahle, C. E., and Kreig, A. M. (1997) Immunostimulatory oligodeoxynucleotides containing the CpG motif are effective as immune adjuvants in tumor antigen immunization. *Proc. Natl. Acad. Sci. USA.* **94,** 10,833–10,837.
26. Sun, S., Kishimoto, H., and Sprent, J. (1998) DNA as an adjuvant: capacity of insect DNA and Synthetic oligodeoxynucleotides to augment T cell responses to specific antigen. *J. Exp. Med.* **187,** 1145–1150.
27. Mor, G., Single, M., Steinberg, D. A., Hoffman, S. L., Okuda, K., and Klinman, D. (1997) Do DNA vaccines induce autoimmune disease? *Human Gene Therapy* **8,** 293–300.
28. Gilkeson, G. S., Ruiz, P., Howell, D., Lefkowith, J. B., and Pisetsky, D. S. (1993) Induction of immune-mediated glomerulonephritis in normal mice immunized with bacterial DNA. *Clin. Immunol. Immunopath.* **68,** 283–292.
29. D'Andrea, A., Rengaraju, M., Valiante, N. M., Chehimi, J., Kubin, M., Aste, M., et al. (1992) Production of natural killer cell stimulatory factor (interleukin 12) by peripheral blood mononuclear cells. *J. Exp. Med.* **176,** 1387–1398.
30. Halpern, M. D., Kurlander, R. J., and Pisetsky, D. S. (1996) Bacterial DNA induces murine interferon gamma production by stimulation of interleukin-12 and tumor necrosis factor alpha. *Cell. Immunol.* **167,** 72–78.
31. Wicks, I. P., Howell, M. L., Hancock, T., Kohsaka, H., Olee, T., and Carson, D. A. (1995) Bacterial lipopolysaccharide copurifies with plasmid DNA: implications for animal models and human gene therapy. *Human Gene Therapy* **6,** 317–323.
32. Sparwasser, T., Miethke, T., Lipford, G., Borschert, K., Hacker, H., Heeg, K., et al. (1997) Bacterial DNA causes septic shock. *Nature* **386,** 336–337.
33. Mouthon, M-A., Mitjavila, M-T., Marquet, J., Vainchenker, W., and Wendling, F. (1994) Erroneous results of ^{3}H-thymidine incorporation are related to position of thymidine residues in oligodeoxynucleotides. *Exp. Hematology.* **22,** 384–387.
34. Manickan, E., Yu, Z., and Rouse, B. T. (1997) DNA Immunization of neonates induces immunity despite the presence of maternal antibody. *J. Clin. Invest.* **100,** 2371–2375.
35. Bot, A., Bot, S., Garcia-Sastre, A., and Bona, C. (1996) DNA immunization of newborn mice with a plasmid-expressing nucleoprotein of influenza virus. *Viral Immunol.* **9,** 207–210.
36. Huygen, K., Content, J., Denis, O., Montgomery, D. L., Yawman, A. M., Deck, R. R., et al. (1996) Immunogenicity and protective efficacy of a tuberculosis DNA vaccine. *Nat. Med.* **2,** 893–898.
37. Hoffman, S. L., Doolan, D. L., Sedegah, M., Gramzinski, R., Wang, H., Gowda, K., et al. (1995) Nucleic acid malaria vaccines. *Ann. NY Acad. Sci.* **772,** 88–94.

38. Xu, D. and Liew, F. Y. (1995) Protection against leishmaniasis by injection of DNA encoding a major surface glycoprotein, gp63, of L.major. *Immunology* **84,** 173–176.
39. Slater, J. E., Perry, J. E., Zhang, Y. J., Arthur-Smith, A., and Colberg-Poley, A. (1997) A DNA vaccine inhibits IgE responses to the latex allergen Hev b 5 in mice. *J. Allergy Clin. Immunol.* **99,** S504.

19

Transcutaneous Immunization

Gregory M. Glenn, Tanya Scharton-Kersten, and Russell Vassell

1. Introduction

Transcutaneous immunization (TCI), the introduction of antigens using a topical application to intact skin, is a new technology that has both practical and immunological merits. Practically speaking, a needle-free method of vaccine delivery will decrease the risk of needle-borne diseases, reduce the complications related to physical skin penetration, improve access to vaccination by eliminating the need for trained personnel and sterile equipment, and provide a simple means for multivalent or multiple boosting immunization. The immunological implications of TCI are profound as this technique appears to target highly accessible antigen presenting cells (APC) in the skin that can be exploited for a variety of immune outcomes. It has been our experience that TCI can be reliably and reproducibly conducted with a variety of antigens to induce potent and functional immune responses. Thus, this new method may significantly impact both the delivery of vaccines and open new possibilities for manipulation of the immune response.

1.1. Background

Our experience with TCI began empirically with the observation that cholera toxin (CT) applied to the skin in a simple saline solution could induce systemic anti-CT antibody responses. Although immunization using the skin is a new and surprising insight, it is based on an amalgam of well-tested science. Our working hypothesis is that TCI utilizes three established paradigms: (1) CT is a potent adjuvant for induction of immune responses to coadministered antigens; (2) the skin is replete with potent APCs, principally Langerhans cells;

From: *Methods in Molecular Medicine, Vol. 42:*
Vaccine Adjuvants: Preparation Methods and Research Protocols
Edited by: D. T. O'Hagan © Humana Press, Inc., Totowa, NJ

(3) the skin can be effectively penetrated using hydration. Each of these elements has been well described in investigations outside of TCI and thus extensive background information can be applied to the experimental questions surrounding TCI. Our hypothesis, that CT penetrates the skin through hydration and activates Langerhans cells, provides a useful guide for the design of experiments using TCI and hopefully will be validated through further research in TCI.

CT and the closely related heat labile enterotoxin from *Escherichia coli* have been extensively studied as adjuvants, providing an enormous fund of knowledge for the development of TCI ***(1,2)***. CT is an 86 kDa heterodimeric protein secreted by the bacterium *Vibrio cholerae* which, when administered perorally or intranasally, induces antibody responses against both itself and coadministered proteins. The strength of the immune enhancement contributed by the use of CT has established CT as the gold standard for mucosal adjuvants ***(2,3)***. However, the perceived toxicity of CT and the LT have limited widespread use of these proteins as vaccine components and adjuvants and has led to mucosal strategies using nontoxic mutants ***(4,5)*** and purified B-subunits ***(6,7)***. Our finding that application of CT to the skin induces robust immune responses without the systemic toxicity that accompanies its use by the oral, nasal, or parenteral routes suggests that TCI allows the safe use of native CT with its unmatched potency as an adjuvant ***(8)***.

Langerhans cells (LCs) were identified in 1886, yet their function as APCs has only been recently appreciated ***(9)***. They are found in the epidermis from the suprabasal layer through the stratum granulosum, i.e., they are almost directly under the stratum corneum. Their superficial location makes these potent APCs attractive targets for vaccine delivery. LCs are thought to phagocytose antigen in the skin and, if activated, will migrate to the draining lymph nodes where they present antigen to T cells. We have proposed that CT activates LCs, which leads to antigen presentation in the draining lymph node, that leads to the induction of a systemic immune response ***(10)***. The remarkable feature of TCI is that systemic immune responses are elicited without signs of systemic or local skin redness or swelling, even in antigen-sensitized mice and humans. The latter clinical observation is highly suggestive that LCs are engaged in this method of immunization, as they are the only APCs in uninflammed skin ***(11)***. Activated LCs can be visualized in split-epidermal sheets from the murine ear after application of CT (*see* **Subheading 3.**), and studies are underway to further define the role of LCs, their fate, and interactions with T cells in the context of TCI.

The stratum corneum is the principal barrier to penetration through the skin. It consists of nonliving keratinized cells and lipids. Although the skin has been traditionally seen as an impervious barrier to the hostile world, the widespread presence of LCs attests to the imperfection of the stratum corneum barrier function, and hydration is one of the processes that can significantly alter this barrier function. Skin hydration, such as that achieved by simple occlusion, alters the barrier function of the stratum corneum and, in fact, is considered to be the best form of skin penetration enhancement ***(12)***. The stratum corneum can increase its water content up to 300%, and 75% of retained water in hydrated skin is free water, which can assist in the passive diffusion of soluble molecules into the skin. It is thought that the free water allows for passive diffusion of soluble vaccine antigens into the living epidermis and to the LCs. Most readers of this chapter will have worn a Band-Aid™ and can attest to the visible swelling and wetness of skin after removal of this semi-occlusive dressing and, thus, can validate the obvious physical changes caused by hydration.

Skin thickness is a further limiting factor for penetration. The human stratum corneum varies in thickness by anatomical site with a range in one study of 8.7–12.9 µm and 18–28 cell layers in subjects with healthy skin ***(13)***. Mouse stratum corneum and epidermis is considerably thinner than human skin, but has more lipid per dry weight of tissue. Obviously, highly keratinized areas such as the palmar and volar surfaces of the hands and feet in humans and the footpad and tail in mice have a far thicker stratum corneum and, not surprisingly, contain more sparse populations of LCs ***(14–16)***.

Whereas transdermal drug delivery typically targets the vasculature in the dermis, TCI is thought to find its target in the epidermal LCs. This may account for the effectiveness of TCI in that only the most superficial layer of the skin, the stratum corneum, needs to be penetrated by antigens to encounter APCs, which then carry out the actual delivery of the vaccine antigens to the lymph nodes. This may explain why large molecules such as CT (86 kDa), and even larger molecules such as diphtheria toxoid and tetanus toxoid so readily traverse the skin. These vaccine antigens induce profound immune responses despite the maxims of skin penetration that would limit the molecular size of molecules that can be effectively used for transdermal application to far smaller molecules in the range of 0.5–1 kDa ***(17)***. Although the role of skin hydration in penetration is well described, the mechanism by which hydration contributes to skin penetration is not well characterized. Thus, the goal of our current immunization protocol is to hydrate the skin as a prelude to penetration of vaccine antigens and adjuvants for the induction of immune responses.

1.2. Immune Responses to TCI

CT and other related ADP-ribosylating exotoxins such as heat-labile enterotoxin from *E. coli* (LT) are in themselves strong immunogens when given by routes other than TCI. In our early experiments, we noted that high levels of anti-CT antibodies could be rapidly induced after one application of CT to the

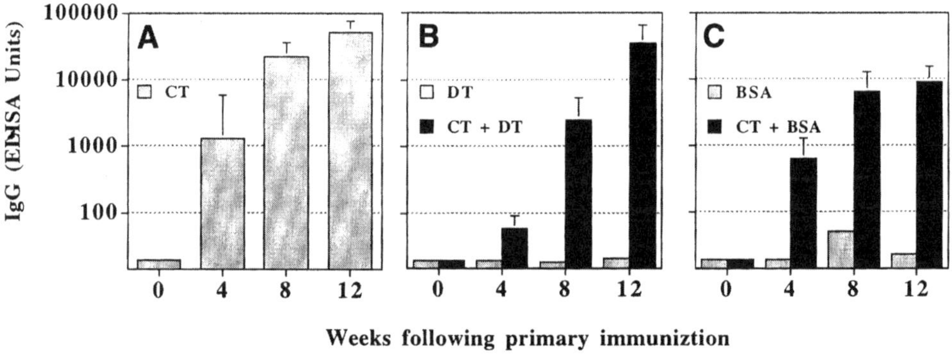

Fig. 1. Kinetics of the serum IgG antibody response to CT (**A**), DT (**B**), or BSA (**C**) in animals immunized (0 wk) and boosted (4 and 8 wk) by the transcutaneous route with CT (100 µg), DT (100 µg) ± CT, or BSA (200 µg) ± CT. Antibodies were measured by enzyme-linked immunosorbent assay (ELISA) at multiple time points. The results are reported as the mean ± SEM in ELISA units, the inverse dilution at which the absorbency at 405 nm is equal to 1.0. Similar results were observed in two independent experiments. Anti-CT antibody titers in CT + DT and CT+BSA groups were not different from the CT alone group.

skin and that these antibodies could be increased in subsequent boosting immunizations (**Fig. 1A**). We have also found that the use of CT as an adjuvant on the skin results in classic priming and secondary antibody responses to coadministered antigens when boosting is conducted using CT as an adjuvant (**Fig. 1B**) *(18)*. Thus, high levels of antibodies to vaccine antigens can be induced, similar to those induced by priming and boosting using intramuscular (im) immunization with alum. In addition, IgG antibodies to coadministered vaccine antigens can be readily detected in the stool and lung washes in mice immunized using TCI (**Fig. 2A**). Anti-CT IgG and IgA can also be detected in mucosal compartments, as well in the serum (**Fig. 2B**, **C**). The serum anti-CT antibodies confirm the proper delivery of the vaccine solution on the skin when CT is used as adjuvant as successful immunization will always produce anti-CT antibodies.

No obvious interference between the immune responses to the adjuvant and the antibody response to coadministered antigen have been observed. The serum antibody response to CT when administered as an adjuvant with coadministered antigens is not diminished compared to the response to CT alone. More importantly, the antibody response to antigens such as DT and BSA can be boosted using CT as an adjuvant despite the presence of high levels of CT antibodies (**Fig. 2**). Reimmunization with a second coadministered antigen in mice previously immunized using CT as an adjuvant has also been

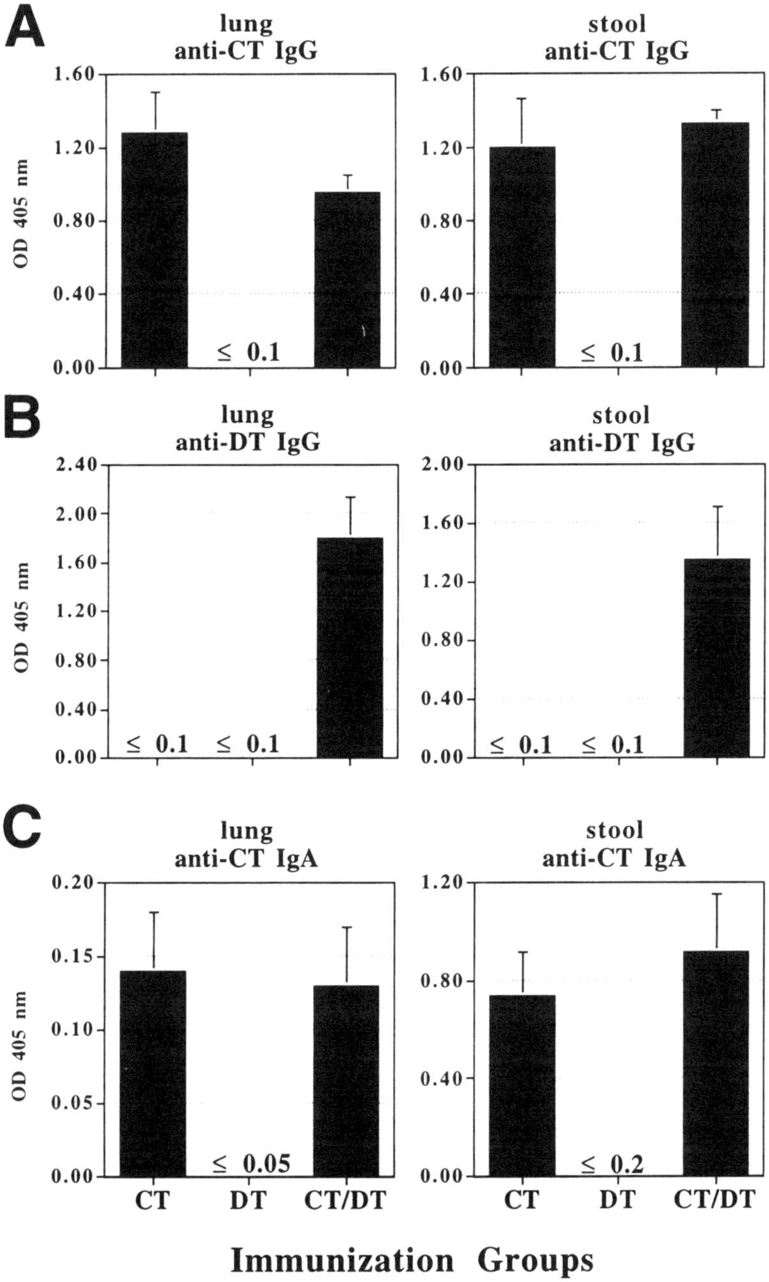

Fig. 2. Antibody responses to CT and DT at the mucosa in TCI mice. Animals were immunized with CT (100 μg), DT (100 μg), or CT and DT (CT/DT) at 0, 8, and 18 wk. Thirty weeks later, stool and lung wash extracts were collected and analyzed for anti-CT IgG (**A**), anti-DT IgG (**B**), or anti-CT IgA (**C**). Antibodies were measured by ELISA and reported as the OD_{405} nm at the following dilutions: lung anti-CT IgG 1 to 320, stool anti-CT IgG 1 to 8, lung anti-DT IgG 1 to 10, stool anti-DT IgG 1 to 4, lung anti-CT IgA 1 to 10, stool anti-CT IgA 1 to 4. Values shown arc the mean ± SEM for groups of five mice.

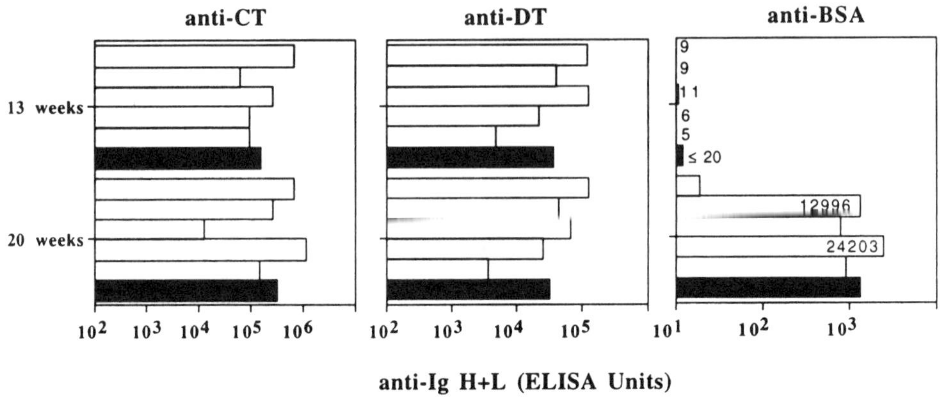

Fig. 3. Reimmunization of mice with preexisting high titer CT responses. Mice were immunized transcutaneously at 0, 4, and 8 wk with CT (100 µg) and DT (100 µg), and then exposed to CT (100 µg) and BSA (200 µg) 13 and 17 wk after the first immunization. Serum was analyzed from animals at 0, 13, and 20 wk. The results are reported for individual mice (white bars) and the geometric mean thereof (black bars) for each group.

shown, without diminution of the antibody responses (**Fig. 3**). Thus, we found that TCI results in classic secondary responses to boosting and that CT can be repeatedly used as an adjuvant on the skin.

The antibodies generated by TCI are functional in vitro and can protect against lethal mucosal cholera toxin challenge ***(19)*** and systemic challenge with tetanus toxin ***(18)***. In the first challenge study, mice immunized a single time with CT transcutaneously developed high levels of serum and mucosal anti-CT antibodies. They were then challenged intranasally with doses of CT, which could induce a fatal pulmonary hemmorrhagic pneumonia. Eighty percent of singly immunized mice vs 11% of control mice, survived the challenge and, 100% of mice immunized twice were protected. These data suggest that TCI can be used for protection against toxin-mediated diseases such as diphtheria, pertussis, or enteric diseases such as cholera and entertoxogenic *E. coli*. In another study, mice were immunized with CT and a papain derivative of tetanus toxin, fragment C from tetanus toxin (tetC) that has been shown to be a protective antigen against tetanus toxin challenge in other vaccine models ***(20)***. Mice immunized with tetC plus CT produced anti-tetC and antitetanus toxoid antibodies and were fully protected against tetanus toxin challenge.

The aforementioned models were selected to evaluate whether TCI could produce a protective immune response against a vaccine preventable disease or mucosal toxin-mediated disease. The correlate for systemic protection against tetanus is known to be serum antitoxin IgG ***(21)***. Both functional antigen-specific IgG against tetanus and IgG against CT induced via TCI have been shown to be protective ***(18,19)***. Although the correlates for protection from other vaccine preventable diseases, such as diphtheria and Haemophilus influenza B, are also known to be serum antigen-specific IgG ***(11,22)***, the presence of mucosal IgG induced by TCI (**Fig. 2**) may enhance protection and thus improve vaccine efficiency against pathogens with mucosal entry points or in which mucosal pathology plays a central role.

The doses of antigen and adjuvant used in our studies have been determined empirically. Initial studies using CT as an immunogen indicated that 100 μg of antigen was sufficient to induce high levels of serum antibodies ***(19)***. There is a dose–response relationship for CT and the humoral response. Varying doses of CT (1–300 μg) in a fixed volume of a saline solution (i.e., different concentrations) applied to the skin indicate that there is a plateau at 0.5–1 mg/mL. Mice that were immunized with less than 0.5–1 mg/mL respond less uniformly. Nonetheless, a clearly detectable response has been observed in doses as low as 3 μg. Similarly, LT antigen-specific antibody titers were induced in a dose-dependent manner and 10 μg in 100 μL (0.1 μg/μL) was clearly immunogenic. These data suggest that lower doses of CT or other adjuvants may be effective for TCI and further studies are needed to determine the optimal adjuvant doses.

TCI is a new technique and little specific information has been published. There have been reports of the use of a mixture of phospholipids and bile salts ***(24)*** to immunize using topical application, as well as live adenoviruses carrying foreign genes after disrupting the stratum corneum with potasium hydroxide (NAIR™) ***(25)***. In the latter case, immune responses were demonstrated using Western blot, but quantitative and qualitative data have not been shown and adjuvants were not used. We have found that simple application of proteins themselves on intact hydrated skin (controls in our experiments) will result in occasional modest immune responses. However, such responses cannot be construed as useful unless they are of sufficient magnitude and quality to result in protection. To make skin immune responses useful, for example, in the form of serum IgG against tetanus toxin, the TCI response requires the use of an adjuvant active on the skin.

Although human skin immune responses have been described for many decades, they have been associated with skin pathology and/or serum IgE and not the systemic IgG responses to TCI that can confer protection against vaccine preventable disease. Experimentally, pathologic skin immune responses and antigen-specific serum IgE have been induced by prolonged application of very large doses of OVA on mouse skin, under occlusion for extended periods of time ***(26)***. Antigen-specific IgE has not been observed in the context of TCI ***(19)***.

At this stage, it appears that adjuvants are crucial to inducing sufficiently potent and functional immune responses on the skin. The use of adjuvants have recast the fields of vaccine research for injectable, oral, and nasal immunization. We believe that adjuvants, such as CT and LT and other adjuvants, and delivery techniques that can target LCs may revolutionize the future delivery of vaccines. It is to this end that we have provided our most current information on TCI to encourage other researchers to further this concept.

2. Materials

1. CT, Pseudomonas exotoxin A, diphtheria toxoid (DT), tetanus fragment "C" (tetC), and tetanus toxoid were obtained from List Biologicals (Campbell, CA).
2. Bovine serum albumin (BSA), heat labile toxin from *E. coli* (LT), and sterile water were obtained from Sigma (St. Louis, MO).
3. Clippers and blades were obtained from Wahl Clipper Corp. (Sterling, IL).
4. Ketamine, xylazine, and artificial tears were obtained from Phoenix Pharmaceuticals (St. Joseph, MO).

3. Methods

3.1. TCI on the Back (*see* Note 1)

1. Shave mice 2 d prior to immunizing. Using clippers with a No. 40 blade, gently shave a 2-cm-wide area on the back from approximately 1.0 cm above the base of the tail to the distal aspect of the scapula. Care should be taken not to injure the skin and any visibly nicked mice should not be used (*see* **Note 2**).
2. Just prior to immunizing, anesthetize the mice with a cocktail of ketamine (64 mg/mL) and xylazine (6.4 mg/mL) intramuscularly or intraperitoneally to give a final dose of 110 mg/kg ketamine and 11 mg/kg xylazine. Return mice to cage until anesthesia takes effect (3–5 min) and mice are no longer mobile (*see* **Note 3**).
3. Coat eyes with artificial tears to prevent drying.
4. Place mice on a clean surface such as a diaper with a heating pad underneath to control temperature (*see* **Note 4**).
5. Prepare the skin for immunization by saturating a clean gauze pad with sterile water and gently rubbing an approximately 4-cm^2 area on the dorsum until the skin becomes moist (5–10 passes). Alternatively, this technique may be preceeded by the same procedure using isopropanol to remove lipids at the site and followed by hydration *(27)*. Allow approximately 0.5 mL of water to remain on the skin for 5 min (*see* **Note 5**).
6. Blot excess water with a clean gauze pad before immunizing.
7. Immunize mice by applying 25–100 µL of the antigen solution to the prepared skin using a pipetor. Spread the solution over the prepared area using the rounded barrel of the pipet tip, rather than the end to avoid scratching the skin surface. Do not scrape the skin with the end of the tip (*see* **Note 6**).
8. It may be desirable to rewet the skin at 30–45 min (when immunizing solution appears mostly absorbed) with a volume of sterile water equal to that of the immunizing solution used (*see* **Note 7**).

9. Allow antigen to remain on the skin a total of up to 2 h (Note: the minimum time for optimal immunization may be as little as 15 min).
10. Blot excess antigen solution with a clean gauze pad.
11. Rinse the back of the mice under a lukewarm stream of tap water. Blot dry with a clean gauze pad. Repeat rinse and blot. The rinse should be collected in a basin for proper disposal by local regulations (*see* **Note 8**).
12. Return mice to their cage with a heating pad underneath and cover the mice with bedding to warm the animals. Ensure that all mice are ambulatory before returning to the housing room.

3.2. TCI on the Ear (*see* Note 9)

1. Anesthetize the mice as in the TCI on the back (procedure above).
2. Lay mice on their backs with the head slightly tilted toward the ear to be immunized so that the *ventral* surface of this ear presents a relatively flat surface on which to apply the antigen solution.
3. Wet the ventral surface of the ear by pipeting 25 μL of sterile water to the center of the surface.
4. Saturate a cotton-tipped applicator with sterile water and gently spread the water over the ventral surface, being careful not to spread the water to the edge of the ear or into the ear canal.
5. Allow the water to remain on the ear for 5 min, then blot dry with a clean applicator.
6. Apply antigen solution to the prewetted area using a pipetor. Do not scrape the skin with the tip. A volume of 25–50 μL is recommended for the ears.
7. Allow antigen solution to remain on the ear 1–2 h until mostly absorbed.
8. Blot excess antigen solution with a clean applicator.
9. Rinse and blot the ears twice, as in TCI, on the back.
10. Post immunization care is the same as for TCI on the back.

4. Notes

1. We have successfully immunized mice (Balb/C, C57Bl/c, Swiss Webster, and C3H), guinea pigs, rabbits [New Zealand White (NZW)], sheep, and pigs *(28)*. The detailed procedure addresses the immunization of mice on which the majority of our work has been conducted. Guinea pigs present particular problems in that their hair is coarse and grows rapidly. Thus, shaving guinea pigs should be done immediately before immunization, being careful to avoid nicking. Swab with isopropanol to remove lipids.
2. In our experience, the best way to shave mice is to hold the mouse by the tail allowing the mouse to grab a wire mesh with its front feet only so that the mouse is at approximately a 45° angle. The clippers are then held perpendicular to the back and passed over the back from approximately 1.0 cm above the tail to the scapula several times. Balb/c mice can easily be shaved in this manner, but more aggressive mice such as C57Bl/6 should be lightly anesthetized to avoid nicking.

3. A dose of 110 mg/kg ketamine and 11 mg/kg xylazine will typically yield 1–2 h anesthesia. If mice begin to wake too early (e.g., before 1 h and 45 min after application of antigen) they can be safely reanesthetized with another one-quarter to one-half dose.
4. During anesthesia, the mice may become cold. We typically do not warm them until the end of the procedure because this may cause them to wake early, however, it may be necessary to warm them sooner.
5. We have also used other means to prepare the skin for immunization, such as rubbing with a 70% isopropyl alcohol pad, rubbing with an alcohol pad followed by hydration, or hydration followed by an alcohol rub. These techniques are believed to enhance antigen penetration.
6. We typically immunize with an antigen concentration of 0.5–2.0 mg/mL (CT and admixed antigen) corresponding to a dose of 10–100 μg each of adjuvant and antigen. We believe that a dose given at a high concentration and low volume is likely more effective than the same dose delivered at a low concentration. We have typically administered antigen dissolved in PBS, but have also had success with gels and emulsions.
7. The time and necessity of rewetting will depend on the volume of antigen used, the ambient humidity and on the method used to prepare the skin. Large antigen volumes may not require rewetting. Skin prepared with an alcohol rub will require rewetting early (e.g., before 30 min).
8. When rinsing mice, they should be held in such a way that the rinsate comes into contact as little as possible with areas other than the skin used for immunization. The rinsate should not contact mucosal sites such as the face, anus, or genitalia.
9. Immunizing on the ear affords a good method for studying the role of LCs because epithelial cell suspensions and epithelial sheets are easily prepared from ears. *See* **refs.** ***3*** and ***12*** for a description of procedures.

References

1. Lycke, N. (1997) The mechanism of cholera toxin adjuvanticity. *Res. Immunol.* **148,** 504–520.
2. Snider, D. P. (1995) The mucosal adjuvant activities of ADP-ribosylating bacterial enterotoxins. *Crit. Rev. Immunol.* **15,** 317–348.
3. Elson, C. O. and Ealding, W. (1984) Cholera toxin feeding did not induce oral tolerance in mice and abrogated oral tolerance to an unrelated protein antigen. *J. Immunol.* **133,** 2892–2897.
4. Dickinson, B. L. and Clemens, J. D. (1995) Dissociation of *Escherichia coli* heat-labile enterotoxin adjuvanticity from ADP-ribosyltransferase activity. *Infect. Immun.* **63,** 1617–1623.
5. Lobet, Y., Cluff, C. W., and Cieplak, W. (1991) Effect of site-directed mutagenic alterations on ADP-ribosyltransferase activity of the A subunit of *Escherichia coli* heat-labile enterotoxin. *Infect. Immun.* **59,** 2870–2879.

6. Holmgren, J., Svennerholm, A-M., Jertborn, M., Clemens, J., Sack, D. A., Salenstedt, R., and Wigzell, H. (1992) An oral B subunit: whole cell vaccine against cholera. *Vaccine* **10,** 911–914.
7. Tamura, S., Funato, H., Nagamine, T., Aizawa, C., and Kurata, T. (1989) Effectiveness of cholera toxin B subunit as an adjuvant for nasal influenza vaccination despite pre-existing immunity to CTB. *Vaccine* **7,** 503–505.
8. Glenn, G. M., Rao, M., Matyas, G. R., and Alving, C. R. (1998) Skin immunization made possible by cholera toxin. *Nature* **391,** 851.
9. Kripke, M. L., Munn, C. G., Jeevan, A., Tang, J. M., and Bucana, C. (1990) Evidence that cutaneous antigen-presenting cells migrate to regional lymph nodes during contact sensitization. *J. Immunol.* **145,** 2833–2838.
10. News and views (1998) *Nature Medicine* **4,** 672.
11. Udey, M. C. (1997) Cadherins and Langerhans cell immunobiology. *Clin. Exp. Immunol.* **107 (Suppl. 1),** 6–8.
12. Roberts, M. S. and Walker, M. (1993) Water the most natural penetration enhancer, in *Pharmaceutical Skin Penetration Enhancement* (Walters, K. A. and Hadgraft, J., eds.), Marcel Dekker, New York, pp. 1–30.
13. Holbrook, K. A. and Odland, D. F. (1974) Regional differences in the thickness (cell layers) of the human stratum corneum: an ultrastructural analysis. *J. Invest. Dermatol.* **62,** 415–422.
14. Berman, B., Chen, V. L., France, D. S., Dotz, W. I., and Petroni, G. (1983) Anatomical mapping of epidermal Langerhans cells densities in adults. *Br. J. Dermatol.* **109,** 553–558.
15. Bergstresser, P. R., Fletcher, C. R., and Streilein, J. W. (1980) Surface densities of Langerhans cells in relation to rodent epidermal sites with special immunological properties. *J. Invest. Dermatol.* **74,** 77–80.
16. Schweizer, J. (1980) Langerhans cell-free regions in orthokeratinizing sole-of-foot epidermis of the adult mouse. *Arch. Dermatol. Res.* **268,** 157–166.
17. *Fisher's Contact Dermatitis*, 4th ed. (1995) (Rietschel, R. L. and Fowler, J. F., eds.), Williams & Wilkins, Baltimore, MD, p. 2.
18. Glenn, G. M., Scharton-Kersten, T., Vassell, R., Matyas, G. R., and Alving, C. R. (1999) Transcutaneous immunization using bacterial ADP-ribosylating exotoxins as antigens and adjuvants. *Infect. Immun.* **67,** 1000–1006.
19. Glenn, G. M., Scharton-Kersten, T., Vassell, R., Mallet, C. P., Hale, T. L., and Alving, C. R. (1998) Transcutaneous immunization with cholera toxin protects mice against lethal mucosal toxin challenge. *J. Immunol.* **161,** 3212–3214.
20. Fairweather, N. F., Lyness, V. A., and Maskell, D. J. (1987) Immunization of mice against tetanus with fragments of tetanus toxin synthesized in *Escherichia coli*. *Infect. Immun.* **55,** 2541–2545.
21. McComb, J. A. (1964) The prophylactic dose of homologous tetanus antitoxin. *N. Engl. J. Med.* **270,** 175–178.
22. Schneerson, R., Robbins, J. B., Taranger, J., Lagergard, T., and Trollfors, B. (1996) A toxoid vaccine for pertussis as well as diphtheria? Lessons to be relearned. *Lancet* **348,** 1289–1292.

23. Goldblatt, D., Vaz, A. R., and Miller, E. (1998) Antibody avidity as a surrogate maker of successful priming by Haemophilus influenzae type b conjugate vaccines following infant immunization. *J. Infect. Dis.* **177,** 1112–1115.
24. Paul, A. and Cevc, G. (1995) Noninvasive administration of protein antigens: Transdermal immunization with bovine serum albumin in transferasomes. *Vaccine Res.* **3,** 145–164.
25. Tang, D. C., Shi, Z., and Curiel, D. T. (1997) Vaccination onto bare skin. *Nature* **388,** 729–730.
26. Wang, L., Lin, J., Hsieh, K., and Lin, R. (1996) Epicutaneous exposure of protein antigen indices a predominant Th2-like response with high IgE production in mice. *J. Immunol.* **156,** 4077–4082.
27. Scharton-Kersten, T., Glenn, G. M., Vassell, R., Yu, J., Walwender, D., and Alving, C. R. (1999) Principles of transcutaneous immunization using cholera toxin as an adjuvant. *Vaccine* **17(Suppl),** 537–543.
28. Hammond, S. A., Tsonis, C., Sellins, K., Rushlow, K., Scharton-Kersten, T., Colditz, I., and Glenn, G. M. (2000) Transcutaneous immunization of domestic animals: opportunities and challenges. *Adv. Drug Delivery Rev.,* in press.

20

Mutant Heat-Labile Enterotoxins As Adjuvants for CTL Induction

Jason A. Neidleman, Gary Ott, and Derek O'Hagan

1. Introduction

Heat-labile enterotoxin (LT) from *Escherichia coli* and Cholera toxin (CT) from *Vibro cholerae* are known to be potent mucosal immunogens. These toxins have 80% sequence homology and a similar tertiary structure ***(1–4)***, and both elicit potent serum IgG and mucosal IgA responses ***(5,6)***. Moreover, both also serve as excellent adjuvants for coadministered antigens. However, they are toxic in their native state and both produce accumulation of intestinal fluid and watery diarrhea ***(7)***. LT is the cause of traveler's diarrhea, whereas CT causes cholera. In order to make use of the adjuvanticity of these molecules but reduce their toxicity, several mutants have been generated by site-directed mutagenesis. Of these, there are two mutants of the enzymatic A subunit, LTK63 and LTR72, that maintain a high level of immunogenicity and have significant potential as adjuvants. This chapter will focus on the use of LTK63 and LTR72 as intramuscular and intranasal adjuvants for the induction of cytotoxic T lymphocytes (CTL) activity against coadministered protein immunogens.

LT and CT belong to the family of adenosine 5′-diphosphate (ADP)-ribosylating bacterial toxins. The toxins in this family have an A-B structure. The A subunit is enzymatically active, binds nicotinamide adenine dinucleotide (NAD) and transfers the ADP ribose group to a guanosine 5′-triphosphate (GTP)-binding protein, which regulates the activity of adenylate cyclase and increases intracellular accumulation of cyclic adenosine monophosphate (cAMP). Accumulation of cAMP is thought to be responsible for the toxicity of both LT and CT. The pentameric B subunit of LT and CT binds the A sub-

From: *Methods in Molecular Medicine, Vol. 42:*
Vaccine Adjuvants: Preparation Methods and Research Protocols
Edited by: D. T. O'Hagan © Humana Press, Inc., Totowa, NJ

unit to cell membrane surface receptors by its receptor-binding site, through interaction mainly with GM1 ***(1,8,9)***. In addition, the B subunit allows the transfer of the A subunit to the cytoplasm of the cell. The challenge in developing safe mutants has been to modify them to make them sufficiently nontoxic, while maintaining the molecule's capacity to act as an adjuvant ***(10)***.

The mechanism of the adjuvant activity of these LT and CT remains poorly defined. Some have reported that it is based on enzymatic activity ***(11)***. However, others have reported adjuvant effects with mutants that lack ADP-ribosyltransferase activity ***(6,12)***. There is evidence that ADP-ribosylation is at least a contributor to adjuvanticity. In a preliminary study, LTK63 has been shown to be a potent mucosal adjuvant for inducing CTL with a coadministered peptide immunogen ***(13)***. LTR72, which maintains a small amount of enzymatic activity, has shown improved mucosal adjuvanticity for antibody induction compared to LTK63, which lacks enzymatic activity ***(6)***.

The mutants LTK63 and LTR72 were generated by site-directed mutagenesis. LTK63 is the result of a substitution of serine 63 in the A subunit with a lysine which renders it enzymatically inactive ***(14–17)***. LTR72 is derived from a substitution of alanine 72 with an arginine in the A subunit and has about 0.6% of the enzymatic activity of wild-type LT. In addition, LTR72 is 100,000-fold less toxic than wild-type LT in Y1 cells in vitro and 25–100 times less toxic than wild-type LT in rabbit ileal loops. LTR72 has also been reported to have superior mucosal adjuvanticity to LTK63 by measurement of antibody and antigen-specific T-lymphocyte priming ***(18)***. LT mutants have been described previously as adjuvants for the induction of antibodies through both the oral and nasal routes of immunization ***(18)***.

In this chapter, the ability of LT mutants to induce CTL in combination with yeast-derived human immunodeficiency virus (HIV) *p55* and *p24* gag will be discussed. The procedure for assaying CTL activity in immunized mice will be provided. In this procedure, mice are immunized according to a standard schedule and splenocytes are harvested and prepared for stimulation. The splenocytes are restimulated and assayed by ^{51}chromium release to determine the ability of the vaccine of interest to elicit a *p55* gag-specific CTL response.

2. Materials

2.1. Stimulation of Splenocytes

1. Screens and syringe plungers (5 mL) for disrupting spleens.
2. Sterile surgical instruments for removal of spleens.
3. Splenocyte culture medium: RPMI-1640 (with 100 m*M* L-glutamine)/α-Mem (Minimum Essential Medium Alpha Medium with L-glutamine, deoxyribonucleosides or ribonucleosides) (1 : 1) supplemented with 10% heat-inactivated fetal calf serum (inactivated in a 56°C water bath for 30 min), 100 U/mL penicillin,

100 μg/mL streptomycin, 10 μl/L of 100 m*M* sodium pyruvate and 50 μ*M* 2-mercaptoethanol. Sterile filtered (0.2 μm).

4. Interleukin 2 (IL-2). (T-stim culture supplement Rat without Con A. Cat. # 40116, Collaborative Biomedical Products). Add IL-2 after sterile filtration. Do not filter IL-2 media.
5. Peptide for stimulation of splenocytes and target: p7g is an H-$2K^d$ restricted HIV-1_{SF2}p24gag CTL epitope and is a synthetic 9 mer peptide: (aa, 199-AMQMLKETI-207) ***(21)***. $pGag^b$ is an H-$2D^b$-restricted HIV-1_{SF2} *p55*gag CTL epitope and is a synthetic 9 mer peptide: (aa, 390-SQVTNPANI-398) ***(19,20)***.
6. 24-well plates.

2.2. Chromium Release Assay

1. Acetic acid (2%)
2. Trypan blue (0.4% solution).
3. DMEM high glucose (Dulbecco's modified Eagle's medium) with 4.5 g/L of glucose, supplemented with 1% sodium pyruvate and 10% heat-inactivated fetal calf serum. Sterile filtered.
4. Cell-lifting media for adherent targets (0.25% STV). For 1 L of 0.25% STV: Potassium chloride (0.4 g), sodium chloride (8 g), glucose (1 g), sodium bicarbonate (0.58 g), trypsin (2.5 g), ethylenediamine tetraacetic acid (EDTA) (0.2 g) phenol red (0.004 g), hydrochloric acid, 6 *N* as required, sterile H_2O up to 1 L. Add each chemical to the solution in the order listed, stir each component except for trypsin one at a time for at least 10 min. Stir trypsin for at least 30 min. Keep solution covered after adding phenol. Adjust pH to 7.05 ± 0.05 using HCl 6 *N*. Sterile filter (0.22 μm). Store at 4°C, expires in 6 mo.
5. Triton lytic mix. For 1 L of triton lytic mix: Triton, 10% (in 0.01 *M* Tris-HCl, pH 8.0) (10 mL), 1 *M* Tris-HCl, pH 8.0 (50 mL), 0.25 *M* EDTA, pH 8.0 (250 mL), sterile H_2O up to 1 L. Store at 2–30°C. Expires in 1 yr.
6. ^{51}Cr (Sodium Chromate (Na_2CrO_4) in normal saline at 1.00 mCi/mL). ^{51}Cr used has an approximate specific activity of 543 mCi/mg. Ordered from NEN Life Science Products, Inc., Boston, MA.
7. 96-well plates (u or v-bottom).

3. Methods

3.1. Immunization of Mice

Follow all institutional guidelines for working with mice.

3.1.1. Intraperitoneal (ip) for Vaccinia Immunization (Positive Control Group in Assays)

1. Fill syringe with injectate and remove bubbles.
2. Manually restrain animal by exposing abdomen and pointing the head downward.
3. Insert needle into lower left or right quadrant of abdomen (avoid abdominal midline).
4. Inject with moderate pressure and speed.

5. Vaccinia virus is administered at 100–200 μL per animal and 1×10^7 plaque forming units (pfu) per injection. The virus used in these experiments is a recombinant vaccinia virus vector that expresses *p55* gag and pol proteins derived from HIV-1_{SF2} (vv gag-pol) ***(19,21)***.

3.1.2. Intramuscular (im)

1. Fill syringe with injectate and remove bubbles.
2. Manually restrain the animal.
3. Insert the needle into heavy musculature of the quadriceps or posterior thigh (<23 guage needle and ≤ 0.05 mL per site). The same muscle should be used for all immunizations.
4. Aspirate briefly and ensure correct placement of needle (i.e., to prevent intravenous or intra-arterial injection).
5. Inject with moderate pressure and speed to prevent tissue damage.

3.1.3. Intranasal (in)

1. Manually restrain the nonanesthetized animal in an upright position so that the nose is pointed upwards.
2. Drop the vaccine into the nose slowly and dropwise with a pipet tip. Allow each drop to disperse before proceeding to the next drop.

3.1.4. Immunization Schedule

1. 18–22 g mice are purchased (CB6F1 in this experiment from Charles River Breeding Laboratories).
2. Animals are quarantined for 1 wk.
3. Animals are vaccinated at day 0, 7, and 14 (except for mice immunized with vaccinia virus, which are immunized only once at d 0).
4. Spleens are harvested on d 28.
5. Spleens may be used individually or as pools in restimulation cultures. We generally use five spleens as a pool because this was determined to be the minimum for statistically significant results. The number of splenocytes harvested from a single spleen vary widely, but 8×10^7 to 1.2×10^8 cells may be expected.

3.2. Preparation of Mouse Spleens for Bulk Culture Stimulation

1. Spleens are placed in the top of a 100-mm dish in 5 mL of splenocyte culture media.
2. A screen is placed into the bottom of the 100-mm dish with sterile forceps and 10 mL of mouse media are added to the dish.
3. Spleens are transferred onto the screen to be dispersed (*see* **Note 1**).
4. After the spleens from a group have been mashed, the cells are pipeted through the screen to break up any large clumps.
5. The cell mix is pipeted into a 15-mL tube and the clumps are allowed to settle by gravity for about 2 min.

6. The cell suspension above the clumps is removed and transferred to another 15-mL tube (usually 8 mL or less is taken).
7. Before these samples are spun down (at 300*g*), a 50-μL sample is taken and added to 50 μL of trypan blue in a counting tube. Next, 400 μL of 2% acetic acid is added to the tube to lyse red blood cells. The cells surviving treatment with acetic acid are nucleated splenocytes and will appear clear (*see* **Note 2**).
8. The cells are then resuspended in a volume that will yield 3×10^7 cells/mL.
9. In order to set up the responder cells, 3×10^7 cells will be taken (1 mL and 5×10^6 cells per well) and added to 5 mL of mouse media in a 15-mL tube. Next, 1 mL will be dispensed in each of 6 wells of a 24-well plate. Note that 12 wells may be set up to allow for a second experiment if desired (or necessary!) by simply doubling the number of cells used here and in the pulse step. This plate may then be incubated at 37°C, 7% CO_2 until the antigen-presenting cells (APC) are ready.
10. To prepare the APC to be pulsed, 1×10^6 cells per well to be stimulated are taken and added to 2 mL of media (to facilitate centrifugation) in a 15-mL tube.
11. The cells are centrifuged for 8 min at 300*g*, the media is poured off and the cells are resuspended in 1 mL of media containing the epitopic peptides at 10 μ*M* to sensitize the cells. The cells are incubated for 1 h at 37°C (with intermittent shaking).
12. The cells are then washed three times and added to the responder cells prepared in **step 10** at 1×10^6 cells/mL in media containing Rat T-Stim IL-2 at 10%. This will give a final IL-2 concentration of 5%.
13. The cultures are then incubated at 37°C for 6–7 d.

3.3. Chromium Release Assay

1. Target cells are prepared before the chromium release assay. Several flasks of cells should be grown to near confluence in preparation for assay day.
2. Target cells are lifted with 0.25% STV and are counted and washed. Cells are resuspended at 2.5×10^6 cells/mL and 0.5 mL are aliquoted into tubes for each target. The tubes are then centrifuged and the media is removed by aspiration.
3. 10 μL of peptide at 1 μ*M* concentration and 50–100 μCi of ^{51}Cr is added to the target cells and the cells are then incubated for 1.5 h at 37°C with agitation every 30 min.
4. When the target cells are being incubated, the effector cells are prepared. The cells are recovered from the 24-well plates, counted, washed, and resuspended at 3×10^6 cells/mL. This is in anticipation of an initial E:T ratio of 60:1. However, initial E:T ratios may range from 50 to 100:1. The cells are then plated in duplicate wells and are serially diluted 1:3 to achieve E:T ratios of 60:1, 20:1, and 6.7:1.
5. Target cells are washed three times and resuspended at a concentration of 5×10^4 cells/mL. The cells are then added to the effector cells in 100 μL. Cells (100 μL) are also dispensed into wells containing 100 μL of media alone for spontaneous release or an empty well to which 100 μL of triton lytic solution will subsequently be added to give the total release. Duplicate wells are typically used.

Table 1
Intramuscular Immunization With *p55* Gag and LTK63 and LTR72

Antigen adjuvant	E:T ratio	SV/B p7g	MC57 p7g
p55 gag (25µg)	60:1	49	3
LTK63 (10µg)	15:1	19	4
	4:1	8	1
p55 gag (25µg)	60:1	44	3
LTR72 (10µg)	15:1	20	3
	4:1	9	4
p55 gag (25µg)	60:1	17	4
	15:1	7	4
	4:1	5	2
Vv gag-pol	60:1	59	2
	15:1	27	0
	4:1	11	0

p55 gag protein alone (the negative control) was compared to formulations including the adjuvants LTK63 and LTR72. All vaccinations were intramuscular (im). The negative control is unadjuvanted protein administered at a dosage equivalent to that of the adjuvanted vaccines in the experiment. There is a weak cytotoxic response indicated by the SV/B-p7g targets which is higher than the irrelevant cell/peptide pair. This weak specificity for protein alone is a typical result and gives a benchmark with which to compare the adjuvanted protein. Vaccination with vv-gag-pol typically results in a very strong cytotoxic response and therefore, is used as the positive control to judge the quality of the assay (because the % release is expected to fall in a certain range in a successful ^{51}Cr-release assay) and as a benchmark for a very strong cytotoxic response. Typical values range from 50–80% lysis and may be less or more in some circumstances. A value below 40% may call the experiment into question or suggest the need for a repeat. Formulations of *p55* gag protein (25 µg) with 10 µg of either LTK63 or LTR72 induced potent, titratable cytotoxic T-cell responses.

6. The plates are incubated for 4 h (37°C, 7% CO_2) and then a sample of the supernatant is taken to measure the ^{51}Cr released as described ***(22)***.

3.4. Conclusions

In conclusion, we have demonstrated that LT mutants are capable of inducing potent CTL responses following coadministration with *p55* or *p24* gag proteins by both the im and in routes. In contrast, alternative adjuvants were not effective for CTL induction to *p24* by the in route. In addition, although the data is not presented here, we have also seen strong CTL responses to LT mutants and *p55* gag protein administered orally.

Table 2
Intranasal Immunization With *p55*gag and LTK63 and LTR72

Antigen adjuvant	E:T ratio	SV/B p7g	MC57 p7g
p55 gag (25μg)	60:1	43	5
LTK63 (10μg)	15:1	14	2
	4:1	5	0
p55 gag (25μg)	60:1	31	12
LTR72 (1μg)	15:1	14	7
	4:1	6	4
p55 gag (25μg)	60:1	21	16
	15:1	8	7
	4:1	4	3
Vv gag-pol	60:1	69	3
	15:1	41	3
	4:1	14	1

p55 gag protein alone (the negative control) was compared to formulations including the adjuvants LTK63 and LTR72 by the intranasal route. Specific ^{51}Cr releases are significantly higher for both adjuvant formulations than for protein alone at the highest E:T ratio. In this experiment, there were higher levels of nonspecific background in the *p55* gag alone and the LTR72 group than in the im experiment. Vv gag-pol is used as a positive control and was administered by the ip route.

4. Notes

1. Some hairs from the dissection step may be visible in the media and should be separated from the spleens before they are transferred. The plunger from a 5-cc syringe is used to force the spleens contents through the screen until only the white connective tissue remains on the upper side of the screen.
2. If a hemocytometer with a 0.1 μL/small box capacity is used, the total number of cells is arrived at by dividing the number of cells counted by the number of squares counted and multiplying by 1×10^5 (1×10^4 for hemocytometer and 10 for sample dilution). This value is then multiplied by the volume of cells in the sample. Thus if a sample was taken from 8 mL and 375 cells were counted in 1 box: $375 \times 1 \times 10^5 \times 8 = 3.0 \times 10^8$ total cells.
3. CTL experiments involving HIV-1 *p55*gag are set up with a positive control (vv gag-pol), a negative control (protein alone), and the formulations of interest. The target cells are SV/Balb (H-2^d) derived from the Balb/c mouse line and MC57 (H-2^b) derived from the C57BL/6 mouse line. Mice used for immunization were CB6F1 (H-2^{bxd}) which are an F1 cross between Balb/c and C57BL/6 mice. The peptides used are p7g and pgag^b described in **Subheading 2.**

Table 3
Intranasal Immunization With *p24* gag and a Range of Adjuvants, Including LTK63

Antigen adjuvant	E:T ratio	SV/B p7g	MC57 p7g
PLG/*p24* gag	60:1	1	<1
entrapped (25μg)	12:1	4	<1
	2.4:1	5	<1
p24 gag ISCOM	60:1	8	2
(25μg)	12:1	6	<1
	2.4:1	7	1
p24 gag (25μg)	60:1	5	<1
Matrix (6μg)	12:1	5	2
	2.4:1	4	1
p24 gag (25μg)	60:1	70	<1
LTK63 (10μg)	12:1	39	<1
	2.4:1	13	<1
p24 gag protein	60:1	10	1
(25μg)	12:1	<1	<1
	2.4:1	3	1
Vv gag-pol	60:1	64	<1
	12:1	27	<1
	2.4:1	12	1

p24 gag protein alone was compared to immunization by the intranasal route with a range of potent adjuvants. This study demonstrated the ability of LTK63 to induce CTL in contrast to alternative adjuvants by this route. Although the other adjuvants have been shown to induce CTL by the intramuscular route of immunization (data not shown), LTK63 is able to induce CTL by both routes. All of the formulations in this experiment include 25 μg of *p24* protein. The preparation of microparticles is described in Chapter 5, while the preparation of ISCOMS® and Iscomatrix is described in Chapter 14.

4. The percent specific lysis shown in **Tables 1**, **2**, and **3** was calculated using the formula:

$$\% \text{ specific release} = \frac{(\text{avg. cpm released} - \text{avg. spontaneous release}) \times 100}{(\text{avg. total release} - \text{avg. spontaneous release})}$$

5. The specific response is shown in the SV/p7g cell/peptide combination, with MC57/p7g being a cell line pulsed with an irrelevant peptide. Percent spontaneous release values indicate the amount of ^{51}Cr that is in the supernatant of the targets alone wells divided by the amount of ^{51}Cr in the supernatant of the total release wells. Values are typically under 20%, a value higher than this is indicative of a problem with the target cells or the assay. (Value not shown in tables.)

References

1. Magagnoli, C., Manetti, R., Fontana, M. R., Giannelli, V., Giuliani, M. M., Rappuoli, R., et al. (1996) Mutations in the A subunit affect yield, stability, and protease sensitivity of nontoxic derivatives of heat labile enterotoxin. *Infection and Immunity* **64,** 5434–5438.
2. Dallas, W. S. and Falkow, S. (1980) Amino acid homology between cholera toxin and *Escherichia coli* heat labile toxin. *Nature* **288,** 499–501.
3. Spicer, E. K., Kavanaugh, W. M., Dallas, W. S., Falkow, S., Konisberg, W. H., and Shafer, D. (1981) Sequence homologies between A subunits of *E. Coli* and *V. cholerae* enterotoxin. *Proc. Natl. Acad. Sci. USA* **78,** 50–54.
4. Yamamoto, T., Tamura, T., and Yokota, T. (1984) Primary structure of heat-labile enterotoxin produced by *Escherichia coli* pathogenic for humans. *J. Biol. Chem.* **259,** 5037–5044.
5. Clements, J. D. and Dickinson, B. L. (1996) Use of *Escherichia coli* heat-labile enterotoxin as an oral adjuvant, in *Mucosal Vaccines* (Kiyono, H., Ogra, P. L., and McGhee, J. R., eds.), Academic, London and New York, pp. 73–87.
6. Douce, G., Turcotte, C., Cropley, I., Roberts, M., Pizza, M., Domenighini, M., et al. (1995) Mutants of *Escherichia coli* heat-labile toxin lacking ADP-ribosyltransferase activity act as nontoxic, mucosal adjuvants. *Proc. Natl. Acad. Sci. USA* **92,** 1644–1648.
7. Pizza, M., Fontana, M. R., Giuliani, M. M., Domenighini, M., Magagnoli, C., Giannelli, V., et al. (1994) A genetically detoxified derivative of heat-labile *Escherichia coli* enterotoxin induces neutralizing antibodies against the A subunit. *J. Exp. Med.* **180,** 2147–2153.
8. Holmgren, J., Lonnroth, I., and Svennerholm, L. (1973) Tissue receptor for cholera exotoxin: postulated structure from studies with GM1-ganglioside and related glycolipids. *Infect. Immun.* **8,** 208–214.
9. Sugii, S. T. (1989) Binding specificities of heat-labile enterotoxins isolated from porcine and human enterotoxigenic *Escherichia coli* heat-labile toxin and cholera toxin. *Can. J. Microbiol.* **35,** 670–673.
10. Pizza, M., Fontana, M. R., Scarlato, V., and Rappuoli, R. (1996) Genetic detoxification of bacterial toxins in, *Methods in Molecular Medicine: Vaccine Protocols* (Robinson, A., Farrar, G., and Wiblin, C., eds.), Humana, Totowa, NJ, pp. 91–109.
11. Lycke, N. and Holmgren, J. (1992) The adjuvant effect of *Vibro cholerae* and *Escherichia coli* heat-labile enterotoxins is linked to ADP-ribosyltransferase activity. *Eur. J. Immunol.* **22,** 2277.
12. Di Tommaso, A., Saletti, G., Pizza, M., Rappuoli, R., Dougan, G., Abrignani, S., et al. (1996) Induction of antigen specific antibodies in vaginal secretions by using a nontoxic mutant heat-labile enterotoxin as a mucosal adjuvant. *Infect. Immun.* **64,** 974–979.
13. Partidos, C. D., Pizza, M., Rappuoli, R., and Steward, M. W. (1996) The adjuvant effect of a non-toxic mutant heat-labile enterotoxin of *Escherichia coli* for the induction of measles virus-specific CTL responses after intranasal co-immunization with a synthetic peptide. *Immunology* **89,** 483–487.

14. Clements, J. D. and Finkelstein, R. A. (1979) Isolation and characterization of homogeneous heat-labile enterotoxin with high specific activity from *Escherichia coli* cultures. *Infect. Immun.* **24,** 760–769.
15. Clements, J. D., Yancy, R. J., and Finkelstein, R. A. (1980) Properties of homogeneous heat-labile enterotoxin from *Escherichia coli. Infect. Immun.* **29,** 91–97.
16. Pizza M., Domenighini M., Hoi, W., Giannelli, V., Fontana, M. R., Giuliani, M. M., et al. (1994) Probing the structure-activity relationship of *Escherichia coli* LT-A by site-directed mutagenesis. *Mol. Microb.* **14,** 51–60.
17. Pizza, M., Fontana, M. R., Giuliani, M. M., Domenighini, M., Magagnoli, C., Giannelli, V., et al. (1994) A genetically detoxified derivative of heat-labile *Escherichia coli* enterotoxin induces neutralizing antibodies against the A subunit. *J. Exp. Med.* **180,** 2147–2153.
18. Giuliani, M. M., Del Giudice, G., Giannelli, V., Dougan, G., Douce, D., Rappuoli, R., et al. (1998) Mucosal adjuvanticity and immunogenicity of LTR72, a novel mutant of *Escherichia coli* heat-labile enterotoxin with partial knockout of ADP-ribosyltransferase activity. *J. Exp. Med.* **187,** 1–10.
19. Doe, B. and Walker, C. M. (1996) HIV-1 p24 gag-specific cytotoxic T-lymphocyte responses in mice. *Correspondence, AIDS* **10,** 793–806.
20. Elvin, J., Cerundolo, V., Elliott, T., and Townsend, A. (1991) A quantitative assay of peptide-dependant class I assembly. *Eur. J. Immunol.* **21,** 2025–2031.
21. Paliard, X., Doe, B., and Walker, C. M. (1998) The T cell repertoire primed by antiviral vaccination is influenced by self-tolerance. *Cellular Immunol.* **188,** 73–79.
22. Doe, B., Steimer, K. S., and Walker, C. M. (1994) Induction of HIV-1 envelope (gp120)-specific cytotoxic T lymphocyte responses in mice by recombinant CHO-derived gp120 is enhanced by enzymatic removal of N-linked glycans. *Euro. J. Immunol.* **24,** 2369–2376.

Index

From: *Methods in Molecular Medicine, Vol. 42: Vaccine Adjuvants: Preparation Methods and Research Protocols*
Edited by: D. T. O'Hagan © Humana Press Inc., Totowa, NJ

L

M